Great advances have been made in recent years towards a better understanding of the healthy brain and the physical basis of psychiatric disorder. This text brings together contributions from leading international authorities to provide a timely and multidisciplinary overview of this fast-developing area. Its broad coverage ranges from epilepsy and schizophrenia to basal ganglia disorder and brain lesions. In many cases, a clinically oriented chapter is paired with one that describes the basic science that underpins it and considerable attention is given to the impact of the new technologies – structural and functional neuroimaging. In highlighting the basic pathophysiological mechanisms of multifaceted clinical manifestations, this book serves as a valuable review of current neuropsychiatry. It will be welcomed by clinicians, researchers and students alike from neuroscience through to neuropsychology and psychiatry.

DISORDERS OF BRAIN AND MIND

DISORDERS OF BRAIN AND MIND

Edited by

MARIA A. RON
Professor of Neuropsychiatry, Institute of Neurology, London

and

ANTHONY S. DAVID
Professor of Cognitive Neuropsychiatry, King's College School of Medicine & Dentistry and Institute of Psychiatry, London

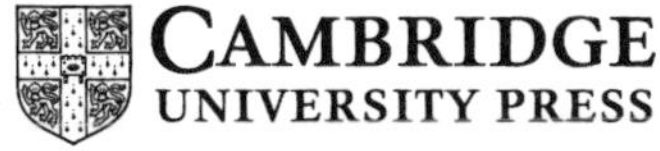

PUBLISHED BY THE PRESS SYNDICATE OF THE UNIVERSITY OF CAMBRIDGE
The Pitt Building, Trumpington Street, Cambridge CB2 1RP, United Kingdom

CAMBRIDGE UNIVERSITY PRESS
The Edinburgh Building, Cambridge CB2 2RU, United Kingdom
40 West 20th Street, New York, NY 10011–4211, USA
10 Stamford Road, Oakleigh, Melbourne 3166, Australia

First published 1998

Printed in the United Kingdom at the University Press, Cambridge

Typeset by 10/13 Times New Roman [SE]

A catalogue record for this book is available from the British Library

Library of Congress Cataloguing in Publication data

Disorders of brain and mind / edited by Maria A. Ron and Anthony S. David.
p. cm.
Includes index.
ISBN 0 521 47306 3 (hardback)
1. Neuropsychiatry. 2. Brain – Diseases. 3. Psychology, Pathological. I. Ron, Maria A. II. David, Anthony S.
[DNLM: 1. Neuropsychology. 2. Brain Diseases – physiopathology. 3. Mental Disorders – physiopathology. 4. Memory Disorders – physiopathology. WL 103.5 D6115 1997]
RC343.D57 1997
616.8 – dc21
DNLM/DLC
for Library of Congress 97–7309 CIP

ISBN 0 521 47306 3 hardback

Contents

Contributors

D. Frank Benson
Professor of Neurology, Augustus S. Rose Department of Neurology, University of California School of Medicine, Centre for Health Sciences, Los Angeles, California 90024, USA

Geraldo Busatto
Lecturer, Department of Psychological Medicine, Institute of Psychiatry, De Crespigny Park, Denmark Hill, London SE5 8AF, UK

Tyrone D. Cannon
Assistant Professor, Department of Psychology, University of Pennsylvania, 3815 Walnut Street, Philadelphia, PA 1904, USA

Jeffrey L. Cummings
Professor of Neurology and Psychiatry, Department of Neurology , Reed Neurological Research Centre, UCLA School of Medicine, 710 Westwood Plaza, Los Angeles, California 90024, USA

Anthony S. David
Professor of Cognitive Neuropsychiatry, Department of Psychological Medicine, Institute of Psychiatry, De Crespigny Park, Denmark Hill, London SE5 8AF, UK

Sam Hutton
Research Fellow, Queen Mary's University Hospital, Roehampton Lane, London SW15 5PN, UK

John G.R. Jefferys
Professor of Neuroscience, Department of Physiology, University of Birmingham, Birmingham B15 2TT, UK

Eileen Joyce
Senior Lecturer in Psychiatry, Queen Mary's University Hospital, Roehampton Lane, London SW15 5PN, UK

Michael D. Kopelman
Reader, United Medical and Dental School, St Thomas's Hospital, Lambeth Palace Road, London SE1 7EH, UK

Shôn Lewis
Professor, Department of Psychiatry, University of Manchester, Withington Hospital, West Didsbury, Manchester M20 8LR, UK

Michael Maier
Senior Lecturer, Charing Cross and Westminster Medical School, London W6 8RP, UK

Andrew R. Mayes
Professor of Cognitive Neuroscience, Royal Hallamshire Hospital, Sheffield University, Glossop Road, Sheffield S10 2JF, UK

Susan E. McPherson
Assistant Clinical Professor, Department of Psychiatry and Biobehavioural Sciences, UCLA School of Medicine, Los Angeles, California 90024, USA

J. Megginson Hollister
Post-doctoral Fellow, Department of Psychiatry, University of Pennsylvania, 3815 Walnut Street, Philadelphia, PA 1904, USA

Jane Mellanby
Lecturer, Department of Experimental Psychology, University of Oxford, Oxford OX1 3UD, UK

Adrian M. Owen
Senior Research Associate, Department of Psychiatry, University of Cambridge, Addenbrooke's Hospital, Cambridge CB2 2QQ

Trevor W. Robbins
Professor in Cognitive Neuroscience, Department of Experimental Psychology, University of Cambridge, Downing St, Cambridge CB2 3EB, UK

Maria A. Ron
Professor of Neuropsychiatry, Institute of Neurology, Queen Square, London WC1N 3BG, UK

Barbara J. Sahakian
Lecturer in Clinical Neuropsychology, Department of Psychiatry, University of Cambridge, School of Clinical Medicine, Addenbrooke's Hospital, Cambridge CB2 2QQ, UK

Eric Taylor
Professor of Developmental Neuropsychiatry, Department of Child Psychiatry, Institute of Psychiatry, De Crespigny Park, Denmark Hill, London SE5 8AF, UK

Brian K. Toone
Consultant Neuropsychiatrist, Department of Psychological Medicine, Kings College Hospital, Denmark Hill, London SE5 8AF, UK

Michael R. Trimble
Professor of Behavioural Neurology, Department of Neurology, Institute of Neurology, Queen Square, London WC1N 3BG, UK

Preface

The description and categorisation of mental phenomena has been the traditional métier of psychiatry. Much of this painstaking work was done without reference to the brain, which, by implication, was perceived as largely irrelevant or else too forbidding and inaccessible. In parallel with this brainless psychiatry, the neurosciences largely contrived to bypass the study of mental phenomena in favour of more accessible areas of research. The brain and the mind thus remained apart.

A dramatic change in this desolate situation has taken place in the last two decades. Neurobiologically based models of behaviour have sprung from new theoretical concepts of brain function such as parallel distributed processing, which leave behind the limited traditional localisationist approach. New neuropsychological tools to analyse behavioural components have been designed and finely tuned and meanwhile considerable progress has been made in elucidating the neurochemical underpinnings of normal and abnormal behaviour. Among these developments, neuroimaging occupies a central place. The advent of computerised tomography (CT) in the mid-seventies, followed by magnetic resonance imaging (MRI) a decade later allowed the visualisation and quantification of subtle structural brain abnormalities in the major psychoses bringing in its wake a renewed interest in the neuropathology of mental illness. Magnetic resonance spectroscopy (MRS) has recently opened a window into the living chemistry of the brain and functional imaging using PET and fMRI has given us much information about the neural systems involved in cognitive processes. These latter techniques are only beginning to make the transition from research to the clinical arena.

The idea behind this book was to gather salient examples of this coming together of brain and mind, focusing on some areas where clinically relevant progress has been made. In a rapidly evolving discipline attempts at comprehensive coverage would have almost certainly led to failure. Our intention was to illustrate these points of convergence and not to produce a comprehensive textbook or exhaustive compilation of activity in the field. Our personal interests have inevitably coloured the choice of topics and we therefore must accept the blame for what some may see as important omissions.

A further reason for producing *Disorders of Brain and Mind* was to find a suitable way to mark the retirement of Professor Alwyn Lishman and we dedicate this book to him. From his position as Professor of Neuropsychiatry at the Institute of Psychiatry, Alwyn Lishman has provided the leading inspiration to generations of psychiatrists, neurologists and psychologists in the UK and abroad. His contribution to neuropsychiatry goes well beyond the impact of his original research, although many areas from memory, to head injury, to alcoholic brain damage and imaging have benefited from his work. For those who had the fortune to work with him, his unrivalled clinical skill and teaching ability are a lasting example and, for the less fortunate, his book *Organic Psychiatry*, now in its third edition, is an invaluable source of information and distilled clinical wisdom.

For the two of us the association with Alwyn Lishman has been a very close and fruitful one and our debt to him therefore greater. It would come as no surprise to our readers to know that many of those who have contributed to the book have also been associated with Alwyn Lishman and their willingness to participate in this small tribute has made our task that much easier. Unfortunately this introduction has to end on a sad note by mentioning the recent death of Professor Frank Benson, a close colleague and friend of Alwyn Lishman who wrote the foreword for *Disorders of Brain and Mind.*

Maria A. Ron
Anthony S. David

London, January 1997

Introduction

D. FRANK BENSON

I consider it a great privilege to present an introduction to the volume entitled *Disorders of Brain and Mind*. The topic has been a lifelong interest of mine and the format devised for this volume by the editors, Maria Ron and Anthony David, holds great promise. By matching cutting-edge reports from the basic sciences with the experiences of seasoned clinicians, this volume helps bridge the chasm separating the two. Through presentations in this volume the editors and their chosen contributors provide a rational, scientifically validated base for the re-emerging subspecialty of neuropsychiatry. It is indeed a privilege to participate in such a challenging and potentially rewarding enterprise.

Appropriately, this volume is dedicated to the pioneering efforts of my true friend and valued colleague, William Alwyn Lishman. Professor Lishman exerted a major influence on my own career, particularly through his attempts to develop for me some sense of the psychiatric approach. More significant, Professor Lishman's seminal contributions and strong influence on the development of contemporary neuropsychiatry deserve recognition. I am pleased to be involved.

To introduce Alwyn Lishman's position requires background concerning the uneven, often unsuccessful, course and current regenesis of neuropsychiatry as a subspecialty. Over the years neuropsychiatry has been used to characterise a number of diverse approaches to the problems of the mentally ill. Instead of a single, widely accepted version, historical neuropsychiatry has multiple versions based on individual interpretations. All are correct. To appreciate the current status of neuropsychiatry and to place Professor Lishman's endeavours in proper perspective, several of the better defined versions deserve review.

In one version, neuropsychiatry can be considered a relatively late development, traced to the origins of neurology and psychiatry as medical specialities that awaited the acceptance of serious mental illness (insanity) into the medical sphere. In a splendid review of the topic, Sir Denis Hill (1964, 1989) stressed that mental illnesses, particularly the most disruptive disorders (psychoses), were not accepted within the province of medicine until the 19th century. Rather, spiritual malfunction, either self-induced (e.g. devil worship, immorality) or externally influenced (e.g. witchcraft, possession states), was the accepted explanation for the genesis of mental illness. The insane were billeted in prison-like structures, incarcerated under cruel, almost routinely inhumane conditions; the few academically inclined individuals who contemplated and discussed the problems of insanity came from the fields of philosophy and theology. Sin, pacts with the Devil, possession by evil spirits, the wages of impure living, and similar states were the topics discussed. Confinement with or without physical punishment was the accepted mode of therapy. Not until the humanitarian aspects of the French Revolution were sufficiently established were the insane accepted and treated as human beings. Phillipe Pinel (1745–1846), the great French psychiatrist, is credited with strong humane influences that improved care of the mentally ill. Attempts to conceptualise the problems of insanity as medical disorders followed.

Slowly, and with an inconsistent progression that continues to the present, physical explanations have been sought, and more than a few put forwards to explain, the problems of the mentally ill. Two totally different approaches to the source of mental illness have been prominent. One is exemplified by the work of Carl Wernicke (1848–1905), the German psychiatrist/investigator, who, following his brilliant demonstration of distinctly different language disorders based on different sites of brain damage, led several generations of Continental investigators in pursuit of neuroanatomical correlates of behavioural disorders. Wernicke and his followers were at least partially successful; their efforts provide a structural groundwork for contemporary neurology of behaviour.

Anatomical–behavioural correlations were often unsuccessful, however. In particular, the genesis of common problems such as the schizophrenias and the affective disorders could not be demonstrated. Relatively replicable distinctions of the major insanities, based on behavioural phenomenology, were recorded and classified by another prominent German psychiatrist–investigator, Emil Kraepelin (1856–1926). He classified observations collected from 19th century psychiatrists and developed a phenomenologically based classification of mental illness that has prevailed throughout the 20th century.

Sir Denis Hill has suggested that neuropsychiatry, as a subspeciality, exists as a bridge between the Wernicke's neuropathologically based and the phenomenologically based Kraepelinian approaches to psychiatry. Those mental illnesses in which both approaches are possible can be incorporated into the province of neuropsychiatry.

A different version of the historical background for neuropsychiatry has been proposed by Michael Trimble (1993). He suggests that neuropsychiatry has an ancient foundation, dating at least to the classical Greek physicians and their concern with epilepsy. Trimble notes that a duality of mental disorder (organic–functional) prevailed from the time of the Greek philosophers through the late 19th century. Localisation of psychological functions in discrete cerebral areas was proposed by Sir Francis Gall (1758–1828), a direct predecessor to the Wernicke localisationist approach. Although ultimately unsuccessful and intellectually debased into the parlour game called phrenology, Gall's initial premise of cortical localisation generated the interest and investigations that eventually led to a localisationist approach to cerebral function.

To develop this version further, Trimble has reviewed ideas developed by the renowned English neurologist, James Hughlings Jackson (1835–1911). Based on Darwinian evolution theories, Jackson posited a hierarchical layering of mental activities with the high-level cognitive functions of human behaviour superimposed over primitive behaviours which, nonetheless, remained active. When correlated with the strong class-structure rankings prevalent at the time, Jackson's postulations implied that mental dysfunctions represented dysfunction at a higher level than other neurological problems. Jackson's views strongly influenced both neurology and psychiatry, particularly in the United Kingdom. Psychiatrists were charged with the care of all mental impairments including those caused by coarse brain disorder. On this basis, neuropsychiatry has long been a recognised subspeciality in the United Kingdom. In sharp contrast, the neurology of behaviour has had few United Kingdom adherents.

In 1989 W.A. Lishman presented yet another version for the genesis of neuropsychiatry. He proposed that currently accepted concepts of neuropsychiatry are of recent origin, derived directly from the serendipitous demonstration that pharmacologic intervention altered the insanities. Successful drug therapy of both schizophrenia and affective disorder provided a scientific approach to mental illness that rivalled that of other medical disciplines. From this psychopharmacologic base psychiatrists have investigated the neuroanatomical structures and the neurophysiologic functions altered by the drugs, coming close, if not truly bridging, the gap between the neuroscientific and phenomenologic descriptions of behaviour. Lishman acknowledges the very real differences between the neurologist and the psychiatrist but finds the two specialities increasingly similar; in his view, the field called neuropsychiatry bridges the two specialised approaches.

Several additional historical facts deserve mention because of their strong influence on the background of neuropsychiatry. The first, easily forgotten by present-day physicians, concerns neurosyphilis, particularly dementia paralytica (general paresis of the insane), a dominant disorder in the practice of both neurology and psychiatry for over a century. Hare (1959) has provided a fascinating description of the history of neurosyphilis. He notes that dementia paralytica was first recognised as a distinct entity in the mental asylums of Paris early in the 19th century. Based on the original, clearly drawn phenomenologic descriptions (Boyle, 1822), the spread of dementia paralytica can be traced along commercial and military routes until recognised throughout the world. Socioeconomically deprived classes (seamen, soldiers, labourers, and their female followers) were most involved, leading to hackneyed aetiological suggestions such as excessive alcoholism, promiscuous sexuality, genetic incompetence, etc. Over the years neurosyphilis increased in frequency, severity and public concern until recognised as a major cause of mental disability.

Dementia paralytica was the first major mental disorder for which a successful treatment (fever therapy: Wagner-Jauregg and Bruetsch, 1946) was developed and the first to have scientific demonstration of a specific disease marker (the Wasserman test). It was among the first mental disorders to have a proven disease-specific aetiology (spirochetes: Noguchi and Moore, 1913), and to have a true cure (pensillin therapy: Mahoney, Arnold and Harris, 1943) discovered. During the century in which these events occurred (first reported in the early 1800s with widespread use of penicillin therapy in the 1940s), numerous physicians specialised in the management and treatment of neurosyphilis. These physicians had to be competent in both neurology and psychiatry and truly deserved the title of neuropsychiatrists. As tertiary syphilis disappeared, specialists in its care were no longer needed and neuropsychiatry, as practiced in the late 19th and the first half of the 20th century, also disappeared.

Another influence that separated neurology and psychiatry, and suppressed interest in neuropsychiatry, developed in the early 20th century. Although dating back to the influences of Mesmer (1734–1815), a purely psychological (non-medical) approach to mental illness was robustly introduced by the efforts of Sigmund Freud (1856–1939) and his many psychoanalytic successors early in the 20th century. 'Dynamic' explanations for mental illness increased in popularity through the early and middle decades of the 20th century until many, quite possibly most, practitioners of psychiatry dealt solely with the 'mind', ignoring disorders of body and brain. Neuropsychiatry had no place in this milieu.

The powerful schism between biological and psychological approaches was enhanced by events preceding World War II. Strong anti-Semitic practices in Nazi Germany compelled migration of many German and Austrian psychiatrists who had practiced in either neuropsychiatry or dynamic psychiatry. Even Sigmund Freud was forced to leave his beloved Vienna. Emigré psychiatrists scattered through the Western world. Those with medical (organic) preferences were comfortable in the tradition established by Hughlings Jackson and tended to migrate to Great Britain. Those favouring a psychological genesis of mental disease, on the other hand, tended to migrate to North America, particularly the United States. Following World War II, psychiatry in the United States was dominated by psychoanalytically oriented psychiatrists while in England a more medical approach had been strengthened by World War II immigrants.

The strong organic–functional dichotomy that had developed in psychiatry was reversed by the demonstration of psychopharmacological influences on the severe mental illnesses. Biological psychiatry and psychopharmacology have produced robust influences on contemporary psychiatry that have led to a tentative rapprochement of neurology and psychiatry. The neuropsychiatry of America remains distinct from that of Great Britain but the interests and goals are similar and the two versions are rapidly integrating.

A number of fundamentally different components make up the current setting of neuropsychiatry. These include basic biological, chemical, pharmacological and anatomical investigations, the field of genetics, and clinical studies (both neurological and psychiatric). Brain imaging by magnetic resonance (MRI), computed tomography (CT), positron and single-photon emission-computed tomography (PET and SPECT), and multiple variations of electroencephalography including evoked responses and quantitative brain mapping, provide vast reservoirs of information for the new neuropsychiatry. Neuropsychiatry has become a diverse, burgeoning field commanding armies of dedicated workers.

One of the most crucial arenas for neuropsychiatric investigation revolves about the phenomenology of mental disorders. In the face of the rapidly progressing scientific techniques, the significance of basic phenomenology is easily overlooked. The symptom clusters identifying the disorders within the domain of neuropsychiatry retain significance. Some, based on structural damage that produces behavioural changes, can be considered hard-wired organic mental states. Others remain descriptions of unique clinical disturbances. the phenomenology that distinguishes the various disorders of classic psychiatry. Through multiple investigations, rapprochement between the hard-wired and descriptive mental states is occurring.

Among the main influences toward the development of contemporary neuropsychiatry, Alwyn Lishman's own *Organic Psychiatry* (Lishman, 1978, 1987) occupies a special position. The broadly based review of the psychiatric and neurologic disorders that encompass the field of neuropsychiatry presented in *Organic Psychiatry* represents an invaluable repository of information. *Organic Psychiatry* has indeed played a major role in the development of contemporary neuropsychiatry.

William Alwyn Lishman was ideally placed to become a leader in the rebirth of neuropsychiatry. Born in 1931 in the north of England, he qualified in Medicine/Surgery in 1956 in Birmingham. From 1957 to 1959, Lishman served as Officer in Charge of the Medical Division of the Army Head Injury Hospital in Oxford, training in Neurology under the tutelage of Ritchie Russell, an acknowledged leader of British neurology of the mid-20th century.

In 1960 Lishman changed hats, starting his psychiatric training at the Maudsley Hospital in London. In 1966 he was appointed Consultant in Psychological Medicine at the National Hospital for Nervous Diseases (now the National Hospital for Neurology and Neurosurgery). He served in this position for only a year to return as Consultant Psychiatrist to the Maudsley and Royal Bethlem Hospitals, and as a Senior Lecturer at the Institute of Psychiatry, part of London University. In 1976 he became the first Professor of Neuropsychiatry, at the Institute of Psychiatry, and in 1985 was awarded a Doctor of Science degree from the University of London. Thus, his career spanned neurology and psychiatry, making important contributions to both.

His contributions are many, from his seminal work on the neuropsychiatric sequelae of head injury to the studies of memory and the application of imaging techniques to the investigation of alcohol addiction and organic psychoses, there is hardly any aspect of the discipline that has not benefited from his pioneering efforts.

Even more important is the influence Lishman has exerted on a generation of psychiatrists, neurologists and psychologists, many of whom have contributed to this book, and this bodes well for neuropsychiatry.

References

Boyle, A.L.J. (1822). *Recherches sur l'arachnitis chronique, la gastrite et la gastro-entérite chronique, et la goutte consideres comme causes de l'aliénation mentale*. Paris: Didot le Jeune.

Hare, E.H. (1959). The origin and spread of dementia paralytica. *Journal of Mental Science*, **105**, 594–626.

Hill, D. (1964). The bridge between neurology and psychiatry. *Lancet*, **i**, 509–14.

Hill, D. (1989). The bridge between neurology and psychiatry. In *The Bridge Between Neurology and Psychiatry* (ed. E.H. Reynolds and M.R. Trimble), pp. 11–23. Edinburgh: Churchill Livingstone.

Lishman, W.A. (1978). *Organic Psychiatry*. Oxford: Blackwell.

Lishman, W.A. (1987). *Organic Psychiatry*, 2nd Edition. Oxford: Blackwell.

Lishman, W.A. (1989). Neurologists and psychiatrists. In *The Bridge Between Neurology and Psychiatry* (ed. E.H. Reynolds and M.R. Trimble), pp. 24–37. Edinburgh: Churchill Livingstone.

Mahoney, J.F., Arnold, P.C. and Harris, A. (1943). Penicillin treatment of early syphilis: Preliminary report. *American Journal of Public Health*, **33**, 1387–91.

Noguchi, H. and Moore, J.W. (1913). A demonstration of *Treponema pallidum* in the brain in cases of general paralysis. *Journal of Experimental Medicine*, **17**, 232–8.

Trimble, M.R. (1993). Neuropsychiatry or behavioral neurology. *Neuropsychiatry, Neuropsychology, and Behavioral Neurology*, **6**, 60–9.

Wagner-Jauregg, J. and Bruetsch, W.L. (1946). The history of the malaria treatment of general paralysis. *American Journal of Psychiatry*, **102**, 577–82.

Section I

Frontal lobes and neuropsychiatry

1

The neuropsychology of the frontal lobes

SUSAN E. McPHERSON & JEFFREY L. CUMMINGS

Introduction

The frontal lobes play a major role in cognition and behaviour. Injury to the prefrontal convexity, orbitofrontal, and medial frontal cortex have been found to produce distinctive syndromes (Cummings, 1985). However, behavioural changes similar to those seen in patients with frontal lobe damage have also been observed in patients with injury to other brain regions (Mendez, Adams and Lewandowski, 1989; Strub, 1989; Sandson *et al.*, 1991). These observations have raised questions regarding the anatomic specificity of 'frontal lobe' syndromes. Recent descriptions of several parallel fronto-subcortical circuits linking regions of the frontal lobe to subcortical structures (Alexander, DeLong and Strick, 1986; Alexander and Crutcher, 1990; Alexander, Crutcher and DeLong, 1990) help to provide a framework for understanding the similarity between behavioural changes produced by frontal lobe damage and those produced by lesions in other anatomic regions. This chapter: (1) presents the cognitive and behavioural functions of the frontal lobe, (2) describes the anatomy of each of three frontal-subcortical circuits, (3) discusses the cognitive and behavioural changes associated with damage to each circuit, and (4) demonstrates the similarity of behavioural syndromes occurring with damage to structures participating in the frontal-subcortical circuits.

Frontal lobes and neuropsychological functions

The frontal lobes mediate aspects of attention and concentration, language, motor abilities, and executive functions. In addition, the frontal lobes play an important organisational role in memory functions and visuospatial skills. The following section summarises the functions of the frontal lobes in these cognitive domains.

Attention and concentration

Deficits in attention, concentration, and conceptual tracking are commonly associated with brain damage in general and specifically with frontal lobe dysfunction (Lezak, 1983; Stuss & Benson, 1986). Attention is defined as the capacity for selective perception (Allison, Blatt and Zimet, 1968; Mirsky, 1978). Concentration refers to a sustained, effortful, deliberate, heightened state of attention in which irrelevant stimuli are excluded from awareness (Russell, 1975). Conceptual tracking refers to the ability to maintain a directed train of thought over a period of time (Lezak, 1983), such as the ability to entertain two or more ideas simultaneously and sequentially. Attention disorders manifested by patients with frontal lobe damage include distractibility, inflexibility and inability to shift from one task to another (perseveration). For example, patients with frontal damage do poorly on tests such as the Trail Making Test, Part B (1944), which requires the patient to connect numbers and letters by alternating between the two sequences. Patients with frontal lobe damage are unable to shift between the numbers and letters, exhibiting perseveration, and an inability to shift attention from one set to another.

The specific site of frontal lobe pathology associated with deficits in attention and concentration has been difficult to demonstrate (Stuss and Benson, 1986). Attentional deficits can occur with damage to broad regions within the frontal lobes. Table 1.1 lists the tests most commonly used in the assessment of attention and concentration abilities.

Language

Deficits in speech and language are among the most well recognised disturbances of frontal lobe damage. Language skills are highly lateralised, with the left hemisphere responsible for mediating and planning verbal discourse and the right hemisphere involved in paralinguistic aspects of speech (Grattan and Eslinger, 1991). Language disturbances associated with frontal lobe damage include Broca's aphasia and transcortical motor aphasia (TMA). Broca's aphasia is caused by damage to the left posterior inferior frontal gyrus (Brodmann's areas 44–45) and is characterised by non-fluent, effortful, dysarthric speech that is telegraphic and agrammatic. Poor confrontation naming and intact comprehension of spoken language are also characteristic. Extensive damage to this area may result in total loss of speech with mutism. Transcortical motor aphasia involves the loss of the ability to produce spontaneous speech, with relatively intact comprehension and repetition of spoken language. The clinical pattern of the

Table 1.1. *Tests of frontal function*

Attention and Concentration
*Auditory Consonant Trigrams
*Continuous Performance Test
Digit Span
*Mental Control
Language
Boston Naming Test
*Controlled Oral Word Association Test
Boston Diagnostic Aphasia Exam
Western Aphasia Examination
Reitan Aphasia Screening Exam
Memory
*California Verbal Learning Test
Rey Auditory Verbal Learning Test
Fuld Object Memory Evaluation
Logical Memory (from Wechsler Memory Scale – Revised)
Wechsler Paired Associate Learning Test
Visuospatial Skills
Block Design (from Wechsler Adult Intelligence Scale – Revised)
*Rey–Osterrieth Complex Figure
*Taylor Figure
Executive Functions
Halstead Category Test
Problems of Fact (Stanford–Binet scales)
Tinker Toy Test
Tower of London
Trail Making Test
Stroop Color Interference Test
Wisconsin Card Sorting Test
Motor
Finger Tapping Test
Grooved Pegboard
Purdue Pegboard
Hand Dynamometer

* These tests provide information on executive function as well as on instrumental neuropsychological skills.

disturbance is marked by an initial period of muteness followed by decreased verbal output including both spontaneous and responsive speech. Articulation, confrontation naming and repetition are spared, comprehension is relatively intact, but categorical word-list generation is impaired (Stuss and Benson, 1986). Damage to tissue anterior or superior to Broca's area or damage to medial frontal areas including supplementary motor area (SMA) result in TMA.

Subcortical lesions extending into the frontal lobe may also produce language disturbances. Lesions associated with 'subcortical' aphasias involve the putamen, caudate, and anterior limb of the internal capsule, and extend anteriorly to involve white matter deep to Broca's area (Stuss and Benson 1986). Patients with lesions in these areas typically have good comprehension, impaired articulation, and right hemiparesis, clinically resembling patients with Broca's aphasia. Echolalia, perseveration, and reduction of volume may be present and confrontation naming and word retrieval are reduced.

Poor word-list generation or verbal fluency is also associated with, but not unique to, frontal lobe damage. Decreased fluency is observed in patients with damage to the left frontal lobe (Milner, 1964; Benton, 1968; Perret, 1974); some studies have found decreased fluency with right frontal lesions as well (Hécaen and Ruel, 1981; Ramier and Hécaen, 1970). Although poor word-list generation is present in frontal lobe dysfunction, deficits on tasks of word-list generation are not specific for frontal pathology (Stuss and Benson, 1984) and also occur with aphasia and psychomotor retardation.

Other alterations in verbal output resulting from frontal lobe damage include mutism and hypophonia (lowered volume). Mutism can occur following lesions in the putamen, internal capsule, operculum, or septal area and with damage to the SMA (Stuss and Benson, 1986). Mutism may also occur transiently in patients with lesions of Broca's area.

Right frontal structures have been implicated in controlling the affective components of communication including emotional prosody and gesturing (Heilman, Scholes and Watson, 1975; Tucker, Watson and Heilman, 1977; Larsen, Skinhoj and Lassen, 1978; Ross and Mesulam, 1979).

Memory

Memory impairment commonly occurs with frontal lobe dysfunction. Damage to the frontal lobes does not result in a primary information storage deficit, but instead reflects inefficient performance secondary to poor executive control, self-regulatory impairments, and inefficient search mechanisms (Grattan and Eslinger, 1991). Luria (1971, 1973) suggested that memory disturbance in patients with frontal lobe lesions results from the inability to create a stable intention to remember and an impairment of the ability to shift recall from one memory trace to another. This theory has been referred to as a 'forgetting to remember' in which details have not been forgotten, but cannot be accessed by the patient. Deficits in selective attention and lack of initiative have also been suggested as the source of memory dysfunction in patients with frontal lobe damage (Hécaen and Albert, 1978). Other theories of the cause of frontal memory deficits have included a variety of processes including susceptibility to interference (Brown, 1958; Kimura, 1963; Cermak and Butters, 1972; Stuss and Benson, 1986), difficulty following instructions (Milner, 1965; Walsh, 1978), impaired encoding and registration (Lewinsohn, Danaher and Kikel, 1972), and poor organisation and monitoring of material to be remembered (Lezak, 1983; Milner and Petrides, 1984; Stuss and Benson, 1986; Eslinger and Grattan, 1989). Patients with frontal lobe damage exhibit impairment on both spatial and nonspatial associative-learning tasks (Petrides, 1985) and are impaired on tasks requiring temporal organisation of material such as the temporal order of events (Milner, 1971; Milner, Petrides and Smith, 1985; Shimamura, Janowsky and Squire, 1990). In a study by Incisa dela Rocchetta and Milner (1993) patients with damage to the left frontal lobe exhibited intact recall of a short paragraph, but had impaired free recall when asked to learn a list of words. Performance improved when encoding and retrieval strategies were supplied, suggesting a deficit in organisation of information. The limbic system and thalamic projections into frontal regions may contribute to regulatory processes in retrieval of memory (Squire and Butters, 1984) and damage to these systems may produce frontal dysfunction and memory deficits.

Visuospatial skills

The frontal lobes are not considered essential to visuoperceptual or visuospatial abilities, per se. Whereas deficits on relatively simple tasks are rare following frontal lobe damage, deficits can occur on complex tasks requiring sequencing, rapid switching of concepts, inhibition of interfering stimuli and planning (Stuss and Benson, 1986). Frontal lobe damage rarely affects copying of simple figures (Luria, 1973; Stuss *et al.*, 1985), suggesting that basic visuoconstructive abilities are intact (Stuss and Benson, 1986). However, copying of complex figures, such as the Rey–Osterrieth Complex Figure (Osterrieth, 1944), is impaired because of poor planning with segmentation, distortion of the figure, unnecessary intrusions and over attention to specific details (Taylor, 1969, 1979).

Executive functions

Executive functions are comprised of four principal neuropsychological components: (1) goal formulation, (2) planning, (3) carrying out goal-directed behaviour, and (4) the ability to monitor effective performance (Lezak, 1983). Deficits in executive functions are cardinal signs of damage to the prefrontal areas. The assessment of executive functions should include tests that allow for the assessment of these four abilities.

Goal formulation

One of the most difficult areas to assess using standardised measures is goal formulation. Patients with mild deficits in goal formulation may be able to carry out simple tasks such as completing chores and engaging in familiar activities without prompting, but they may be unable to formulate new activities spontaneously, or develop and carry out a novel plan. The best sources of information regarding the patient's capacity for goal formulation come from direct observation of the patient's daily activities and information from family members. The 'Problems of Fact' items of the Stanford–Binet scales (Terman and Merrill, 1973) and the 'Cookie Theft' picture of the Boston Diagnostic Aphasia examination (Goodglass and Kaplan, 1972) have both been used to determine if the patient can benefit from and attend to situational cues in the course of goal formulation.

Planning

Planning includes the capacities to conceptualise change from present circumstances, deal objectively with the environment and with the self in relationship to the environment, conceive alternatives, weigh and make choices, and evolve a framework or structure for carrying out a plan (Lezak, 1983). The Porteus Maze Test (Porteus, 1959) is hypothesised to assess planning and foresight, as opposed to other maze tests that are thought to measure spatial learning (Stuss and Benson, 1986). However, recent investigations raise questions regarding the localisation of functions required by the Porteus Mazes (see below). Although used primarily to test abstract reasoning and the ability to shift set, sorting tests also depend on the patient's ability to change from present circumstances and benefit from environmental cues. The two most well-known sorting tasks are the Wisconsin Card Sorting Test (WCST; Berg, 1948) and the Halstead Category Test (Halstead, 1947). While these tests are sensitive to frontal lobe damage, they are not differentially sensitive to frontal dysfunction, as patients with generalised or diffuse brain damage also perform poorly on these tasks (Robinson *et al.*, 1980; Golden *et al.*, 1981).

The extent to which any of the above tests are related to activation of the frontal lobes has been the subject of recent study. Rezai and colleagues (1993) compared activation of regional cerebral blood flow in normals on four neuropsychological tests used in the assessment of frontal lobe functions: the WCST, the Continuous Performance Test (CPT; Rosvold *et al.*, 1956), the Tower of London (TOL; Shallice, 1982), and the Porteus Mazes. Results of single photon emission computed tomography (SPECT) studies indicated significant increases in cerebral blood flow to the frontal regions during the WCST, CPT, and TOL, but not during the Porteus Mazes. The CPT and TOL increased flow in the frontal mesial cortex bilaterally, suggesting prefrontal activation of the cingulate gyrus activity as compared with pure frontal lobe activity. The WCST, on the other hand, produced activation specifically of the left dorsolateral pre-frontal area. These findings provide support for the hypothesised purpose of the WCST in testing abstraction and ability to shift response set.

Carrying out goal-directed behaviour

The capacity to carry out goal-directed behaviour requires the ability to initiate, maintain, switch, and stop sequences of complex behaviour in an orderly and integrated manner (Lezak, 1983). The inability to programme activities will disrupt carrying the plan to fruition, even when patients are able to verbalise intentions, plans, and actions. Lezak (1982) has developed the Tinkertoy® Test, as one experimental means of assessing the ability to conceive and carry out a goal-directed plan. The task involves the initiation, planning, and structuring of a potentially complex activity and the ability to carry out the plan to completion. The patient is given a standard set of Tinkertoys and is given a minimum of five minutes to 'make something'. Scores are based upon several criteria including the ability to complete a structure and whether the object looks like the one that was intended.

Self-regulation of behaviour is also an important component of the ability to carry out a goal-directed plan. It involves the capacity to switch and stop sequences of complex behaviour based upon the demands of the situation and is assessed using tests of cognitive flexibility. Impaired flexibility results in perseverative, stereotyped behaviours and difficulties in modulation of motor acts. Patients may become 'stimulus-bound' resulting in an inability to dissociate responses or withdraw attention from a perceptual field. Inflexibility may manifest as an inability to shift perceptual organisation or adjust ongoing behaviour to meet the needs of the moment. Tests used to evaluate cognitive flexibility include the WCST, the Trail Making Test (Part B) and the Stroop Color Interference Test (Stroop, 1935).

Effective performance

Effective performance involves the patient's ability to monitor, self-correct, and regulate the intensity, tempo and other qualitative aspects of action (Lezak, 1983). Although effective performance is not readily assessed by standardised measures, abilities for self-correction can be observed during the course of a routine neuropsychological assessment by maintaining awareness of the nature of the patient's errors, attitude toward performance, idiosyncratic distortions and compensatory efforts.

Motor functions

Control of motor abilities is one of the most widely recognised frontal lobe functions. Bilateral frontal lobe damage can result in the emergence of 'release' signs such as grasp, rooting, suck, snout, and palmomental. A decrease in coordinative and integrative motor control can be associated with damage to the pre-frontal cortex. Contralateral hemiparesis reflects damage to either the frontal precentral gyrus or its subcortical white matter projection system.

Fine movements

Damage to the primary motor cortex is associated with a loss of ability to make fine independent finger movements and with a loss of speed and power in both hand and limb movements (Kolb and Whishaw, 1985). In the upper limbs, extensor muscles are more affected than flexor muscles. Assessment of fine motor movements includes tests such as the Finger Tapping Test (Halstead, 1947), the Grooved Pegboard (Kløve, 1963; Matthews and Kløve, 1964) or Purdue pegboard (Purdue Research Foundation, 1948); the Hand Dynamometer provides a measure of hand power. Right and left sides are assessed independently for each measure.

Motor impersistence

Motor impersistence is the term used to describe the inability to sustain simple motor acts such as conjugate gaze, eye fixation, protruding the tongue, keeping the mouth open or keeping the eyes closed (Benton *et al.*, 1983). Motor impersistence is associated primarily with right frontal lesions (Kertesz *et al.*, 1985), but may also occur with lesions to the left frontal lobe or with generalised damage (Bigler, 1988).

Apraxia

Apraxia refers to the inability to carry out purposeful movements by a patient with intact primary motor skills (e.g. strength, reflexes, coordination), sensory function, and comprehension (Hécaen, 1981). The two most commonly assessed forms of apraxia are ideomotor and ideational. Ideomotor apraxia is tested by asking the patient to perform previously learned motor acts such as blowing out a match (buccofacial movement) or hammering a nail (limb movement). Ideational apraxia represents a more complex level of function in that it requires the ability to follow a verbal command to perform a motor task linking various skilled movements, such as pouring coffee into a cup and stirring. Lesions of the deep frontal motor association cortex, parieto-frontal projection fibres, and corpus callosum have been associated with ideomotor apraxia (Kertesz and Ferro, 1984).

Emotional disorders

Patients with medial frontal and orbitofrontal lesions exhibit marked changes in personality. Patients with orbitofrontal tumours (Hunter, Blackwood and Bull, 1968), inferior frontal lobe infarction, and orbitofrontal injury secondary to communicating artery aneurysms (Logue *et al.*, 1968) or trauma exhibit behavioural disinhibition and irritability. Medial frontal lesions have also been associated with marked personality change. For example, patients with lesions to the anterior cingulate gyrus display marked apathy, even when in pain, and exhibit indifference to their circumstances (Neilsen and Jacobs, 1951; Barris and Schuman, 1953; Fesenmeier, Kuzniecky and Garcia, 1990). Depression occurs with increased prevalence among patients with left dorsolateral prefrontal lesions (Starkstein and Robinson, 1994).

Summary

Damage to the frontal lobes may result in any of the above neuropsychological sequelae. Patients with frontal lobe dysfunction exhibit impaired attention and concentration, reduced verbal fluency, poor ability to plan and carry out goal-directed behaviour, and motor disturbances. Deficits in memory may result from an inability to organise the information to be recalled or reproduced, an inability to shift recall from one memory trace to another, or deficits in selective attention. Similarly, abnormalities of visuospatial function observed in patients with frontal lobe damage reflect an inability to generate and implement an adequate constructional strategy.

Caution must be used in the interpretation of so-called 'frontal lobe findings'. Patients with dysfunction in other brain regions also present with deficits on frontal lobe tests. For example, patients with aphasia produce poor word-list generation, but may perform within normal limits on other tests of frontal lobe function. Similarly, although performance on sorting tasks are sensitive to frontal lobe damage, such tasks are not differentially sensitive, as patients with generalised or diffuse damage, such as dementia, also perform poorly (Robinson *et al.*, 1980; Golden *et al.*, 1981). As a result, these tests are sensitive to frontal damage, but are not specific for frontal lobe damage.

The cognitive and behavioural complexes described with frontal dysfunction have also been observed in patients with disorders affecting the basal ganglia and thalamus. The recent description of frontal-subcortical circuits linking these structures provide an anatomic framework for understanding the emergence of similar behaviours with lesions in different member structures of the circuits.

Fronto-subcortical circuits

There are five fronto-subcortical circuits linking regions of the frontal lobes to subcortical structures (Alexander *et al.*, 1986; Alexander and Crutcher, 1990; Alexander, Crutcher and DeLong, 1990). Injury to the structures within these circuits result in behavioural disorders similar to those described with frontal lobe lesions. Thus, these circuits provide a framework for understanding frontal-type behavioural changes associated with injury to non-frontal anatomical regions. The anatomy of each circuit is presented and is followed by a discussion of how disruption of each circuit provides insight into specific cognitive and behavioural disorders.

The five fronto-subcortical circuits are: (1) a motor circuit, with organs in the supplementary motor area, (2) an oculomotor circuit, which originates in the frontal eye fields, and three circuits with origins in the prefrontal cortex: (3) dorsolateral prefrontal cortex, (4) lateral orbital cortex, (5) anterior cingulate cortex (Alexander *et al.*, 1986; Alexander and Crutcher, 1990; Alexander *et al.*, 1990). The circuits are similar in the following ways: (1) all involve the same basic anatomic structures including striatum, globus pallidus, substantia nigra, and thalamus, (2) all circuits are contiguous, but remain anatomically segregated throughout, and (3) all circuits receive input from other brain regions and the regions providing the input are functionally related to the specific circuit to which they project (Cummings, 1993). Direct and indirect pathways exist within each circuit, with both pathways projecting to the thalamus. The direct pathway connects the striatum with the globus pallidus interna/substantia nigra complex (Alexander *et al.*, 1990). The indirect pathway connects striatum with globus pallidus externa followed by projection to subthalamic nucleus, and to the globus pallidus interna/substantia nigra (Alexander *et al.*, 1990). Although there are five fronto-subcortical circuits, only those originating in the prefrontal cortex are thought to be associated with cognitive and behavioural functions. The remainder of this section will focus on detailing each of these circuits.

Dorsolateral prefrontal circuit

The dorsolateral prefrontal circuit projects primarily to the dorsolateral portion of the head of the caudate nucleus (Alexander *et al.*, 1986, 1990). This circuit originates in the convexity of the frontal lobe (Broadmann's areas 9 and 10), projects to the caudate, and connects the caudate to the dorsomedial globus pallidus interna and rostral substantia nigra through the direct pathway. Connections through the indirect pathway link the globus pallidus externa to subthalamic nucleus, and back to the globus pallidus interna and substantia nigra. Neurons of the globus pallidus interna and substantia nigra project to the ventral anterior and medial dorsal thalamic nuclei, which in turn connect with the dorsolateral prefrontal region.

Lateral orbitofrontal circuit

The lateral orbitofrontal circuit originates in the inferolateral prefrontal cortex (Broadmann's area 10) and projects primarily to ventromedial caudate nucleus (Alexander *et al.*, 1986, 1990). The direct pathway of this circuit begins in the caudate region and projects to the dorsomedial pallidum and the rostromedial substantia nigra, medial to the area receiving projections from the dorsolateral caudate. The globus pallidus externa and subthalamic nucleus receive connections from the caudate and project to globus pallidus interna/substantia nigra forming the indirect pathway. Projection back to the orbito-frontal cortex occurs via pallidal and nigral connections to medial portions of the ventral anterior and medial dorsal thalamic nuclei.

Anterior cingulate circuit

This circuit begins in the cortex of the anterior cingulate gyrus, also known as Brodmann's area 24. Projections from the anterior cingulate include the nucleus accumbens, olfactory tubercle, and the ventromedial portions of the caudate and putamen (Alexander *et al.*, 1986, 1990; Parent, 1990). Neurons from the hippocampus, amygdala, and entorhinal and peripheral cortices also project to this ventral striatal area. Efferent connections exist between ventral striatum and ventral and rostrolateral globus pallidus and rostrodorsal substantia nigra. Direct and indirect pathways have not been identified but are thought likely to exist (Alexander *et al.*, 1990). Globus pallidus and substantia nigra efferents project to specific regions of the medial dorsal nucleus of the thalamus as well as to the ventral tegmental area, habenula, hypothalamus, and amygdala. Projections from medial dorsal thalamic neurones back to anterior cingulate cortex complete the circuit.

The neuropsychology of the fronto-subcortical circuits

As stated above, each of the fronto-subcortical circuits projects through the striatum, globus pallidus and thalamus. Dysfunction of any of these anatomical structures may produce behavioural and neuropsychological changes similar to those observed with damage to the region of prefrontal cortex to which they are connected.

The neuropsychology of caudate dysfunction

There are few reports of focal caudate lesions. One study, however, found patients with dorsal caudate lesions to be confused and disinterested, while patients with ventral caudate lesions were more disinhibited, euphoric and inappropriate (Mendez *et al.*, 1989). All patients exhibited deficits in memory, attention, and set shifting. Studies of animals with caudate lesions have demonstrated impaired performance on tasks involving spatial choice and memory and disruption of responses to reinforcement and conditioning (Oberg and Divac, 1979). These same changes are also produced with ablation of the corresponding frontal cortical areas projecting to the caudate nucleus (Corbett, McCusker and Davidson, 1986).

Patients with Huntington's disease (HD) provide the best example of the cognitive and behavioural symptoms associated with damage to the caudate nucleus. Neuropsychologically, patients with HD exhibit cognitive and behavioural deficits similar to patients with dorsolateral prefrontal dysfunction. Impaired verbal fluency is one of the earliest abnormalities of cognitive function in HD, preceding the declines in memory and other cognitive functions (Butters *et al.*, 1978). Patients with middle and advanced stages of HD perform poorly on naming tests that demand retrieval of low frequency words and language tests requiring organisation and sequencing of information (Kennedy *et al.*, 1981; Podoll *et al.*, 1988). Other language disturbances such as paraphasias do not occur, although dysarthria is a prominent feature. Patients with HD perform poorly on card-sorting tests (Weinberger *et al.*, 1988), exhibit deficits in concentration and judgment, and are unable to initiate problem-solving behaviour (Cummings and Benson, 1992). They have difficulty with tasks that require organisation, planning, and sequential arrangement of information and perform badly on some visuospatial tasks (Caine *et al.*, 1978; Brandt, Folstein and Folstein, 1988). In addition, they have difficulty on tasks which require sequential motor programming, such as alternating hand sequences; these deficits go beyond those ascribed to their movement disorder (Cummings and Benson, 1992). The above deficits reflect the involvement of the head of the caudate nuclei, which receives lateral prefrontostriatal projections.

An important differentiation between patients with HD and those with frontal lobe damage is that in the former, long-term memory and new learning are equally impaired and there is a marked deficit in retrieval (Caine, Ebert and Weingartner, 1977; Butters, Albert and Sax, 1979; Weingartner, Caine and Ebert; 1979; Albert, Butters and Brandt, 1981; Butters *et al.*, 1986), whereas in the latter long-term memory is intact.

Behavioural manifestations may include apathy, mood disorder, irritability, explosive disorder, and obsessive-compulsive disorder (Folstein, 1989; Cummings and Cunningham, 1992). Alterations in personality occur early in HD, corresponding to initial involvement of medial caudate regions, particularly those that receive projections from the orbitofrontal and anterior cingulate circuits. These circuits mediate limbic system functions and emotion (Vonsattel *et al.*, 1985).

Behavioural changes associated with lesions to the ventromedial striatum/nucleus accumbens area have not been studied extensively and are limited primarily to case studies. Phillips, Sangalang and Stern (1987) observed apathy, withdrawal, and loss of initiative in a patient with a posteriorly located, anterior communicating artery aneurysm. Memory deficits and confabulation were observed on testing. Performance on tests of intellectual ability, constructions, verbal fluency and card-sorting were normal. Autopsy revealed bilateral lesions confined to the rostroventral globus pallidus, nucleus accumbens, septal grey matter, and nucleus of the diagonal band of Broca. Conditions involving the ventral striatum, ventral globus pallidus, and medial thalamus, such as craniopharingiomas, obstructive hydrocephalus, and tumours in the region of the third ventricle have all been linked to akinetic mutism (Lavy, 1959; Klee, 1961; Messert, Henke and Langheim, 1966).

Taken together the above observations suggest that caudate/striatal dysfunction is associated with behavioural disorders similar to those seen with damage to the frontal lobes. Lesions of the dorsal caudate result in impaired executive functions, implicating the dorsolateral prefrontal circuit. Ventral caudate lesions are associated with disinhibition and inappropriate behaviour such as is seen in the orbitofrontal circuits. Lesions to the nucleus accumbens produce apathy and lack of initiative that are characteristic of damage to the anterior cingulate circuit.

The neuropsychology of pallidal dysfunction

Each of the fronto-subcortical circuits projects from the striatum to the globus pallidus and substantia nigra. Reports of focal damage to the globus pallidus are also rare and are limited to case studies or multi-case reports. Focal insults have been reported following carbon monoxide poisoning, manganese intoxication, and occasionally in the course of vascular disease. In one case study of bilateral globus pallidus haemorrhages, the patient exhibited changes in personality marked by prominent apathy, withdrawal and loss of interest, and deficits on tests of memory and set shifting (Strub, 1989). Laplane and colleagues (1984) observed reduced spontaneous activity, impaired initiative and diminished ability to conceive new thoughts following bilateral globus pallidus lesions secondary to carbon monoxide poisoning. These patients exhibited impaired memory functions, with normal language, reasoning, and mental control. Reports of manganese toxicity have been associated with increased irritability, compulsions, depression, apathy, and withdrawal (Schuler *et al.*, 1957; Mena *et al.*, 1967).

Discrete frontal-subcortical syndromes are not easily identifiable in the literature on strategic globus pallidus lesions. However, behavioural manifestations of irritability and apathy and cognitive abnormalities affecting memory and executive functions are similar to those seen in patients with frontal lobe damage, suggesting involvement of all the fronto-subcortical circuits.

The neuropsychology of thalamic dysfunction

The effect of thalamic infarcts on cognitive and behavioural functions has been studied extensively. Patients with bilateral paramedian thalamic infarction can present with cognitive and behavioural deficits similar to those seen in patients with frontal lobe damage. Behavioural changes observed have included dysphoria, irritability and disinhibition, apathy, utilisation behaviour, and distractibility (Gentilini, De Renzi and Crisi, 1987; Bogousslavksy *et al.*, 1988; Eslinger *et al.*, 1991). Cognitive deficits observed have included poor memory (Gentilini *et al.*, 1987; Stuss *et al.*, 1988; Eslinger *et al.*, 1991), reduced verbal fluency, decreased mental control, and intact language (Eslinger *et al.*, 1991). Stuss and colleagues (1988) found that patients with asymmetrical bilateral paramedian thalamic infarctions had deficits in memory and set shifting and changes in personality including apathy. There was some variability in the pattern of deficits, dependent upon the predominant site of injury to the thalamus.

Case studies of patients with thalamic infarction have reported deficits on tests of frontal lobe function. Sandson and coworkers (1991) reported a case of left medial dorsal thalamic infarction in which the patient exhibited apathy, memory impairment, poor word-list generation and poor executive functions, findings similar to those seen in patients with frontal lobe damage. Pepin and Pepin (1993) reported three patients with unilateral thalamic ischemic lesion (two left, one right). Although only two of the three patients exhibited memory changes characteristic thalamic dysfunction, all three exhibited deficits on tasks of verbal fluency, made a significant number of perseverative errors on a task of set shifting ability (WCST), and exhibited susceptibility to interference and an inability to inhibit inappropriate responses as measured by the Stroop procedure. In comparison, patients with lesions of the temporal lobes exhibited similar impairments on tasks of memory, but no impairment on tests of frontal functions. These authors suggested that the selective deficits in frontal functions in these patients was secondary to a loss of thalamocortical afferents. Eslinger and coworkers (1991) reported perseveration, impaired verbal fluency, poor sequential reasoning, and poor motor programming in a patient with a paramedian thalamic infarct. Similarly, Mennemeier and colleagues (1992) found reduced verbal fluency, poor sequential reasoning, decreased unilateral motor performance, and poor performance on a task of motor persistence, sustained attention and response speed (Digit Symbol from WAIS-R) in a patient with a left thalamic infarction, one year after the event. Damage to the thalamus therefore appears to interfere with projections to the frontal lobes resulting in a pattern of frontal deficits.

Memory impairment and poor insight are characteristic of thalamic degenerative diseases, and apathy and disinhibition have also been described (Moossy *et al.*, 1987; Deymeer *et al.*, 1989). Discrete syndromes corresponding to the three frontal-subcortical syndromes are rarely described with lesions at the thalamic level and disorders with mixed features are the rule.

Fronto-subcortical circuits: neuropsychological and behavioural implications

The observations cited above of cognitive and behavioural syndromes associated with damage to frontal, striatal, pallidal, and thalamic structures support the concept of the existence of frontal-subcortical circuits and circuit-specific behaviours. Three frontal lobe symptom complexes are recognisable, each of which corresponds to a different fronto-subcortical circuit. Damage to the dorsolateral prefrontal circuit results primarily in neuropsychological deficits. Disruption of the lateral orbitofrontal circuit produces disinhibition and irritability, and damage to the anterior cingulate circuit results in apathy.

Dorsolateral prefrontal dysfunction

Deficits in executive functions and abnormalities in motor programing characterise the dorsolateral prefrontal syndrome and disruption of the related subcortical circuit. Neuropsychologically, the syndrome is marked by an inability to shift set required by changing task demands, reduced verbal fluency, poor organisational strategies on tests of learning, poor constructional strategies for copying complex designs (Benton, 1968; Jones-Gotman and Milner, 1977), and poor performance on reciprocal and sequential motor tests (Cummings, 1985). Patients with dorsolateral prefrontal lesions may exhibit normal performance on standard tests of new learning capacity such as word recognition, cued recall, and paired-associate learning (Janowsky *et al.*, 1989*a*). Performance on tests of free recall, temporal order, source memory, and metamemory is impaired (Milner, 1971; Janowsky *et al.*, 1989; Janowsky, Shimamura and Squire, 1989*b,c*; Shimamura, Janowsky and Squire, 1991). Shimamura and colleagues (1992) found that patients with dorsolateral prefrontal lesions were not impaired on a task of implicit memory, as assessed by a word-stem completion test but were impaired on the Wisconsin Card Sorting Test and a test of verbal fluency.

Orbitofrontal dysfunction

The primary feature of orbitofrontal dysfunction is a marked change in personality including loss of tact, irritability, apathy, loss of initiative, and elevated mood. These symptoms have been found in patients with anterior communicating artery aneurysms with orbito-frontal injury (Logue *et al.*, 1968), orbitofrontal tumours (Hunter *et al.*, 1968), and inferior frontal lobe infarction (Bogousslavsky and Regli, 1990). Imitation and utilisation behaviours have been observed in patients with anterior orbitofrontal lobe lesions (Lhermitte, Pillon and Serdaru, 1986). These behaviours, which are a form of stimulus-boundedness, reflect enslavement to environmental cues, enforced utilisation of objects in the environment, or automatic imitation of the gestures and actions of others. Disruption to the orbitofrontal circuit may be responsible for the stimulus-bound behaviour associated with frontal lobe syndromes. Patients with orbitofrontal damage may have relatively few neuropsychological deficits and have been found to perform card sorting tasks normally (Laiacona *et al.*, 1989).

Anterior cingulate dysfunction

Anterior cingulate injury has been associated with akinetic mutism when bilateral lesions are present. Symptoms include profound apathy, lack of spontaneous speech, and monosyllabic or no answers to questions. There is a lack of emotion, even when in pain, and indifference to the marked impairment (Nielsen and Jacobs, 1951; Barris and Schuman, 1953; Fesenmeier *et al.*, 1990). Transient akinetic mutism has been observed when unilateral lesions are present (Wyszynski *et al.*, 1989). Medial frontal lobe lesions have been associated with failure to inhibit responses on go–no go tests (Drewe, 1974; Leimkuhler and Mesulam, 1985).

Summary

Fronto-subcortical circuitry provides a framework for linking cognitive and behavioural changes generally associated with frontal lobe damage to alternate but related anatomic structures. Three behaviourally relevant

frontal-subcortical circuits have been described. A
involves identical anatomic structures, the circuits re
tion, simultaneous lesions within the circuits produc
additive effects. Identifiable circuit-specific behaviou
each circuit; changes that are similar cognitively and be
seen in patients with frontal lobe dysfunction. These
dysfunction and motor programming deficits for th
frontal-subcortical circuit; irritability and agitation for
subcortical circuit; and apathy for the anterior cin
circuit.

This model provides insight into and possible explanati
physiology of neuropsychiatric as well as neurobehaviour
example, the precise anatomic correlates of conditions su
compulsive disorder (OCD) and mood disorders are not f
and require further study. However, conditions such as de[illegible] might be explained by the disruption of the dorsolateral or orbitofrontal-subcortical circuits, and the anterior cingulate and orbito-frontal circuits have been implicated in conditions such as OCD (Cummings, 1993). The framework provided here requires further study and validation. However, it facilitates hypothesis generation and can help to guide research exploring the relationship between cognitive and behavioural disorders and fronto–subcortical circuits.

Acknowledgements

This project was supported by the Department of Veteran Affairs and a National Institute on Aging Alzheimers's Disease Core Center grant (AG10123).

References

Albert, M.S., Butters, N. and Brandt, J. (1981). Patterns of remote memory in amnestic and demented patients. *Archives of Neurology*, **38**, 495–500.

Alexander, G.E. and Crutcher, M.D. (1990). Functional architecture of basal ganglia circuits: neural substrates of parallel processing. *Trends in the Neurosciences*, **13**, 26–271.

Alexander, G.E., DeLong, M.R. and Strick, P.L. (1986). Parallel organization of functionally segregated circuits linking basal ganglia and cortex. *Annual Review of Neuroscience*, **9**, 357–81.

Alexander, G.E., Crutcher, M.D. and DeLong, M.R. (1990). Basal ganglia-thalamocortical circuits: Parallel substrates for motor, oculomotor, prefrontal and limbic functions. *Progress in Brain Research*, **85**, 119–46.

Allison, J., Blatt, S.J. and Zimet, C.N. (1968). *The Interpretation of Psychological Tests*. New York: Harper & Row.

Barris, R.W. and Schuman, H.R. (1953). Bilateral anterior cingulate gyrus lesions. *Neurology*, **3**, 44–52.

Beatty, W.W., Salmon, D.P., Butters, N. *et al.* (1988). Retrograde amnesia in patients with Alzheimer's disease or Huntington's disease. *Neurobiology of Aging*, **9**, 181–6.

Benton, A.L. (1968). Differential behavioral effects in frontal lobe disease. *Neuropsychologia*, **6**, 53–60.

Benton, A.L., Hamsher, K. de S., Varney, N.R. and Spreen, O. (1983). *Contributions in Neuropsychological Assessment*. New York: Oxford University Press.

Berg, E.A. (1948). A simple objective technique for measuring flexibility in thinking. *Journal of General Psychology*, **39**, 15–22.

Bigler, E.D. (1988). *Diagnostic Clinical Neuropsychology*. Austin: University of Texas Press.

Bogousslavsky, J., Ferrazzini, M., Regli, F. *et al.* (1988). Manic delirium and frontal lobe syndrome with paramedian infarction of the right thalamus. *Journal of Neurology, Neurosurgery and Psychiatry*, **51**, 116–19.

Bogousslavsky, J. and Regli, F. (1990). Anterior cerebral artery territory infarction in the Lausanne Stroke Registry. *Archives of Neurology*, **47**, 144–50.

Brandt, J., Folstein, M.E. and Folstein, M.F. (1988). Differential cognitive impairment in Alzheimer's disease and Huntington's disease. *Annals of Neurology*, **23**, 555–61.

Brown, J. (1958). Some tests of decay theory of immediate memory. *Quarterly Journal of Experimental Psychology*, **10**, 12–21.

Butters, N., Sax, D., Montgomery, K. *et al.* (1978). Comparison of the neuropsychological deficits associated with early and advanced Huntington's disease. *Archives of Neurology* **35**, 585–9.

Butters, N., Albert, M.S. and Sax, D. (1979). Investigations of the memory disorders of patients with Huntington's disease. *Advances Neurology*, **23**, 203–13.

Butters, N., Wolfe, J., Granholm, E. *et al.* (1986). An assessment of verbal recall, recognition and fluency abilities in patients with Huntington's disease. *Cortex*, **22**, 11–32.

Caine, E.D., Ebert, M.H. and Weingartner, H. (1977). An outline for the analysis of dementia: the memory disorder of Huntington's disease. *Neurology*, **27**, 1087–92.

Caine, E.D., Hunt, R.D., Weingartner, H. *et al.* (1978). Huntington's dementia: clinical and neuropsychological features. *Archives of Neurology*, **35**, 377–84.

Cermak, L.S. and Butters, N. (1972). The role of interference and encoding in short-term memory deficits of Korsakoff's patients. *Neuropsychologia*, **10**, 89–95.

Corbett, A.J., McCusker, E.A. and Davidson, O.R. (1986). Acalculia following a dominant-hemisphere subcortical infarct. *Archives of Neurology*, **43**, 964–6.

Cummings, J.L. (1985). *Clinical Neuropsychiatry*. New York: Grune & Stratton, Inc.

Cummings, J.L. (1993). Frontal-subcortical circuits and human behavior. *Archives of Neurology*, **50**, 873–80.

Cummings, J.L. and Benson, D.F. (1992). *Dementia: A Clinical Approach*. Boston: Butterworth-Heinemann.

Cummings, J.L. and Cunningham, K. (1992). Obsessive-compulsive disorder in Huntington's disease. *Biological Psychiatry*, **31**, 263–70.

Deymeer, F., Smith, T.W., DeGirolami, U. *et al.* (1989). Thalamic dementia and motor neuron disease. *Neurology*, **39**, 58–61.

Drewe, E.A. (1974). Go-no go learning after frontal lobe lesions in humans. *Cortex*, **11**, 8–16.

Eslinger, P.J. and Grattan, L.M. (1989). Specialization for memory in the frontal lobes. *The Clinical Neuropsychologist*, **3**, 287–8.

Eslinger, P.J., Warner, G.C., Grattan, L.M. *et al.* (1991). 'Frontal lobe' utilization behavior associated with paramedian thalamic infarction. *Neurology*, **41**, 450–2.

Fesenmeier, J.T., Kuzniecky, R. and Garcia, J.H. (1990). Akinetic mutism caused by bilateral anterior cerebral tuberculous obliterative arteritis. *Neurology*, **30**, 1005–6.

Folstein, S.E. (1989). *Huntington's Disease: A Disorder of Families*. Baltimore, MD: Johns Hopkins University Press.

Gentilini, M., De Renzi, E. and Crisi, G. (1987). Bilateral paramedian thalamic artery infarcts: Report of eight cases. *Journal of Neurology, Neurosurgery and Psychiatry*, **50**, 900–9.

Geschwind, N. (1967). The apraxias. In *Phenomenology of Will and Action*, (ed. E.W. Straus and R.M. Griffith). Pittsburgh: Duquesne University Press.

Golden, C.J., Osmon, D.C., Moses, J.A., Jr, *et al.* (1981). *Interpretation of the Halstead-Reitan Neuropsychological Test Battery: A Casebook Approach*. New York: Grune & Stratton Inc.

Goodglass, H. and Kaplan, E. (1972). *Assessment of Aphasia and Related Disorders*. Philadelphia: Lea & Febiger.

Grattan, L.M. and Eslinger, P.J. (1991). Frontal lobe damage in children and adults: a comparative review. *Developmental Neuropsychology*, **7**, 283–326.

Halstead, W.C. (1947). *Brian and Intelligence*. Chicago: University of Chicago Press.

Hécaen, H. (1981). Apraxias. In *Handbook of Clinical Neuropsychology* (ed. S.B. Filskov and T.J. Boll), New York: Wiley.

Hécaen, H. and Albert, M.L. (1978). *Human Neuropsychology*. New York: Wiley.

Hécaen, H. and Ruel, J. (1981). Sièges lésionnels intrafrontaux et déficit au test de 'fluence verbale'. *Revue Neurologique* (Paris), **137**, 277–84.

Heilman, K.M., Scholes, R. and Watson, R.T. (1975). Auditory affective agnosia: disturbed comprehension of affective speech. *Journal of Neurology, Neurosurgery and Psychiatry*, **38**, 69–72.

Hunter, R., Blackwood, W. and Bull, J. (1968). Three cases of frontal meningiomas presenting psychiatrically. *British Medical Journal*, **3**, 9–16.

Incisa della Rocchetta, A. and Milner, B. (1993). Strategic search and retrieval inhibition: the role of the frontal lobes. *Neuropsychologia*, **31**, 503–24.

Janowsky, J.S., Shimamura, A.P., Kritchevsky, M. *et al.* (1989*a*). Cognitive impairment following frontal lobe damage and its relevance to human amnesia. *Behavioral Neuroscience*, **103**, 548–60.

Janowsky, J.S., Shimamura, A.P. and Squire, L.R. (1989*b*). Memory and metamemory: comparisons between patients with frontal lobe and amnesic patients. *Psychobiology*, **17**, 3–11.

Janowsky, J.S., Shimamura, A.P. and Squire, L.R. (1989*c*). Source memory impairment in patients with frontal lobe lesions. *Neuropsychologia*, **27**, 1043–56.

Jones-Gotman, M. and Milner, B. (1977). Design fluency: The invention of nonsense drawings after focal cortical lesions. *Neuropsychologia*, **15**, 653–74.

Kennedy, J., Fisher, J., Shoulson, I. *et al.* (1981). Language impairment in Huntington disease. *Neurology*, **31**, 81–2.
Kertesz, A. and Ferro, J.M. (1984). Lesion size and location in ideomotor apraxia. *Brain*, **107**, 921–33.
Kertesz, A., Nicholson, A., Cancelliere, K. *et al.* (1985). A right-hemisphere syndrome. *Neurology*, **35**, 662–6.
Kimura, D. (1963). Right temporal-lobe damage. *Archives of Neurology*, **8**, 264–71.
Klee, A. (1961). Akinetic mutism: review of the literature and report of a case. *Journal of Nervous and Mental Disease*, **133**, 536–53.
Kløve, H. (1963). Clinical neuropsychology. In *The Medical Clinics of North America*. (ed. M. Forster). New York: Saunders.
Kolb, B. and Whishaw, I.Q. (1985). *Fundamentals of Human Neuropsychology*. New York: W.H. Freeman & Co.
Laiacona, M., De Santis, A., Barbarotto, R. *et al.* (1989). Neuropsychological follow-up of patients operated for aneurysms of anterior communicating artery. *Cortex*, **25**, 261–73.
Laplane, D. Baulac, M., Widlocher, D. *et al.* (1984). Pure psychic akinesia with bilateral lesions of basal ganglia. *Journal of Neurology, Neurosurgery and Psychiatry*, **47**, 377–85.
Larsen, B., Skinhoj, J. and Lassen, N.A. (1978). Variations in regional cortical blood flow in the right and left hemispheres during automatic speech. *Brain*, **101**, 193–209.
Lavy, S. (1959). Akinetic mutism in a case of craniopharyngioma. *Psychiatric Neurology*, **138**, 369–74.
Leimkuhler, M.E. and Mesulam, M.-M. (1985). Reversible go-no go deficits in a case of frontal lobe tumor. *Annals of Neurology*, **18**, 617–19.
Lewinsohn, P.M., Danaher, B.G. and Kikel, S. (1972). Visual imagery as a mneumonic aid for brain injured persons. *Journal of Consulting and Clinical Psychology* **45**, 717–23.
Lezak, M.D. (1982). The problem of assessing executive functions. *International Journal of Psychology*, **17**, 281–97.
Lezak, M.D. (1983). *Neuropsychological Assessment*. New York: Oxford University Press.
Lhermitte, F., Pillon, B. and Serdaru, M. (1986). Human anatomy and the frontal lobes. Part I: Imitation and utilization behavior: a neuropsychological study of 75 patients. *Annals of Neurology*, **19**, 326–34.
Logue, V., Dunward, M., Pratt, R.T.C. *et al.* (1968). The quality of survival after an anterior cerebral aneurysm. *British Journal of Psychiatry*, **114**: 137–60.
Luria, A.R. (1971). Memory disturbance in local brain lesions. *Neuropsychologia*, **9**, 367–76.
Luria, A.R. (1973). *The Working Brain: An Introduction to Neuropsychology* (trans. B. Haigh). New York: Basic Books.
Matthews, C.G. and Kløve, H. (1964). *Instruction Manual for the Adult Neuropsychological Test Battery*. Madison, WI: University of Wisconsin.
Mena, I., Marin, O., Fuenzalida, S. *et al.* (1967). Chronic manganese poisoning. *Neurology*, **17**, 128–36.
Mendez, M.F., Adams, N.L. and Lewandowski, K.S. (1989). Neurobehavioral changes associated with caudate lesions. *Neurology*, **39**, 349–54.
Mennemeier, M., Fennell, E., Valenstein, E. and Heilman, K.M. (1992). Contributions of the left intralaminar and medial thalamic nuclei to memory. Comparisons and report of a case. *Archives of Neurology*, **49**, 1050–8.

Messert, B., Henke, T.K. and Langheim, W. (1966). Syndrome of akinetic mutism associated with obstructive hydrocephalus. *Neurology*, **16**, 635–49.
Milner, B. (1964). Some effects of frontal lobectomy in man. In *The Frontal Granular Cortex and Behavior* (ed. J.M. Warren and K. Akert). New York: McGraw-Hill.
Milner, B. (1965). Visually guided maze learning in man: effects of bilateral hippocampal, bilateral frontal, and unilateral cerebral lesions. *Neuropsychologia*, **3**, 317–88.
Milner, B. (1971). Interhemispheric differences in the location of psychological processes in man. *British Medical Bulletin*, **27**, 272–7.
Milner, B. and Petrides, M. (1984). Behavioral effects of frontal lobe lesions in man. *Trends in the Neurosciences*, **7**, 403–7.
Milner, B., Petrides, M. and Smith, M.L. (1985). Frontal lobes and the temporal organization of memory. *Human Neurobiology*, **4**, 137–42.
Mirsky, A.F. (1978). Attention: a neuropsychological perspective. In *Education and the Brain*. Chicago: National Society for the Study of Education.
Moossy, J., Martinez, J., Hamin, I. *et al.* (1987). Thalamic and subcortical gliosis with dementia. *Archives of Neurology*, **44**, 510–13.
Nielsen, J.M. and Jacobs, L.L. (1951). Bilateral lesions of the anterior cingulate gyri. *Bulletin of the Los Angeles Neurological Society*, **16**, 231–4.
Oberg, R.G.E. and Divac, I. (1979). Cognitive functions of the neostriatum. In *The Neostriatum* (ed. I. Divac and R.E.G. Oberg). New York: Pergamon.
Osterrieth, P.A. (1944). Le test de copie d'une figure complexe. *Archives de Psychologie*, **30**, 206–356.
Parent, A. (1990). Extrinsic connections of the basal ganglia. *Trends in the Neurosciences*, **13**, 254–8.
Pepin, E.P. and Pepin, A.P. (1993). Selective dorsolateral frontal lobe dysfunction associated with diencephalic amnesia. *Neurology*, **43**, 733–41.
Perret, E. (1974). The left frontal lobe of man and the suppression of habitual responses in verbal categorical behavior. *Neuropsychologia*, **12**, 323–30.
Petrides, M. (1985). Deficits on conditional associative-learning tasks after frontal- and temporal-lobe lesions in man. *Neuropsychologia*, **23**, 601–14.
Phillips, S., Sangalang, V. and Stern, G. (1987). Basal forebrain infarction: A clinicopathologic correlation. *Archives of Neurology*, **44**, 1134–8.
Podoll, K., Caspary, P., Lange, H.W. *et al.* (1988). Language functions in Huntington's disease. *Brain*, **11**, 1475–503.
Porteus, S.D. (1959). *The Maze Test and Clinical Psychology*. Palo Alto: Pacific Books.
Purdue Research Foundation (1948). *Examiners Manual for the Purdue Pegboard*. Chicago: Science Research Associates.
Ramier, A.-M. and Hécaen, H. (1970). Rôle respectif des atteintes frontales et de la latéralisation lésionnelle dans les défecits de la 'fluence verbale'. *Revue Neurologique* (Paris), **123**, 17–22.
Rezai, K., Andreasen, N.C., Alliger, R. *et al.* (1993). The neuropsychology of the prefrontal cortex. *Archives of Neurology*, **50**, 636–42.
Robinson, A.L., Heaton, R.K., Lehman, R.A.W. *et al.* (1980). The utility of the Wisconsin Card Sorting Test in detecting and localizing frontal lobe lesions. *Journal of Consulting and Clinical Psychology*, **48**, 605–14.
Ross, E.D. and Mesulam, M.-M. (1979). Dominant language functions of the right hemisphere? Prosody and emotional gesturing. *Archives of Neurology*, **36**, 144–8.

Rosvold, H.E., Mirsky, A.F., Sarason, I., *et al.* (1956). A continuous performance test of brain damage. *Journal of Consulting and Clinical Psychology*, **20**, 343–50.

Russell, E.W. (1975). A multiple scoring method for the assessment of complex memory function. *Journal of Consulting and Clinical Psychology*, **43**, 800–9.

Sandson, T.A., Daffner, K.R., Carvalho, P.A. *et al.* (1991). Frontal lobe dysfunction following infarction of the left-sided medial thalamus. *Archives of Neurology*, **48**, 1300–3.

Schuler, P., Oyanguren, H., Maturana, V. *et al.* (1957). Manganese poisoning. *Indian Medicine and Surgery*, **26**, 167–73.

Shallice, T. (1982). Specific impairments of planning. *Philosophical Transactions of the Royal Society, London*, **298**, 199–209.

Shimamura, A.P., Gershberg, F.B., Jurica, P.J. *et al.* (1992). Intact implicit memory in patients with frontal lobe lesions. *Neuropsychologia*, **30**, 931–7.

Shimamura, A.P., Janowsky, J.S. and Squire, L.R. (1990). Memory for the temporal order of events in patients with frontal lobe lesions and amnestic patients. *Neuropsychologia*, **28**, 803–13.

Shimamura, A.P., Janowsky, J.S. and Squire, L.R. (1991). What is the role of frontal lobe damage in amnesic disorders? In *Frontal Lobe Function and Dysfunction*. (ed. H.S. Levin, H.M. Eisenberg and A.L. Benton). New York: Oxford University Press.

Squire, L.R. and Butters, N. (1984). *Neuropsychology of Memory*. New York: Guilford Press.

Starkstein, S.E. and Robinson, R.G. (1994). Neuropsychiatric aspects of stroke. In *Textbook of Geriatric Neuropsychiatry* (ed. C.D. Coffey and J.L. Cummings). Washington, DC: American Psychiatric Press.

Stroop, J.R. (1935). Studies of interference in serial verbal reactions. *Journal of Experimental Psychology*, **18**, 643–62.

Strub, R.L. (1989). Frontal lobe syndrome in a patient with bilateral globus pallidus lesions. *Archives of Neurology*, **46**, 1024–7.

Stuss, D.T. and Benson, D.F. (1984). Neuropsychological studies of the frontal lobes. *Psychological Bulletin*, **95**, 3–28.

Stuss, D.T. and Benson, D.F. (1986). *The Frontal Lobes*. New York: Raven.

Stuss, D.T., Ely, P., Hegenholtz, *et al.* (1985). Subtle neuropsychological deficits in patients with good recovery after closed head injury. *Neurosurgery*, **17**, 41–7.

Stuss, D.T., Guberman, A., Nelson, R. *et al.* (1988). The neuropsychology of paramedian thalamic infarction. *Brain and Cognition*, **8**, 348–78.

Taylor, L.B. (1969). Localization of cerebral lesions by psychological testing. *Clinical Neurosurgery*, **16**, 269–87.

Taylor, L.B. (1979). Psychological assessment of neurosurgical patients. In *Functional Neurosurgery*. (ed. T. Rasmussen and R. Marino). New York: Raven Press.

Terman, M.L. and Merrill, M.A. (1973). *Stanford-Binet Intelligence Scale. Manual for the Third Revision, Form L-M*. Boston: Houghton-Mifflin.

Trail Making Test (1944). *Army Individual Test Battery. Manual of directions and scoring*. Washington DC: War Department.

Tucker, D.M., Watson, R.T. and Heilman, K.M. (1977). Discrimination and evocation of affectively intoned speech in patients with right parietal disease. *Neurology*, **27**, 947–50.

Vonsattel, J.-P., Myers, R.H., Stevens, T.J. *et al.* (1985). Neuropathological classification of Huntington's disease. *Journal of Neuropathology and Experimental Neurology*, **44**, 559–77.

Walsh, K.W. (1978). *Neuropsychology: A Clinical Approach*. New York: Livingston.

Weinberger, D.R., Berman, K.F., Ladorola, M. *et al.* (1988) Prefrontal cortical blood flow and cognitive function in Huntington's disease. *Journal of Neurology, Neurosurgery and Psychiatry*, **51**, 94–104.

Weingartner, H., Caine, E.D. and Ebert, E.H. (1979). Encoding processes, learning, and recall in Huntington's disease. *Advances in Neurology*, **23**, 215–26.

Wyszuynski, B., Marriam, A., Medalia, A. *et al.* (1989). Choreoacanthocytosis: Report of a case with psychiatric features. *Neuropsychiatry, Neuropsychology and Behavioural Neurology*, **2**, 137–44.

2

Frontal lobe structural abnormalities in schizophrenia: evidence from neuroimaging

BRIAN K. TOONE

Introduction

The granular prefrontal cortex, situated principally on the lateral aspect of the frontal lobes, is unique in primates and reaches its largest expansion in humans. The prefrontal cortex and its connections exercise a central executive control over the direction and co-ordination of such higher cognitive functions as planning, temporal sequencing and conceptual flexibility. Early theorists (e.g. Kraepelin, 1971), recognising this, identified the frontal lobe as a likely candidate for neuropathological change in schizophrenia. Later commentators (Parfitt, 1956) noted similarities between some of the clinical features of frontal lobe damage and the negative symptoms of schizophrenia, while others (Levin, 1984) have been impressed by what has seemed at times to be a selective impairment in the performance of psychological tests of frontal lobe function.

However, frontal lobe dysfunction is unlikely to account for the entire spectrum of schizophrenic phenomenology and the frontal lobes may seem an improbable site for the primary locus of neuropathology. A secondary, or symptomatic, schizophrenia is only rarely attributable to frontal lobe damage or disease (Girgis, 1971). Davidson and Bagley (1969), in their copious review, failed to detect any association between psychotic phenomenology and frontal lobe pathology, although it must be said that these authors took little account of negative symptoms. Histological evidence of frontal lobe pathology is sparse (see below) and the case for frontal lobe involvement in the schizophrenic process leans heavily on neuropsychological and neuroimaging data, suggesting a disturbance in function. This has led some authorities (e.g. Weinberger *et al.*, 1992) to consider the possibility that frontal lobe dysfunction arises out of a disturbance in the prefrontal-limbic network and is secondary to damage to mesial temporal structures. The presence of structural abnormalities in the prefrontal regions is critical to this argument. This chapter will review those neuroimaging studies that contain data relating to this issue. An association might be anticipated between gross morphological changes, as demonstrated by conventional neuroimaging methods, and tissue-level changes detectable by morphometric techniques. A brief account of the latter is therefore included.

The neuropathology of the frontal lobe

A detailed account of the neuropathology would unduly extend the scope of this chapter, but a brief description of, in particular, some of the more recent developments will provide a complementary and even, perhaps, an explanatory subtext to the structural neuroimaging review that will follow. When due account is taken of agonal hypoxia, post-mortem autolysis, tissue shrinkage and other confounding influences, some degree of broad parallelism between macroscopic neuropathological and structural neuroimaging morphometric findings might be expected. Similarly, macrostructural abnormalities so identified should be associated with, and interpreted in terms of, histological and neurochemical changes.

Those studies (Stevens, 1982; Bruton *et al.*, 1990) that carried out gross and microscopic examination of the frontal cortex as part of an examination of the whole brain were unimpressed by any obvious abnormalities. Brown *et al.*'s (1986) planimetric measurement of cingulate cortex thickness was also negative.

In the past decade, attention has turned to the study of neuronal size and cell density and to the cytoarchitecture of the cortex and subcortex. Attempts have been made to relate such abnormalities as have been described to changes in neurotransmitter function, notbly the GABA and glutamate systems, and to explain these changes in terms of disturbed neuronal development, either during the neuronal migration that occurs during the second trimester of intra-uterine life or to the pattern of programmed cell death that occurs later. Benes *et al.* (1986) reported reduced neuronal density in most layers of the prefrontal (Brodmann area 10) and primary motor cortices and significant reductions in layers v and vi of areas 4 and 10 respectively. Neuronal density was also significantly reduced in layer v of the anterior cingulate cortex (area 24). Glial densities were also reduced and the neurone:glial ratio unchanged. In a further study Benes *et al.* (1991) again examined areas 10 and 24, and found a reduction in density of small interneurones in layer ii of area 10. Pyramidal cell density, on the other hand, was increased in layer v of area 10. The same group reported other abnormal cytoarchitectural variants in the cingulate cortices, including the presence of smaller neuronal aggregates in layer ii and increased numbers of vertical axons in layers ii and iiia (Benes and Bird, 1987).

Other studies have failed to replicate Benes *et al.*'s findings. Akbarian *et al.* (1995) also examined the prefrontal cortex (area 9) and found no differences in the total number of neurones nor in the sub-population of small neurones that include most of the GABA-containing cells. They did find a non-significant 10% reduction in cortical volume in the schizophrenic group. Pakkenberg *et al.* (1993) sampled from frontal, temporal, parietal and occipital regions to obtain whole-brain and regional estimates of neocortical neuronal numbers and density. Temporal neocortical cell numbers were significantly increased and cortical volumes reduced. The parietal and frontal cortices showed a similar pattern, but failed to achieve significance. Frontal cortical neuronal numbers differed only slightly from controls, but cell density was increased by 13% and cortical volume decreased by 18%.

More recent studies have replicated and strengthened these findings. Daviss and Lewis (1995) used two calcium-binding proteins to identify separate sub-populations of cortical local circuit neurones in areas 9 and 46. The density of one of the proteins, calbindin, was 50–70% greater in the schizophrenic subjects in both prefrontal areas. The density of the other protein, calretinin, was increased by 10–20%, an increase that the authors attributed to the 10–15% decrease in cortical thickness. Selemon, Rajowska and Goldman-Rakic (1995) studied areas 9 and 17 (occipital cortex). In the schizophrenic group, neuronal density was increased by 17% and 10% and cortical thickness decreased by 8% and 5% respectively. The two measures were inversely correlated. The increase in cell density was shown to be due to both pyramidal cells and interneurones.

Several studies therefore have reported cell density increases in total or sub-populations of cortical neurones, accompanied by a modest decrease in cortical volume or thickness of 10–20%. These changes appear not to be restricted to the prefrontal cortex but to reflect a global cortical phenomenon. No study has reported a diminution in neuronal cell volume and a reduction in the neuropil seems most likely. Decreased synaptophysin immunoreactivity in areas 9 and 46 (Glantz and Lewis, 1993), loss of dendritic spines from cortical pyramidal cells (Garey, Patel and Ong, 1994) and loss of cortical neuropil (Selemon *et al.*, 1995) lend support to this interpretation.

Post-mortem pharmacological research has developed rapidly since 1979. Receptor studies complement and assist in the interpretation of microstructural observations. Uptake sites are of interest because, traditionally, their density may be taken as a broad indication of the neurotransmitter-specific innervation of a particular region. Unfortunately, positive results have been difficult to replicate and no clear pattern has emerged. The reported changes in interneurone cell density (Benes *et al.*, 1991) have led to increased interest in gabaergic neurotransmission. Increased $GABA_A$ receptor binding in the cingulate cortex (Benes *et al.*, 1992), reduced GABA uptake (Simpson *et al.*, 1992), defective GABA release (Sherman *et al.*, 1991) and reduced GAD mRNA are each consistent with a reduced gabaergic activity. Whether such changes are primary or occur in response to alterations in adjacent systems, e.g. glutamate, is a matter for speculation (Lewis, 1995).

In summary, the evidence for a prefrontal neuropathology in schizophrenia is at present only fragmentary and susceptible to a range of interpretations. A modest reduction in cortical volume, accompanied by an increase in cell density, is noted in several studies, though this is likely to be a global rather than a regional phenomenon. Less attention is paid to subcortical structures, though Akbarian *et al.* have reported a maldistribution of interstitial neurones in prefrontal (1993*a*, 1996) and in temporal (1993*b*) white matter.

Structural neuroimaging of the prefrontal regions

Although early studies (e.g. Haug 1962), employing now largely obsolete neuroimaging techniques, had already demonstrated abnormalities in schizophrenia, it was not until the introduction and clinical development of computer-assisted tomography (CT), a relatively non-invasive technique, that controlled studies of the major psychoses became a feasible proposition.

Computer-assisted tomography

The first CT study of schizophrenic subjects was reported by Johnstone *et al.* in 1976. Within a decade-and-a-half, CT was to be more or less superseded by magnetic resonance imaging (MRI), a more complex, but far more flexible and informative technique. Computerised tomography is limited by its comparatively weak spatial resolution and by its inability to differentiate grey from white matter. Regions of interest, other than the ventricular system, are not easy to define, and few researchers have attempted to do so. The presence of frontal or anterior 'atrophy' is usually inferred from measures of frontal sulci, together with measures of the anterior interhemispheric fissure (Raz and Raz, 1990). Studies that have addressed the issue of structural changes in the frontal regions are summarised in Table 2.1. Choice of measurement and criteria for sulcal enlargement vary. Most have

Table 2.1. *CT studies that report measures of frontal lobe structure*

Study	Sample	Diagnostic criteria & clinical characteristics	Sex (M:F)	Age	Mean duration of illness (years)	Measurement criteria	Findings & comments
Pandurangi *et al.*, 1984	23 patients 23 controls	DSM-III Neurological patients with normal scans	23:0 23:0	28 34	2–19	Maximum width of largest frontal lobe sulcus	No significant differences
Oxenstierna *et al.*, 1984	30 patients No controls	RDC (26 patients)	17:13	M: 32 F: 35	8		Atrophic changes in 10 patients. Four had wide hemispheric and inter-hemispheric sulci in the frontal region
Otta *et al.*, 1987	25 patients No controls	RDC	13:12	32.4	7.6	0–3 ratings	Trend for negative symptom score to be positively correlated with frontal lobe atrophy
Pfefferbaum *et al.*, 1988	45 patients 57 controls	RDC 38 chronic; 6 subchronic; 1 acute Normal volunteers	45:0 57:0	34 20–82	11	Semi-automated volume measures	Frontal sulcal enlargement in patient group
Shelton *et al.*, 1988	71 patients 30 controls	DSM-III 31 paranoid; 30 undifferentiated; 6 disorganised Normal volunteers	49:22 14:16	28.7 28.7	9.7	0–3 ratings	Frontal sulcal enlargement in patient group, particularly women
Williamson *et al.*, 1991	20 patients 20 controls	DSM-III	16:4 15:5	30.9 30.3		0–3 ratings	Four schizophrenic and 6 controls had ratings of 1

rated cortical surface markings on a scale of 0–3 from 0 (fissures and sulci not visualised) to 3 (fissures and sulci evident with fluid-filled spaces visible), but others used linear measurement (Pandurangi *et al.*, 1984) or semi-quantitative techniques (Pfefferbaum *et al.*, 1988). No studies attempted to define the frontal or prefrontal regions in precise neuroanatomical terms. Two studies merit additional comment. Shelton *et al.* (1988) compared a schizophrenic cohort with normal volunteers. Significant differences were detected in both ventricular:brain ratio (VBR) and third ventricular width, but not in a generalised atrophy score. A prefrontal atrophy score, however, indicated marked differences between the samples: 49% of the patients compared with 20% of the control subjects had scores of one or more. No relationship was detected between measures of frontal and general sulcal enlargement or between either of these two measures and VBR and third ventricular width. Pfefferbaum *et al.* (1988) were the first to use semi-automated techniques to quantify sulcal size. An increase in frontal sulcal size was demonstrated, but only as part of an overall pattern of sulcal enlargement; in fact, there was a trend for occipito-parietal atrophy to be more marked.

Several studies (Golden *et al.*, 1981; Largen, Calderon and Smith, 1983; Rossi *et al.*, 1989; Pearlson *et al.*, 1989) have compared CT density measurements, but results have been inconsistent.

The contribution of computerised tomography to the issue of structural frontal lobe changes in schizophrenia is necessarily limited. In only two studies did the size of the patient cohort exceed 30. Most studies were rated according to visual inspection only. Even so, only one study was entirely negative; each of the others found some evidence of sulcal enlargement, although whether this was limited to the frontal regions or was part of a pattern of global atrophy was not resolved.

Magnetic resonance imaging

The introduction of MRI technology into clinical and research practices marks a sea change in our capacity to represent visually and to measure the details of cerebral structure. Magnetic resonance imaging techniques, far more so than CT, are complex and dynamic, and therefore possess the greater potential to evolve. The power of the present generation of scanners is as far removed from early MRI as the latter was from CT. The greater magnetic field strength and the ever-growing variety and precision of image sequencing have led to increased spatial resolution and improved tissue definition. Volume estimate has replaced the less informative linear and area measurements (Raz and Raz, 1990). The availability of pulse sequences that may be chosen respectively to optimise anatomical detail or to characterise lesional abnormalities, and the opportunity to image in coronal and sagittal as well as in transverse (as CT is largely restricted to) planes, and to assemble a three-dimensional reconstruction enhances MRI's flexibility and diversity. This has led to methodological advances. MRI does not use ionising radiation, and the apparent lack of bio-hazard has largely resolved concerns about the use of normal volunteer controls and has opened the way for longitudinal studies using repeat scans. Both spatial resolution and tissue demarcation now permit more precise, valid and reliable operational distinctions of regions of interest (ROI). However, because of the greater range and complexity of MRI, studies from different centres are not always readily comparable. They may differ not only in size and patient selection, but in the field strength of magnet, choice of imaging sequences, ROI definition, etc. (Table 2.2). The following is intended as a brief guide to technical and methodological variations and developments.

Group characteristics

Almost all of the published studies have provided the basic demographic and clinical details that have now come to be expected. All have used internationally recognised diagnostic criteria (usually DSM-III/DSM-IIIR); most supplied evidence of sub-category status, chronicity and severity. Most of the cohorts reported were made up of the chronically ill, undergoing long-term treatment, but De Lisi *et al.* (1991) studied first-episode schizophrenia-like psychoses. Patients were invariably on treatment at the time of examination, but this is of less significance than in functional neuroimaging studies and, although there is some evidence to suggest that treatment with antipsychotic drugs may contribute to the variance in size of basal ganglial structures (Chakos *et al.*, 1994), there is, as yet, little reason to suppose that this is so for frontal lobe structure. Although the importance of heterogeneity in schizophrenia is frequently stressed, in practice less attention is paid to this, either in the selection or in the characterisation of patient cohorts. De Lisi *et al.* (1991) identified first-episode and chronic schizophrenics, Schwarzkopf *et al.* (1991) family-history positive and negative groups. Others included deficit and non-deficit (Buchanan *et al.*, 1993) and drug-responsive and drug-resistant (Lawrie *et al.*, 1995) samples. Some studies carried out a *post hoc* analysis of the association between socio-clinical variables and neuroimaging measurements (Zipursky *et al.*, 1992; Harvey *et al.*, 1993; Schlaepfer *et al.*,

Table 2.2. *MRI structural studies that report frontal lobe data in schizophrenia*

Study	Sample	Diagnostic criteria & clinical characteristics	Sex (M:F) Age	Mean duration of illness (years)	Tesla strength	Regional definition	Measurement criteria	Imaging protocol	Findings & comments
Andreasen *et al.*, 1986	38 patients, 49 normal controls	DSM-III	28:10 23 28:21 28	11	0.5	Undefined	Area (cm^2) using planimetry	Mid-sagittal section	Frontal area reduced in patients
Besson *et al.*, 1987	23 patients 15 normal, controls	DSM-III	20:3 36 12:3 36	12	0.08	Undefined	RIO T1 values	Transverse sections 1 cm thick	Patients vs controls n.s.
Smith *et al.*, 1987	29 patients, 21 normal controls	DSM-III	5:29 30.7 9:12 32.1	6.6	0.3	Undefined	Linear (cm) and area (cm^2) T1 values	12 mm coronal sections	No difference in linear and area measures. T1 values in anterior white matter (left and right) and anterior grey matter (left) in schizophrenics
Kelsoe *et al.*, 1988	24 patients, 14 normal controls	DSM-III	22:5 29 10:4 31	8	0.5	Anterior to genu of corpus callosum	Area	1 cm coronal sections	No difference
De Myer *et al.*, 1988	25 patients, 25 normal controls	DSM-III	12:13 28.7 12:13 28.5	6.5	0.15	Anterior to the anterior horns of lateral ventricles	Area	1 cm transverse slices at level of (1) foramen of Monroe and (2) widest part of lateral ventricles	Frontal area reduced in patients on superior slice only, especially on left

Suddath *et al.*, 1989	17 patients, 17 normal controls	DSM-III Chronic 12 undifferentiated	10:7 30.6 10:7 33.2		0.5	3–4 coronal slices anterior to the corpus callosum genu	Volume	Contiguous 1 cm coronal slices	No differences in total, grey or white matter
Uematsu and Kaiya, 1989	40 patients, 17 normal controls	DSM-IIIR	40:0 32.2 17:0 31.5			None given	Area	1 cm sagittal slices	No difference in frontal lobe or frontal/brain ratio measurements
Andreasen *et al.*, 1990	55 patients, 47 normal controls	DSM-III	37:18 32.5:35.4 28:19 32.9:36.6	11.3:13.5	0.5	Undefined	Area (cm^2) using planimetry	1 cm thick mid-saggital slice	No differences
Dauphinais *et al.*, 1990	28 patients, normal controls (1)21 (2)21	All DSM-III RDC 10 schizophrenics 18 schizoaffective	15:13 32.4 (1)12:9 36.5 (2)11:10 33.3	12.8	0.5	Slices measured insufficiently anterior to impinge on prefrontal cortex	Area (cm^2)	1 cm thick coronal slices	No differences
Suddath *et al.*, 1900	15 discordant monozygotic twin pairs	DSM-IIIR chronic	16:14 32.4	10.5	1.5	All slices (7–8) anterior to the genu of corpus callosum	Vol (cm^2)	5 mm contiguous coronal slices	No differences
De Lisi *et al.*, 1991	(1)30 patients (2)15 patients (3)20 normal controls	(1)First-episode schizophrenia-like psychosis (2)DSM-IIIR chronic schizophrenics	(1)3:7 27 (2)9:6 33 (3)12:8 29	(2)9.0	1.5	Frontal pole to slice that includes optic chiasma and sella turcica	Vol (cm^2)	5 mm coronal slices. 2 mm spacing	No differences
Jernigan *et al.*, 1991	42 patients, 24 normal controls	DSM-IIIR chronic schizophrenics, 10 disorganised 24 undifferentiated	19:24 30 19:5 32	10.6	1.5	Quadrant defined with reference to mid-point of corpus callosum	Volume measurements. Grey/white/CSF distinction using thresholding techniques	5 mm transverse sections. 2.5 mm spacing	Reduction in anterior inferior and posterior inferior mesial cortex

Table 2.2. (*cont.*)

Study	Sample	Diagnostic criteria &clinical characteristics	Sex (M:F) Age	Mean duration of illness (years)	Tesla strength	Regional definition	Measurement criteria	Imaging protocol	Findings & comments
Schwarzkopf *et al.*, 1991	31 patients, 14 normal controls	DSM-IIIR stable outpatients FH+16 FH−15	31:0 31.6 14:0 29.6	9	1.5	Anterior to mid-point of corpus callosum		Average of two parasaggital slices immediately adjacent to mid-sagittal slice, thickness 3 mm	No differences between patients and controls or between F+ and F−
Young *et al.*, 1991	31 patients, FH-, 33 normal controls	RDC			0.08	Rostral to anterior commissure and optic chiasma	Area (cm^2). Cortical boundaries traced by hand	2 series of 8 mm and 12 mm thick coronal slices	No differences in frontal cortical areas
Breier *et al.*, 1992	44 patients, 29 normal controls	Stable outpatients		14.7	1.5	Anterior to genu of corpus callosum	Volume measurements, grey/white distinctions using thresholding techniques	3 mm contiguous coronal sections	Reduced total prefrontal volume on left and right due to white matter reduction
Raine *et al.*, 1992	17 schiz. patients, 18 psych. controls, 19 normal controls	DSM-IIIR 14 paranoid, psych, controls, neurotic	10:7 35.1 12:6 35.6 10:9 33.9	9.9	0.15	Anterior to (coronal and saggital) corpus collosum genu and (transverse) anterior horns of lateral ventricle	Area	10 mm coronal, transverse and mid-sagittal slices	Reduced pre-frontal areas on all slices

Zipursky *et al.*, 1992	22 patients, 20 normal controls	DSM-IIIR 19 chronic	22:0 34.1 20:0 36.2	11	1.5	Anterior to genu of corpus callosum	Volume thresholding distinction between grey/white matter	5 mm transverse slices, 2.5 mm intervals	Generalised reduction in cortical grey matter
Buchanan *et al.*, 1993	41 patients, 30 normal controls	DSM-IIIR Deficit 17 Non-deficit 24	12:5 35 14:10 36 20:10 34	15 14	1.5	Anterior to genu of corpus calossum	Volume (thresholding)	3 mm contiguous coronal slices	Deficit>non- deficit, controls> non-deficit
Harvey *et al.*, 1993	48 patients, 36 normal controls	RDC	37:11 31.1 19:15 31.6	9	1.5	No clear distinction	Volume grey/white distinction by region growing techniques	5 mm contiguous coronal slices	Generalised reductions in cortical grey matter
Schlaepfer *et al.*, 1994	46 patients, 27 bipolar, 60 normal controls	DSM-IIIR	32:14 32 16:11 32 43:17 35		1.5	Dorsolateral prefrontal cortex identified	Volume grey/white matter segmented	5 mm contiguous transverse slices	Dorsolateral prefrontal cortex reduced in volume
Seidman *et al.*, 1994	17 schiz. patients	DSM-IIIR	14:3 33.6	11	1.5	Anterior to genu of corpus callosum	Area	5–6 mm contiguous coronal slices	Significant cor- relation between neuropsychologi- cal performance and DLPF cortex area
Lawrie *et al.*, 1995	40 patients,	DSM-IIIR 20 responsive 20 resistant to treatment	 36 36	 11.6 12.6	1.0	Anterior to genu of corpus callosum	Volume	1.56 mm contiguous coronal slices	No group difference
Maher *et al.*, 1995	18 patients	DSM-IIIR	34		1.5	Anterior to genu of corpus callosum	Area	5–6 mm contiguous coronal slices	Recall correlation with volume of DLPF cortex
Wible *et al.*, 1995	14 patients, 15 normal controls	DSM-IIIR chronic			3 slices anterior to temporal stem	Volume grey white matter segmentation	1.5 mm contiguous coronal slices	1.5	No group difference

1994). Several have included a more detailed neuropsychological assessment (Seidman *et al.*, 1994; Maher *et al.*, 1995; Lawrie *et al.*, 1995), but it is a feature of the latter studies that none employed a control group. Elsewhere, normal controls were employed but only two studies (Raine *et al.*, 1992; Schlaepfer *et al.*, 1994) included psychiatric control groups. The most powerful design was employed by Suddath *et al.* (1990), who compared monozygotic twins discordant for schizophrenia. Statistical power is compromised by small group size. In comparison with CT studies of the psychoses (Raz and Raz, 1990), few publications based on MRI include patient cohorts greater than 50 (Andreason *et al.*, 1990, 1994; Harvey *et al.*, 1993), and of the 25 studies cited here, six had fewer than 20.

The need to correct estimates of ventricular volume for brain size was recognised early on, but the inadequacy of the ratio measurements and the dependence of brain size on a multiplicity of contributory factors were slow to be acknowledged (Harvey *et al.*, 1993) and, even then, not always taken into sufficient account. The importance of controlling for years in education was made clear by the studies by Andreason *et al.* (1986, 1990). Gender, ethnicity and height may be related to intra-cranial volume (Harvey *et al.*, 1993); yet very few studies have taken account of all of these variables.

Magnetic resonance imaging technology has advanced rapidly. Imaging procedures that at first were varied, and at times idiosyncratic, have converged towards a largely standardised protocol. The coronal plane is preferred, and slices that do not exceed 5 mm in thickness and are contiguous reduce error due to partial volume and provide superior spatial resolution. Structural MRI studies of the prefrontal region are summarised in Table 2.2. They vary considerably, both in statistical power and in technical sophistication. Studies published since 1990 are more likely to have used magnets of adequate field strength, fine coronal slicing, volume measurements, and to have defined a region of interest in relation to the genu of the corpus callosum, an easily identifiable and anatomically appropriate reference point. But some earlier studies, notably those by Andreason *et al.* (1986, 1990) and by Suddath *et al.* (1990) merit particular mention.

Early studies (1986–1990)

With the exception of the above-mentioned, studies during this early period employed magnets of weak field strength (0.5 T or less), thick slices (1 cm or more) and linear or area units of measurement. Regions of interest were ill-defined. Two studies (Andreason *et al.*, 1986; de Myer *et al.*,

1988) reported reduced frontal area in the patient group. Eight studies were essentially negative. Andreason *et al.* used as a control group normal volunteers who had, on average, spent more years in education than the patients. A later, and larger, study (Andreason *et al.*, 1990) used a similar methodology and the same rater, but took account of years in education. The control group, compared with that in the earlier study, was less well-educated and showed a reduction in cranial, cerebral and frontal area measurements. The patient and control groups no longer differed. Frontal lobe area and years of education were positively and significantly correlated in both studies.

Suddath *et al.*, in the second of two structural MRI studies (1990), used a superior methodology and an ideal matching paradigm. Fifteen monozygotic twin pairs, discordant for chronic schizophrenia, were studied. Frontal grey and white matter volumes were measured. No significant differences were detected. The direction of the early studies was therefore conclusively negative, with only one group (de Meyer *et al.*, 1988) reporting reductions in frontal lobe size.

Later studies

In this period 14 studies were reported, 11 of which used matched control groups. Six reported reductions in frontal lobe measurements; four failed to detect significant differences. No obvious methodological differences account for this discrepancy. The larger and more recent studies (Jernigan *et al.*, 1991; Breier *et al.*, 1992; Harvey *et al.*, 1993; Schlaepfer *et al.*, 1994; Andreason *et al.*, 1994) tend to report positive findings. One negative study (Young *et al.*, 1991) was technically less advanced; another (de Lisi *et al.*, 1991) employed as the main patient group first-episode schizophrenia-like psychotics, and it may be argued that this group was diagnostically less robust and less likely to show frontal lobe abnormalities.

Among those studies that reported positive findings, four (Jernigan *et al.*, 1991; Zipursky *et al.*, 1992; Harvey *et al.*, 1993; Schlaepfer *et al.*, 1994) found reductions in cortical volume. One (Breier *et al.*, 1992) found reduction in white matter volume and one (Raine *et al.*, 1992) did not make a distinction between grey and white matter. The first four studies are of particular interest. One group (Jernigan *et al.*, 1991; Zipursky *et al.*, 1992) used a particularly sophisticated technical approach. Another (Harvey *et al.*, 1993) used a multiple regression analysis to control for variables such as height and ethnicity, frequently ignored in other studies. All identified widespread reductions in cortical volume well beyond the confines of the prefrontal regions. Jernigan *et al.* (1991) reported a reduction in anterior–inferior quadrantic cortical grey matter. This would include temporal as well as mesial and lateral orbito-frontal cortex, and it is possible that the differences noted were due to the former.

The relationship between MRI, structural and clinical variables

Most studies took some account of the clinical variation. Most recorded the simple parameters of clinical course and outcome and included these in their analysis. Some sub-typing was attempted, e.g. the presence or absence of family history (Schwarzkopf *et al.*, 1991), the chronic schizophrenia sub-types, e.g. paranoid, undifferentiated, disorganised, etc. (Suddath *et al.*, 1989). A number of studies explored and recorded negative and positive symptomatology and used standardised measures of symptomatology such as the BPRS (Young *et al.*, 1991; Zipursky *et al.*, 1992). Only a minority of studies, most notably Schwarzkopf *et al.* (1991) and Buchanan *et al.* (1993) appear to have designed studies with the express intention of studying clinical heterogeneity. *A priori*, an association between frontal abnormalities and negative symptomatology might be predicted, and a number of studies have explored this possibility. Cortical grey matter overall was negatively correlated with the BPRS withdrawal–retardation factor, though a more specific negative correlation with prefrontal grey matter narrowly failed to achieve significance (Zipursky *et al.*, 1992). Reduced anterior cortical volume was related to unemployment (Harvey *et al.*, 1993). Others also reported an association in the same direction, but this must be balanced against the number of negative studies (De Meyer *et al.*, 1988; Andreason *et al.*, 1990; Young *et al.*, 1991; Raine *et al.*, 1992). The one study that set out to explain frontal structural abnormalities/negative symptomatology relationships (Buchanan *et al.*, 1993) reported data that they would hardly have predicted. Deficit and non-deficit groups were compared with normal controls; sample sizes were adequate. Both patient groups showed the anticipated reduction in volume of mesial temporal structures, but only the non-deficit group showed frontal abnormalities, total left and right prefrontal volumes being reduced in comparison with each of the other groups.

An association between prefrontal structural abnormalities and performance in putative tests of frontal lobe function might also be predicted, and several studies have investigated this. Seidman *et al.* (1994) reported a strong correlation between left dorso-lateral prefrontal cortex area and the Wisconsin Card Sort Test (both categories attained and perseverative error scores). Other, less impressive, associations between the same cortical areas and other cognitive measures, e.g. general IQ, Similarities and various tests of memory, were also demonstrated. The same group (Maher *et al.*, 1995) discovered a relationship between the dorso-lateral area of the prefrontal cortex and the capacity to use context as an aid to recall in a verbal memory task. However, these studies were based on a limited number of subjects and lacked controls. Lawrie *et al.*'s (1995) findings suggest that cognitive performance is positively correlated with measures of frontal lobe volume in both schizophrenia and normals.

How consistent is quantification across studies? An examination of data drawn from studies comparable in terms of definition of regions of interest, technique and use of volumetric measures reveals a wide scatter of values, but the expected direction of asymmetry (right larger than left) is found in most instances.

Conclusion

Some of the earlier CT studies of schizophrenia reported a very substantial increase in size of the ventricular system (e.g. Johnstone *et al.*, 1976). Subsequently, over time, this effect has diminished (Van Horn and McManus, 1992), a decline that may be attributable to refinements in methodology, in particular greater care in the selection of more representative samples and use of unbiased normal control subjects rather than negatively investigated neurological patients (Smith and Iacono, 1986). It is perhaps yet too early to be certain that the same trend will not emerge in MRI schizophrenia research, but methodological lessons have been well learnt and MRI data analysis has shown a greater awareness of its multivariate nature. The evolving pattern of MRI research has been characterised less by refinements in methodology, more by improvements in technique. The CT findings of third and lateral ventricular enlargement and (less robustly) sulcal enlargement have been largely confirmed; early MRI findings of mesial temporal volume loss have usually been replicated. MRI studies of frontal lobe structure have been less consistent, but there has been a trend whereby the larger, more recent, and technically more advanced, studies are more likely to report positive findings. The ability to distinguish and to measure separately white and grey matter volume has enabled recent studies (Zipursky *et al.*, 1992; Harvey *et al.*, 1993) to identify a reduction in the latter as the critical frontal lobe abnormality. It appears that cortical thinning may be a global rather than simply a regional phenomenon. Recent neuropathological findings (Selemon *et al.*, 1995) also suggest a generalised reduction in thickness of the cortical mantle, perhaps accompanied by increased neuronal density. This effect was seen to be small, and in this respect it is noteworthy that few of the MRI studies approach the magnitude of some of the larger CT studies. Further progress will be favourably influenced by technical advance, but will depend to an even greater extent on the use of larger patient cohorts and the selection of subgroups that can be characterised in a clinically and neuropsychologically meaningful way.

References

Akbarian, S., Bunney, W.E., Potkin, S.G. *et al.* (1993*a*). Altered distribution of nicotinamide adenine dinucleotide phosphate-diaphorase cells in the frontal lobe of schizophrenics implies disturbance of cortical development. *Archives of General Psychiatry*, **50**, 169–77.

Akbarian, S., Viñuela, A., Kim, J.J. *et al.* (1993*b*). Distorted distribution of nicotinamide adenine dinucleotide phosphate-diaphorase neurons in temporal lobe of schizophrenics implies anomalous cortical development. *Archives of General Psychiatry*, **50**, 178–87.

Akbarian, S., Kim, J.J., Potkin, S.G. *et al.* (1995). Gene expression for glutamic acid decarboxylase is reduced without loss of neurons in the prefrontal cortex of schizophrenics. *Archives of General Psychiatry*, **52**, 258–66.

Akbarian, S., Kim, J.J., Potkin, S.G. *et al.* (1996). Maldistribution of interstitial neurons in prefrontal white matter of the brains of schizophrenic patients. *Archives of General Psychiatry*, **53**, 425–36.

Andreasen, N., Nasrallah, H.A., Dunn, V. *et al.* (1986). Structural abnormalities in the frontal system in schizophrenia. *Archives of General Psychiatry*, **43**, 136–44.

Andreasen, N., Ehrhardt, J.C., Swayze, V.W. *et al.* (1990). Magnetic resonance imaging of the brain in schizophrenia: the pathophysiologic significance of structural abnormalities. *Archives of General Psychiatry*, **47**, 35–46.

Andreasen, N.C., Flashman, L., Flaum, M. *et al.* (1994). Regional brain abnormalities in schizophrenia measured with magnetic resonance imaging. *Journal of the American Medical Association*, **272**, 1763–9.

Benes, F.M. and Bird, E.D. (1987). An analysis of the arrangement of neurons in the cingulate cortex of schizophrenic patients. *Archives of General Psychiatry*, **44**, 608–16.

Benes, F.M., Davidson, J. and Bird, E.D. (1986). Quantitative psychoarchitectural studies of the cerebral cortex of schizophrenics. *Archives of General Psychiatry*, **43**, 31–5.

Benes, F.M., McSparren, J., Bird, E.D. *et al.* (1991). Deficits in small interneurons in prefrontal and cingulate cortices of schizophrenic and schizoaffective patients. *Archives of General Psychiatry*, **48**, 996–1001.

Benes, F.M., Vincent, S.L., Alsterberg, G. *et al.* (1992). Increased GABA receptor binding in superficial layers of cingulate cortex in schizophrenics. *Journal of Neuroscience*, **12**, 924–9.

Besson, J.A.O., Corrigan, F.M., Cherryman, G.R. and Smith, F.W. (1987). Nuclear magnetic resonance brain imaging in chronic schizophrenia. *British Journal of Psychiatry*, **150**, 161–3.

Breier, A., Buchanan, R.W., Elkashef, A. *et al.* (1992). Brain morphology and schizophrenia. *Archives of General Psychiatry*, **49**, 921–6.
Brown, R., Colter, N., Corsellis, J.A.N. *et al.* (1986). Post-mortem evidence of structural brain changes in schizophrenia: differences in brain weight, temporal horn area and parahippocampal gyrus compared with affective disorder. *Archives of General Psychiatry*, **43**, 36–42.
Bruton, C.J., Crow, T.J., Frith, C.D. *et al.* (1990). Schizophrenia and the brain: a prospective post-mortem study. *Psychological Medicine*, **20**, 285–304.
Buchanan, R.W., Breier, A., Kirkpatrick, B. *et al.* (1993). Structural abnormalities in deficit and non-deficit schizophrenia. *American Journal of Psychiatry*, **150**, 59–65.
Chakos, M.H., Lieberman, J.A., Bilder, R.M. *et al.* (1994). Increase in caudate nuclei volumes of first-episode schizophrenic patients taking antipsychotic drugs. *American Journal of Psychiatry*, **151**, 1430–6.
Dauphinais, I.D., De Lisi, L.E., Crow, T.J. *et al.* (1990). Reduction in temporal lobe size in siblings with schizophrenia: a magnetic resonance imaging study. *Psychiatric Research: Neuroimaging*, **35**, 135–47.
Davison, K. and Bagley, C.R. (1969). Schizophrenia-like psychoses associated with organic disorders of the central nervous system: a review of the literature. *British Journal of Psychiatry*, Special Publications, no. 4, 113–84.
Daviss, S.R. and Lewis, D.A. (1995). Local circuit neurons of the prefrontal cortex in schizophrenia: selective increase in the density of calbindin-immunoreactive neurons. *Psychiatry Research*, **59**, 81–96.
De Lisi, L.E., Hoff, A.L., Schwartz, J.E. *et al.* (1991). Brain morphology in first-episode schizophrenic-like psychotic patients: a quantitative magnetic resonance imaging study. *Biological Psychiatry*, **29**, 159–75.
De Meyer, M.K., Gilmor, R.L., Hendrie, H.C. *et al.* (1988). Magnetic resonance brain images in schizophrenic and normal subjects: influence of diagnosis and education. *Schizophrenia Bulletin*, **14**, 21–32.
Garey, L.J., Patel, T. and Ong, W.Y. (1994). Loss of dendritic spines from cortical pyramidal cells in schizophrenia. *Schizophrenia Research*, **11**, 137.
Girgis, M. (1971). The orbital surface of the frontal lobe of the brain and mental disorders. *Acta Psychiatrica Scandinavica*, Supplement 222.
Glantz, L.A. and Lewis, D.A. (1993). Synaptophysin and not RABA3 is specifically reduced in the pre-frontal cortex of schizophrenic subjects. *Society for Neuropsychiatry Abstracts*, **20**, 622.
Golden, C.J., Graber, B., Coffman, J. *et al.* (1981). Structural deficits in schizophrenia: identification by tomographic scan measurement. *Archives of General Psychiatry*, **38**, 1014–17.
Harvey, I., Ron, R.M., Du Boulay, G. *et al.* (1993). Reduction of cortical volume in schizophrenia on magnetic resonance imaging. *Psychological Medicine*, **23**, 591–604.
Haug, J.O. (1962). Pneumoencephalographic studies in mental disease. *Acta Psychiatrica Scandinavica* (supplement), **165**, 1–114.
Jernigan, T.L., Zisook, S., Heton, R.K. *et al.* (1991). Magnetic resonance imaging abnormalities in lenticular nuclei and cerebral cortex in schizophrenia. *Archives of General Psychiatry*, **48**, 881–90.
Johnstone, E.C., Crow, T.J., Frith, C.D. *et al.* (1976). Cerebral ventricular size and cognitive impairment in chronic schizophrenia. *Lancet*, **ii**, 924–6.
Kelsoe, J.R., Cadet, J.L., Pickar, D. and Weinberger, D.R. (1988). Quantitative neuroanatomy in schizophrenia: a controlled magnetic resonance imaging study. *Archives of General Psychiatry*, **45**, 533–41.

Kraepelin, E. (1971). *Dementia Praecox and Paraphrenia* (Facsimile 1919 edition). New York: R.E. Krieger Publishing Company.

Largen, J.W., Calderon, M. and Smith, R.C. (1983). Asymmetries in the densities of white and grey matter in the brains of schizophrenic patients. *American Journal of Psychiatry*, **140**, 1060–2.

Lawrie, S.M., Ingle, G.I., Santosh, C.G. *et al.* (1995). Magnetic resonance imaging and single photon emission tomography in treatment-responsive and treatment-resistant schizophrenia. *British Journal of Psychiatry*, **167**, 202–10.

Levin, S. (1984). Frontal lobe dysfunction in schizophrenia – II. Impairments of psychological and brain function. *Journal of Psychiatric Research*, **18**, 57–72.

Lewis, D.A. (1995). Neural circuitry capacity in prefrontal cortex in schizophrenia. *Archives of General Psychiatry*, **52**, 269–73.

Maher, B.A., Manschreck, T.C., Woods, B.T. *et al.* (1995). Frontal brain volume and context effects in short-term recall in schizophrenia. *Biological Psychiatry*, **37**, 144–50.

Ota, T., Maeshiro, H., Ishido, H. *et al.* (1987). Treatment-resistant chronic psychopathology and CT scans in schizophrenia. *Acta Psychiatrica Scandinavica*, **75**, 415–27.

Oxenstierna, G., Bergstrand, G., Bjerkenstedt, L. *et al.* (1984). Evidence of disturbed CSF circulation and brain atrophy in cases of schizophrenic psychosis. *British Journal of Psychiatry*, **144**, 654–61.

Pakkenberg, B. (1993). Total nerve cell number in neocortex in chronic schizophrenics and controls estimated using optical dissectors. *Biological Psychiatry*, **34**, 768–72.

Pandurangi, A.K., Dewan, M.J., Lee, S.H. *et al.* (1984). The ventricular system in chronic schizophrenic patients: a controlled computed tomography study. *British Journal of Psychiatry*, **144**, 172–6.

Parfitt, D.N. (1956). The neurology of schizophrenia. *Journal of Mental Science*, **102**, 671–718.

Pearlson, G.D., Kim, W.S., Kubos, K.L. *et al.* (1989). Ventricle-brain ratio, computed tomographic density and brain area in 50 schizophrenics. *Archives of General Psychiatry*, **41**, 690–7.

Pfefferbaum, A., Zipursky, R.B., Limb, K.O. *et al.* (1988). Computed tomographic evidence for generalised sulcal and ventricular enlargement in schizophrenia. *Archives of General Psychiatry*, **45**, 633–40.

Raine, A., Lencz, T., Reynolds, G.P. *et al.* (1992). An evaluation of structural and functional prefrontal deficits in schizophrenia: MRI and neuropsychological measures. *Psychiatry Research: Neuroimaging*, **45**, 123–37.

Raz, S. and Raz, N. (1990). Structural brain abnormalities in the major psychoses: a quantitative review of the evidence from computerised imaging. *Psychological Bulletin*, **108**, 93–108.

Rossi, A., Stratta, P., D'Albenzio, L. *et al.* (1989). Quantitative computed tomographic study in schizophrenia: cerebral density and ventricle measures. *Psychological Medicine*, **19**, 337–42.

Schlaepfer, T.E., Harris, G.J., Tien, A.Y. *et al.* (1994). Decreased regional cortical grey matter volume in schizophrenia. *American Journal of Psychiatry*, **151**, 842–8.

Schwarzkopf, S.B., Nasrallah, H.A., Olson, S.C. *et al.* (1991). Family history and brain morphology in schizophrenia: an MRI study. *Psychiatry Research: Neuroimaging*, **40**, 49–60.

Seidman, L.J., Yurgelun-Todd, D., Kremen, W.S. *et al.* (1994). Relationship of prefrontal and temporal lobe MRI measures to neuropsychological performance in chronic schizophrenia. *Biological Psychiatry*, **35**, 235–246.

Selemon, L.D., Rajkowska, G. and Goldman-Rakic, P.S. (1995). Abnormally high neuronal density in the schizophrenic cortex. *Archives of General Psychiatry*, **52**, 805–18.

Shelton, R.C., Karson, C.N., Doran, A.R. *et al.* (1988). Cerebral structural pathology in schizophrenia: evidence for a selective prefrontal cortical defect. *American Journal of Psychiatry*, **145**, 154–63.

Sherman, A.D., Davidson, A.T., Baruah, S. *et al.* (1991). Evidence of glutamatergic deficiency in schizophrenia. *Neuroscience Letters*, **121**, 77–80.

Simpson, M.D.C., Slater, P., Royston, M.C. and Deakin, J.F.W. (1992). Regionally selective deficits in uptake sites for glutamate and gamma-aminobutyric acid in the basal ganglia in schizophrenia. *Psychiatry Research*, **42**, 273–82.

Smith, G.N. and Iacono, W.G. (1986). Lateral ventricular size in schizophrenia and choice of control group. *Lancet*, **i**, 1450.

Smith, R.C., Baumgartner, R. and Calderon, M. (1987). Magnetic resonance imaging studies of the brains of schizophrenic patients. *Psychiatry Research*, **20**, 33–46.

Stevens, J.R. (1982). Neuropathology of schizophrenia. *Archives of General Psychiatry*, **39**, 1131.

Suddath, R.L., Casanova, M.F., Goldberg, T.E. *et al.* (1989). Temporal lobe pathology in schizophrenia: a quantitative magnetic resonance imaging study. *American Journal of Psychiatry*, **146**, 464–72.

Suddath, R.L., Christison, G.W., Torrey, E.F. *et al.* (1990). Anatomical abnormalities in the brains of monozygotic twins discordant for schizophrenia. *The New England Journal of Medicine*, **322**, 789–94.

Uematsu, M. and Kaiya, H. (1989). Mid-sagittal cortical pathomorphology of schizophrenia: a magnetic resonance imaging study. *Psychiatry Research*, **30**, 11–20.

Van Horn, J.D. and McManus, I.C. (1992). Ventricular enlargement in schizophrenia: a meta-analysis of studies of the ventricle:brain ratio (VBR). *British Journal of Psychiatry*, **160**, 687–97.

Weinberger, D.R., Berman, K.F., Suddath, R. and Torrey, E.F. (1992). Evidence of dysfunction of a prefrontal limbic network in schizophrenia: a magnetic resonance imaging and regional cerebral blood flow study in discordant monozygotic twins. *American Journal of Psychiatry*, **149**, 890–7.

Wible, C.G., Shenton, M.E., Hokama, H. *et al.* (1995). Prefrontal cortex and schizophrenia: a quantitative magnetic resonance imaging study, **52**, 279–88.

Williamson, P., Pelz, D., Merskey, H. *et al.* (1991). Correlation of negative symptoms in schizophrenia with frontal lobe parameters on magnetic resonance imaging. *British Journal of Psychiatry*, **159**, 130–4.

Young, A.H., Blackwood, D.H.R., Roxborough, H. *et al.* (1991). A magnetic resonance imaging study of schizophrenia: brain structure and clinical symptoms. *British Journal of Psychiatry*, **158**, 158–64.

Zipursky, R.B., Lim, K.O., Sullivan, E.V. *et al.* (1992). Widespread cerebral grey matter volume deficits in schizophrenia. *Archives of General Psychiatry*, **49**, 195–205.

Section II

Basal ganglia and neuropsychiatry

3

The neuropsychology of basal ganglia disorders: an integrative cognitive and comparative approach

TREVOR W. ROBBINS, ADRIAN M. OWEN & BARBARA J. SAHAKIAN

Introduction

Over the last 30 years or so it has been realised that Parkinson's disease (PD) and other basal ganglia disorders such as Huntington's disease (HD), Steele–Richardson–Olzsewski (SRO) syndrome and the recently characterised multiple system atrophy (MSA) are indeed associated with a quite well-defined profile of intellectual impairment, even in the earliest stages of the disease. The existence of dementia in the later stages of Parkinson's and Huntington's diseases has now largely been accepted (Brown and Marsden, 1988; Brandt and Bylsma, 1993), although its exact neural and neuropathological basis remains a matter for debate (see Quinn, 1993). These dementing signs could be attributed to additional pathology, distinct from the primary pathology of the nigro-striatal dopamine pathway in PD, for example, to degeneration of the basal forebrain or locus ceruleus, or to cortical Lewy bodies (see Agid *et al.*, 1987; Quinn, 1993). In the case of Huntington's disease, it is still unclear just how much of the cognitive impairment can be attributed to striatal degeneration, as distinct from cortical atrophy (see e.g. Starkstein *et al.*, 1992).

Part of the initial reluctance to accept that PD and other conditions have their own collection of cognitive deficits may have stemmed from the prejudice that the basal ganglia are essentially structures with motor functions, notwithstanding early far-sighted theoretical speculations and findings to the contrary (e.g. Hassler, 1978; Divac, Rosvold and Szwarcbart, 1967). Part may have rested on the occasionally well-founded suspicions of confounding measurement of cognitive abilities by the complications of co-existing depression and motor dysfunction (see Marsden, 1980, 1981; and the commentaries by Cools *et al.*, 1981 and Oberg and Divac, 1981).

Increasing sophistication of neuropsychological assessment and a better understanding of functional neuroanatomy have led to a marked reappraisal of the status of cognitive deficits in basal ganglia disease. The accumulation of knowledge about the neuroanatomical organisation of the basal ganglia, largely from animal studies, has prompted new hypotheses about the nature and neural substrates of cognitive deficits in these conditions. For example, on the basis of anatomical, neurophysiological and behavioural evidence, the concept of cortico-striatal loops has evolved, which emphasises the functional inter-relationships between the neocortex and striatum (Alexander, DeLong and Strick, 1986). Of particular note is the fact that the prime target of basal ganglia outflow appears to be the frontal lobes, whether to the premotor regions such as the supplementary motor area, or to discrete regions of the prefrontal cortex, such as dorsolateral prefrontal cortex or orbito-frontal cortex, which receive projections from different loops involving different sectors of the caudate nucleus (see Figure 3.1).

These anatomical facts are compatible with some of the earliest theories of cognitive deficits following basal ganglia malfunction that lumped them together with a diverse collection of other conditions, including hydrocephalus and multiple sclerosis, under the heading 'subcortical dementia' – to differentiate them from the more obviously 'cortical' dementia of Alzheimer's disease (Albert, Feldman and Willis, 1974; McHugh and Folstein, 1975; Cummings and Benson, 1984). The major features of subcortical dementia, of which Steele–Richardson's syndrome (i.e. progressive supranuclear palsy) was a prototypical form, included impaired mood and motivation, altered personality, specific forms of memory disturbance, slowed thinking and impaired reasoning, that were reminiscent of some of the executive deficits produced by frontal lobe damage. In the case of the basal ganglia deficits at least, the revised term 'fronto-subcortical' dementia could readily be reinterpreted as 'fronto-striatal dementia', on the basis of the new anatomical findings. However, relating specific deficits in PD to, say, its non-striatal chemical pathology, to striatal or cortical dopamine loss, or even to medication with L-dopa, has been extremely difficult, just as it has been to decide which of the cognitive features of HD are associated with striatal degeneration and which to cortical atrophy (Brandt and Bylsma, 1993). This chapter summarises the progress made in understanding the cognitive and neural nature of the cognitive deficits in basal ganglia disease, and describes our own strategy of utilising studies from non-human primates in order better to understand these deficits.

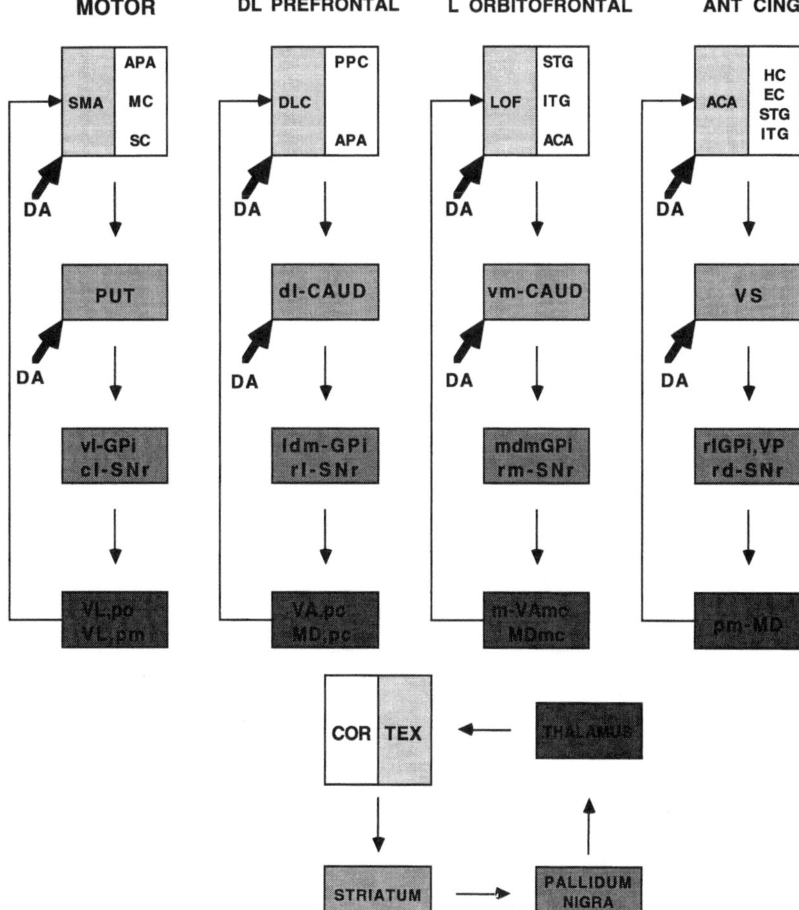

Figure 3.1. Cortico-striatal 'loops' according to the scheme of Alexander *et al.*, 1986. Note DA innervation at both the cortical and striatal levels, indicated by thick black arrows. Those cortical structures innervating the striatum are shown at the top of the diagram. The 'loop' only projects back to a restricted subset of those structures, all of which are in the frontal lobe. Abbreviations: ACA, anterior cingulate region; APA, arcuate premotor area; CAUD, caudate nucleus; DLC, dorsolateral prefrontal cortex; EC, entorhinal cortex; GPi, internal segment of the globus pallidus; HC, hippocampus; ITG, inferior temporal gyrus; LOF, lateral orbitofrontal cortex; MC, motor cortex; MDmc, medialis dorsalis, pars magnocellularis; MD, pc, medialis dorsalis, pars parvocellularis; PPC, posterior parietal cortex; PUT, putamen; SC, somatosensory cortex; SMA, supplementary motor cortex; SNr, substantia nigra, pars reticularis; STG, superior temporal gyrus; VAmc, ventralis anterior, pars magnocellularis; VA, pc, ventralis anterior, pars parvocellularis; VL, pm, ventralis lateralis, pars medialis; VL, po, ventralis lateralis, pars oralis; VP, ventral pallidum; VS, ventral striatum; cl, caudolateral; dl-, dorsolateral; 1-, lateral; ldm-, lateral dorsomedial; m-, medial; mdm-, medial dorsomedial; pm-, posteromedial; rd-, rostrodorsal; rl-, rostrolateral; rm-, rostromedial; vm-, ventromedial; vl-, ventrolateral. The bottom diagram indicates the general organisation of the cortico-striatal–pallidal–thalamic loop.

Origins of the frontal-executive theory of cognitive deficits in basal ganglia disorders

While there is an extensive literature on visuospatial and memory deficits in PD, HD and SRO, much of this can be assimilated to the existence of a specific pattern of deficits that can be related to executive dysfunction. For example, deficits in free recall and conditional learning occur more readily than those in recognition memory (Talland, 1962; Weingartner, Burns and Lewitt, 1984; Moss *et al.*, 1986; Taylor, Saint-Cyr and Lang, 1990; see Brandt and Bylsma, 1993 for a review), and there are severe impairments in certain forms of short-term memory, exemplified especially by the Brown–Petersen test, which are often associated with 'frontal' memory deficits (Sagar *et al.*, 1988; Cooper *et al.*, 1991). Moreover, isolating specific impairments in visuospatial function from such executive requirements as planning, sequencing and attentional set-shifting has been difficult, if not impossible.

Bowen (1976) was one of the first investigators to provide specific information on 'frontal' deficits in PD from studies of the Wisconsin Card Sorting Test (WCST), a traditional means of assessing 'frontal' dysfunction. This classic study was followed by several research initiatives. The first of these was published as a paper in *Brain* in 1986 entitled 'Frontal lobe dysfunction in Parkinson's disease' (Taylor, Saint-Cyr and Lang, 1986). This paper used a number of tests with putative frontal components to test PD patients at several stages of the disease. The tests included not only the WCST, but also the 'Tower of Toronto', related to the well-known Tower of Hanoi, in order to assess planning function, as well as a number of tests of short-term memory. On the basis of results using these tests the authors asserted that the inability to elaborate efficient strategies spontaneously or use internally guided behaviours may explain recall and problem-solving deficits in PD (see also Saint-Cyr, Taylor and Lang, 1988; Taylor *et al.*, 1990). The second approach was derived from a cognitive theory that emphasised the utilisation of processing resources and the internal regulation of attention, in both of which PD patients were found to be deficient (e.g. Brown and Marsden, 1988*b*, 1991; Brown, 1993). The third approach capitalized on the poor performance of PD patients on the WCST first described by Bowen *et al.* (1975), even when unmedicated and early in the course of the disease (Lees and Smith, 1983; Canavan *et al.*, 1989). These deficits are generally categorised as reflecting impairments of set-formation, maintenance and, especially, set-shifting ability, and have now been observed by a number of other investigators in different forms, sometimes with test material not directly related to the WCST (e.g. Cools *et al.*, 1984; Flowers and Robertson, 1985; Downes *et al.*, 1989; Downes *et al.*, 1993; Channon, Jones and Stephenson, 1993). A third perspective was obtained by longitudinal studies using well-established neuropsychological forms of assessment that suggested specific impairments in PD in temporal sequencing on a subtest of WAIS that can be interpreted as reflecting executive deficits (Cooper *et al.*, 1991).

Despite this emphasis on the 'frontal' hypothesis, there has been relatively little direct comparison of those cognitive deficits observed in PD with impairments present in frontal lobe damaged patients within the same study. Moreover, the specificity of deficits seen has seldom also been tested with appropriate comparisons in other relevant groups such as neurosurgical cases of temporal lobe ablation and early cases of dementia of the Alzheimer type. In the latter case, it is particularly important to focus on the performance of patients early in the course of Parkinson's disease, prior to medication. There is a similar dearth of parametric comparisons with other basal ganglia conditions, particularly Huntington's disease and the SRO syndrome (c.f. Brown and Marsden, 1988*a*). In the case of the former, there has been considerable interest in the comparison with organic amnesia, in the context of dissociations of different memory systems, for example for 'declarative' and 'procedural' memory (as assessed by pursuit rotor tasks or by performance on the 'procedural' aspects of Tower of Hanoi performance) (see Brandt and Bylsma, 1993). However, while it has been pointed out that the 'executive' aspects of the intellectual deficit in HD contribute importantly to everyday disability (e.g. Bamford *et al.*, 1989), there has been little formal assessment of the executive problems afflicting patients with this disease, especially early in its course. A few major clinically oriented analyses and surveys have revealed that SRO patients fail classical tests of frontal lobe function such as the Wisconsin Card Sorting Test and verbal fluency, and exhibit frontal lobe 'signs', including enhanced grasp reflexes, motor impersistence and utilisation behaviour. Two studies have shown that, when matched for age and severity of intellectual deterioration, the SRO patients perform worse than PD groups on such tests of frontal lobe dysfunction (Pillon *et al.*, 1986; Dubois *et al.*, 1988). On the other hand, one study has claimed that SRO patients are relatively intact on tests of problem-solving, a classic form of frontal lobe dysfunction (Grafman *et al.*, 1990). Clearly again there is much to be gained from a detailed neuropsychological comparison of basal ganglia disorders with patients with frontal lobe damage.

An integrated cognitive neuroscientific approach

Our own approach has attempted to integrate the cognitive, neuropsychological and neurobiological approaches by using tests or collections of tests that can be theoretically decomposed into their constituent elements at a cognitive level, and which make connections with important animal neuropsychological studies. The latter serve to localise at a neural level elements of executive control that are presumably present in more elaborate forms in humans. The great advantage of animal studies is that it is possible to make highly specific neural or neurochemical interventions to isolate a fraction of the complex patterns of pathology that make difficult the analysis of basal ganglia disorders. Their main disadvantage is the difficulty of relating behavioural deficits in animals to cognitive deficits in man. Thus, it is admittedly difficult to model planning deficits in man that entail the relative evaluation of efficacy of sequences of mental responses in relation to specific goals or outcomes. However, many of the elements of planning can be defined and measured separately; for example, the working memory load, the capacity to sequence responses and to shift set on the basis of reward and the ability to respond according to conditional rules have each been addressed by primate neuropsychological studies, and are included in our own battery of tests for monkeys and human patients (CANTAB) (see Sahakian and Owen, 1992; Roberts and Sahakian 1993; Robbins *et al.*, 1994*a*).

Experimental tests of planning function

Nevertheless, the impetus for one of our main tests for patients was born from a cognitive theory which suggested that a major aspect of executive function was attention to action, especially in novel behavioural circumstances that require planning. The 'Tower of London' test was modified by Shallice and McCarthy (Shallice, 1982) from the earlier Tower of Hanoi puzzle to stress the capacity for mental planning with only a single goal outcome specified. The usual form of the four-disc Tower of Hanoi requires the subject to sort the four discs according to their size from one vertical peg to another in a precise configuration. But this generally requires repeated trials and the subject essentially has to learn the very long effective sequences of responses on a trial and error basis more reminiscent of procedural learning routines than of mental planning, in which the subject visualises the various candidate solutions in advance before selecting the most efficacious one. This confounding between the procedural and executive aspects of problem solving can potentially confuse attempts to isolate 'frontal' deficits, especially when the basal ganglia are often implicated in procedural aspects of memory.

Thus, modified versions of the Tower of London test were developed to compare planning ability in patients with localised frontal lobe excisions and patients with PD, SRO, MSA and, most recently, patients at different stages of HD. In one of the computerised tasks the subject was required to move an arrangement of coloured balls hanging in 'socks' or 'pockets' to match a goal arrangement presented in the top half of the screen (Figure 3.2a). The test incorporated a touch sensitive screen such that a ball could be moved simply by touching it and then by touching an empty position in one of the other pockets. The degree of planning required was manipulated by varying the minimum number of moves required to make the correct match between two and five moves. The proportion of perfect solutions (i.e. solved in the minimum possible number of moves) and the efficiency of planning, as measured by the excess moves used beyond the minimum specified, provide measures of the efficiency of planning. In two versions of the test the relative contributions of initial and subsequent 'thinking' or planning time during the execution of the solution have also been the main performance indices. As the time taken to complete the task was to some extent dependent on movement (i.e. 'motor') time, and basal ganglia damaged patients may be expected to have several disabling forms of motor impediment, a related 'yoked control' condition was also employed to measure motor initiation and motor execution time over an identical series of single moves. By subtracting the latencies for each move in this motor control condition from those of the planning condition, estimates of initial and subsequent 'thinking time' were derived.

The results of our initial study (Owen *et al.*, 1990) both confirmed and extended findings of Shallice (1982) using the original 'pegs and beads' version of the test that showed impairments in a group of patients with 'anterior' cortical damage. Although patients with localised frontal lobe excisions completed even the most difficult problems within the maximum number of moves allowed, they nevertheless required significantly more moves per problem than control subjects, matched for age and premorbid verbal IQ, consequently producing fewer (perfect) minimum move solutions. In addition, although the two groups did not differ in the amount of time spent thinking prior to the first move (Figure 3.3), the frontal lobe patients spent significantly more time thinking during the execution of the problem solution. This pattern of impairment appears to be relatively specific for cortical frontal lesions since no deficits are observed in neurosurgical patients with temporal lobe damage (Owen *et al.*, 1995*a*).

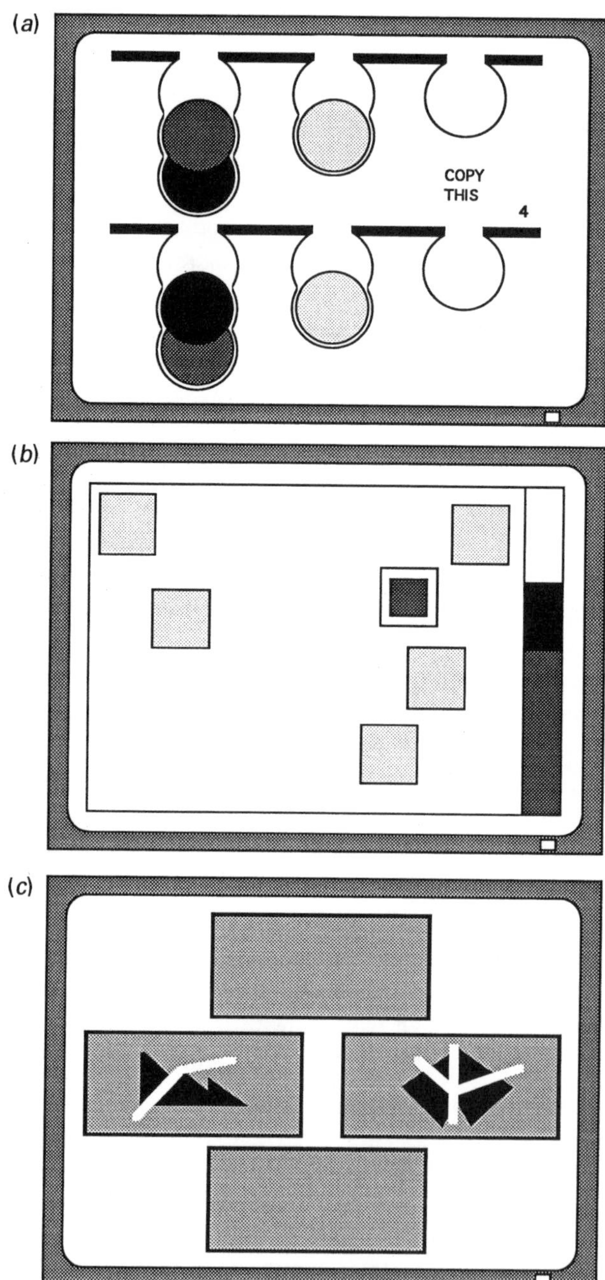

Figure 3.2. The three major computerised neuropsychological tests shown to be sensitive to frontal lobe dysfunction: (a) Tower of London; (b) Spatial Working Memory; (c) Attentional set-shifting (ID/ED test). This shows the general nature

A parallel study of patients with PD (Owen *et al.*, 1992) demonstrated that L-dopa medicated and non-medicated patients at different stages of the disease can be differentiated in terms of their performance on this test of planning. Thus, a 'frontal like' impairment in solution accuracy was only evident in a group of medicated patients with severe clinical symptoms (Hoehn and Yahr stages III–IV). In contrast, medicated patients with both mild (Hoehn and Yahr stages I–II) and severe symptoms were slower than controls to initiate solutions to the planning problems, but *unlike* the frontal lobe patients, neither group was impaired in terms of subsequent 'thinking' time. No impairments were observed in a third group of PD patients who were non-medicated and had relatively mild clinical symptoms. These results indicate that whereas a prominent test of frontal function, the Tower of London test of planning, is quite sensitive to cognitive impairment in PD, the qualitative nature of the deficits appears to be different. The slowed 'initial thinking time' seen in PD was not prominent following frontal lobe damage, and yet is consistent with the cognitive deficits of 'sub-cortical' dementia and the clinical symptom of 'bradyphrenia'. Detailed consideration of its cognitive basis is beyond our present scope (see discussion in Owen *et al.*, 1992 and Morris *et al.*, 1988). However, it seems likely that it can be related quite directly to the dopaminergic deficit in PD, as it was severely exacerbated by L-dopa withdrawal (Lange *et al.*, 1992). Only with severe clinical disability was the 'frontal' pattern of inaccurate solutions evident. Therefore, it appears that the Tower of London deficits in PD show qualitatively distinct features from those seen following frontal lobe damage, which might reflect differences in the operation of different nodes in the fronto-striatal loops (see Figure 3.1) and in their neurochemical modulation.

The comparison between frontal and PD patients has recently been extended using a version of the task that minimises the motor requirement and is amenable to activation paradigms using PET, which confirm a frontal involvement (Owen *et al.*, 1995*b*; Baker *et al.*, 1996). This task does not inform the subjects how many moves are required to solve the problems, requiring them to estimate this instead. This difference not only

Caption for Fig. 3.2 (*cont.*)
and presentation of the pairs of stimuli, which can be composed of any combination of elements of the two dimensions (i.e. lines and shapes). The presentation of the IDS (intra-dimensional shift) and EDS (extra-dimensional shift) stages is preceded by a series of simple tests of simple and compound discrimination learning and reversal. The subject proceeds from one stage to the next by reaching a criterion of 6/6 correct within 50 trials. See text for details, Figure 3.5 for data at the IDS and EDS stages and Figure 3.6 for data showing general performance across stages for clinical groups and controls.

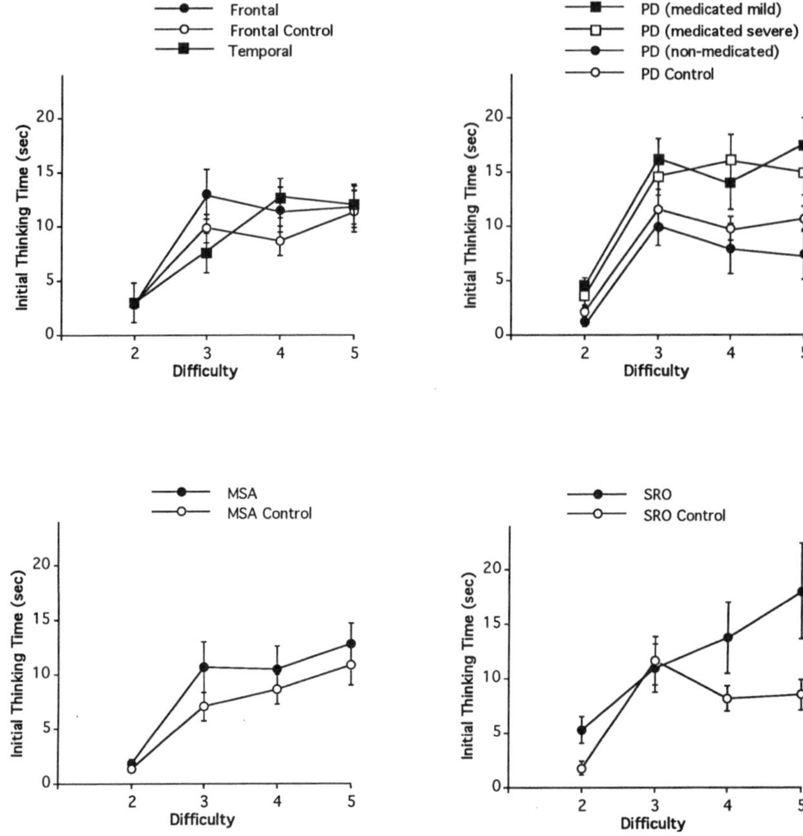

Figure 3.3. Initial thinking time on the Tower of London test for various patient groups with cortical excisions or basal ganglia degeneration, compared to age- and IQ-matched control groups. PD, Parkinson's disease; MSA, multiple system atrophy (of striato-nigral predominance); SRO, Steele–Richardson–Olzsewski syndrome (see Owen *et al.*, 1991, 1992, 1995*a*; Robbins *et al.*, 1994*b*).

makes the task more difficult, but also results in a monotonic increase in thinking time as a function of the number of moves. It is significant that a deficit in unmedicated, early-in-the-course PD patients emerges under these conditions.

Contrasting patterns of impairment on the earlier planning task in which the problems are produced move by move were also found in groups of patients with MSA and SRO who, in terms of their clinical disability, were most similar to the group of medicated PD patients with severe clinical symptoms described above (Robbins *et al.*, 1994*b*). Thus, like the medicated patients with PD, the 18 SRO patients were significantly impaired in terms of their initial thinking time (Figure 3.3) (though not in terms of their subsequent thinking time), and showed a significant decrease in the number of minimum move, or 'perfect' solutions. In contrast with the performance of PD patients, but like the patients with frontal lobe damage, the 16 patients with MSA exhibited significantly prolonged subsequent, but not initial thinking times (Figure 3.3) although this deficit was not accompanied by any significant impairment in performance accuracy.

Another pattern of disability on the same version of the Tower of London test that specifies the number of moves needed to solve the problem and requires their actual enactment, is evident from a recent comparison of performance of patients with relatively late-stage HD with dementia of Alzheimer's type, matched for overall level of dementia, as assessed by the Mini-Mental State examination (Lange *et al.*, 1995). Perhaps surprisingly, the HD patients performed significantly worse in terms of accuracy of planning, although the result is entirely consistent with the hypothesis that there are distinct patterns of deficit in dementia. However, neither group was able to attempt the most difficult problems and it could be conjectured that planning as such was impossible for both. Their partially successful performance on the easier problems might have reflected some of the more automatic features of 'planning' arising from a rapid perceptual identification of the various possibilities, analogous to the 'schema' postulated by Shallice and Norman (see Shallice, 1982), and it is this aspect of performance that appeared to be differentially disrupted in HD. Thus, again it appears that while the basal ganglia damaged patients show impairments on a 'frontal' test of cognitive function, there appear to be major *qualitative* differences in the nature of the deficits between such patients and those with frontal lobe damage that cannot easily be ascribed to the stage of the disease and general intellectual deterioration, and suggest instead that the basal ganglia fulfil quite specific functions within the context of tests of executive function.

Fractionation of component cognitive abilities

The above analysis shows that impaired performance in the Tower of London test may be profitably considered further in terms of the component processes required for accurate planning. For example, given the importance of attentional 'set' for efficient problem solving, the ability to shift between competing possibilities may play a crucial role in the final selection of the most appropriate solution. Consistent with this possibility, Wallesch, Karnath and Zimmerman (1992) found that the performance of

Parkinson's disease patients in a 'covered' maze, presented on a computer screen was markedly disrupted by problems of response shifting; the nature of this deficit contrasted rather sharply with that of patients with frontal lobe excisions, as we would have predicted on the basis of our analysis of the Tower of London task. Cronin-Golomb, Corkin and Growdon (1994) have recently also argued this point in the case of a rather different form of problem solving in patients with PD.

Another possibility is that the planning deficits observed reflect an impairment of memory function. Accurate planning on the Tower of London test requires an active search of possible solutions, placing a significant load on spatial working memory. In fact, a recent large-scale analysis of Tower of London performance has confirmed that the test loads significantly with tests of spatial working memory in factor analyses, which reveal an unprecedentedly high degree of intercorrelation for tests of frontal lobe function (Owen *et al.*, 1992; Robbins *et al.*, 1997).

(i) Spatial working memory

The spatial working memory task is essentially a modification of one used by Passingham to examine the effects of dorsolateral prefrontal cortex lesions in primates (Passingham, 1985) and conceptually similar to the 'radial arm maze', which has been successfully used to assess the role of the hippocampus in working memory in rats (Olton, Becker and Handelman, 1979). The test is open-ended in the sense that the subject is free to produce his or her own 'self-ordered' sequences of responses.

In our version of the task, adapted for humans, subjects were required to 'search through' a number of red boxes presented on the computer screen (by touching each one) in order to find blue 'tokens' that were hidden inside (Figure 3.2b). The object was to avoid those boxes in which a token had already been found. Importantly, the subjects could search through the boxes in any order they wished although the number of boxes visited before a token was found was determined by the computer. The neurosurgical patients with frontal lobe damage were significantly impaired on this task (Figure 3.4), making more returns to boxes ('between search' errors) in which a token had previously been found, at all levels of task difficulty as determined by the number of boxes employed (2, 3, 4, 6 or 8). In addition, these patients were shown to be less proficient in the use of a searching strategy known to improve performance on this task. This strategy retraced previous 'routes' while 'editing' them to exclude previously successful locations. This strategic impairment suggested that at least some of the frontal impairment in spatial

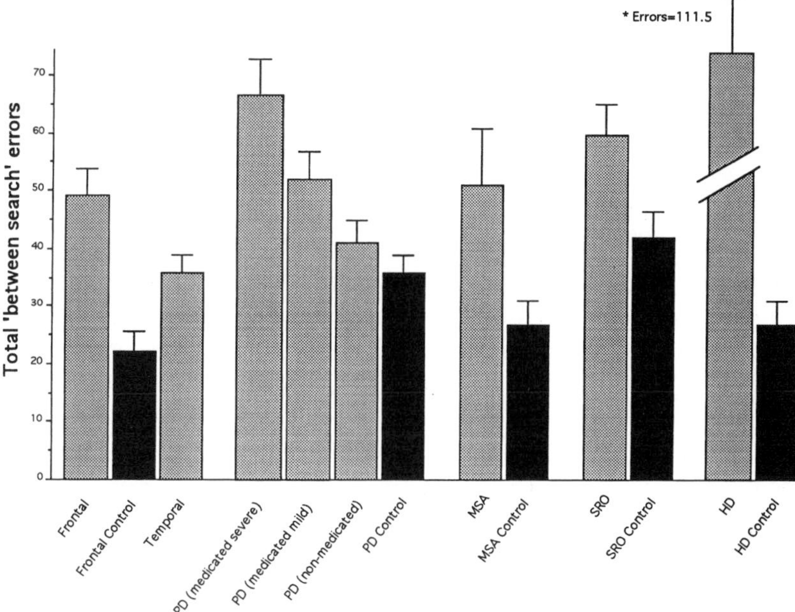

Figure 3.4. Performance on the spatial working memory test, as measured by between search errors. PD, Parkinson's disease; HD, Huntington's disease; MSA multiple system atrophy (of striato-nigral predominance); SRO, Steele-Richardson-Olzsewski syndrome. Data taken from Owen *et al.*, 1992, 1995*a*; Robbins *et al.*, 1994. The HD group were relatively late in the course of disease (see Lange *et al.*, 1995).

working memory arises secondarily from a more fundamental deficit in the use of organisational strategies. This task may also be sensitive to deficits in patients with temporal lobe damage although only at the most extreme level of task difficulty (i.e. 8 boxes). Unlike the frontal lobe patients, however, the temporal lobe group utilises a normal and effective searching strategy (Owen *et al.*, 1995*a*). This test therefore has fundamental mnemonic requirements that interact powerfully with strategic factors, thus requiring the co-ordination of posterior cortical capacities with the executive functions of more anterior zones. As such, the task provides an intriguing challenge for patients with basal ganglia deficits who could be expected to be impaired on the basis either of deficient processing of information carried by temporal lobe afferents to the basal ganglia or by connections to the frontal lobes.

We have found that tests sensitive to temporal, but not frontal lobe damage, such as the capacity to recognise briefly presented patterns, are only sensitive to deficit in PD with severe clinical disability, who are presumably late in the course of the disease. When these deficits in pattern recognition occur, they are also not exacerbated by L-dopa withdrawal (Lange *et al.*, 1992). These observations suggest that the nature of the profile of cognitive deficits in PD is quite distinct from that of Alzheimer's disease, and that tests sensitive to frontal lobe damage are generally also sensitive to deficits in relatively early-in-the-course PD, although the nature of these deficits may not be identical.

In support of the view that patients with basal ganglia disease have a qualitatively distinct cognitive profile of deficits to those of Alzheimer's disease, it has been shown recently that patients with advanced HD are certainly much more severely impaired on the spatial working memory task than those with DAT; indeed the HD group deficit is as great as any we have observed following frontal lesions (Lange *et al.*, 1995 – see Figure 3.4). It seems likely that it results from a combination of memory and strategic deficits. Among groups of patients with PD, an impairment in terms of the accuracy of performance on the spatial working memory task was observed in medicated PD patients with both mild and severe clinical symptoms. However, unlike the frontal lobe patients, neither group was impaired in terms of the strategy adopted to tackle the problem. Non-medicated patients with PD were unimpaired on this task (Owen *et al.*, 1992), but medicated PD patients with either mild or severe clinical disability showed significant impairment.

The spatial working memory task also proved to be most sensitive to deficits in patients with MSA and SRO (Figure 3.4). Both groups were significantly impaired in terms of the number of returns to boxes in which a token had previously been found. Moreover, like the frontal lobe group, this deficit was found to relate directly to the inappropriate use of a repetitive searching strategy in the SRO (though not in the MSA) patients (Robbins *et al.*, 1994*b*).

This form of self-ordered spatial working memory test is known to depend on the integrity of prefrontal lobe function in monkeys, but has not been studied specifically in terms of neurochemical mechanisms within the frontal cortex or via its connections with the basal ganglia. Much better understood is the simpler delayed response task, a test of short-term spatial memory that can be made using either limb movements or delayed saccades (c.f. Goldman-Rakic, 1990). The delayed response task similarly depends on the dorsolateral prefrontal cortex, on the basis of behavioural, electrophysiological and metabolic evidence (Goldman-Rakic, 1990). Some evidence also argues for a role for dopamine D1 receptors (Goldman-Rakic, 1992) and adrenergic alpha-2 receptors (the latter in aged primates, Arnsten, Cai and Goldman-Rakic, 1988). In terms of the basal ganglia, classical studies found that radiofrequency lesions aimed at that region of the head of the caudate nucleus in monkeys that is known to be part of the 'dorsolateral prefrontal cortex loop' in purely anatomical terms (see Figure 3.1) impaired the ability to perform the task, though not as severely as damage to the prefrontal cortex itself (Battig, Rosvold and Mishkin, 1960, 1962). Recent studies have shown that MPTP-treated monkeys resulting in profound striatal dopamine depletion exhibit delayed response deficits (Schneider and Kovelowski, 1990). Therefore, there is a clear anatomical substrate for this type of task that makes it susceptible to striatal, as well as frontal lobe damage. There is considerable evidence for a contribution to inefficient spatial working memory performance in PD, as our study of the effects of controlled L-dopa withdrawal in a small group of patients with marked clinical disability showed a significant further deterioration of performance (Lange *et al.*, 1992). However, the locus of this effect (i.e. frontal or striatal) remains unknown.

(ii) Attentional set-shifting

The third paradigm designed to assess frontal lobe dysfunction in PD was based on similar principles to the Wisconsin Card Sorting Test (WCST), the classic index of frontal lobe dysfunction (Milner, 1963) used in so many of the previous studies of basal ganglia patients. However, in addition to efficient set shifting, successful performance on this test requires a number of other distinct cognitive abilities not directly related to attentional set-shifting ability (for discussion, see Downes *et al.*, 1989). These processes may not depend directly on frontal lobe mechanisms and may independently contribute to some of the deficits observed. For this reason, we devised a computerised test of attentional set-shifting ability, which helps to decompose the WCST into its constituent elements (Figure 3.2c). The test was derived from the animal learning literature and based on the concepts of 'intra' and 'extra-dimensional' shifts. An 'intra-dimensional shift' (IDS) occurs when a subject is required to cease responding to one exemplar of a particular stimulus dimension (e.g. 'blue' from the dimension 'colour') and begins responding to a new exemplar of that same dimension (e.g. 'red'). An 'extra-dimensional shift' (EDS) occurs when the subject is required to switch responding to a novel exemplar of a previously irrelevant dimension (e.g. from the colour 'red' to 'squares' from the dimension 'shape'). In fact, we used shifts between shapes and superimposed lines (Figure 3.2c). If the subject commits more errors when attempting the EDS compared with the IDS, then it can be inferred that he was employing selective attentional processes in solving the task, rather than a somewhat inefficient learning strategy that requires list-learning of different configurations of the test stimuli (see Roberts, Robbins and Everitt, 1988). This pattern of superior IDS performance is found in a variety of species ranging from humans, rhesus monkeys (personal communication from L. Gold and G.F. Koob) and marmosets (see Figure 3.5) to the rat. Thus, this paradigm successfully passes the test of cross-species behavioural homology. There are also neural homologies between monkeys and man in that the EDS component of the test is selectively impaired in both man (Owen *et al.*, 1991) and marmoset (Dias, Roberts and Robbins, 1996) following frontal lobe excisions in neurosurgical cases and excitotoxic lesions, respectively (see Figure 3.5). Current research is seeking to define more clearly those 'cortico-striatal loops' mediating performance in marmosets.

For both monkeys and man, the IDS/EDS test necessarily involves training on a number of more elementary stages (see Downes *et al.*, 1989). For example, initially the subject is required to learn a series of discriminations in which one of two stimuli was correct and the other was not, using feedback provided automatically by the computer. The test was composed of nine stages presented in the same fixed order, beginning with a simple discrimination (SD) and reversal (SDR) for stimuli varying in only one dimension (i.e. two white line configurations). A second, alternative dimension was then introduced (purple filled shapes) and compound discrimination (CD) and reversal (CDR) were tested. To succeed, subjects had to continue to respond to the previously relevant stimuli (i.e. white lines), ignoring the presence of the new, irrelevant dimension (shapes). At the intra-dimensional shift (IDS) stage new exemplars were introduced from each of the two dimensions (new lines and new shapes) and subjects were required to transfer the previously learnt rule to a novel set of exemplars from the same stimulus dimension. Thus, to succeed, they had to continue to respond to one of the two exemplars from the previously relevant dimension (lines). Following another reversal of contingencies (IDR) the extra-dimensional shift (EDS) and reversal (EDR) was presented and again, novel exemplars from each of the two dimensions were introduced. However, at this stage, the subject was required to shift 'response set' to the alternative (previously irrelevant) stimulus dimension and ignore the previously relevant dimension.

At each stage, a change in contingencies would occur once the subject had learnt the current rule to a criterion of six consecutive correct responses. The subject was only allowed to proceed to each successive stage of the test if he or she reached criteria at the previous stage. This permits a

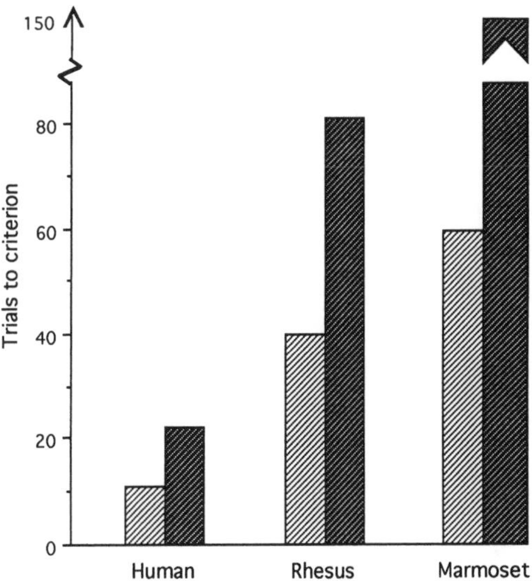

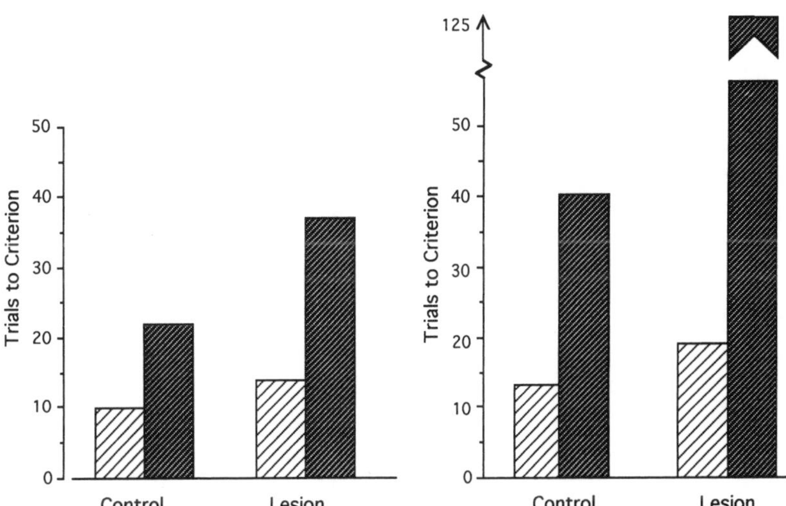

Figure 3.5. Light cross-hatching is IDS (intra-dimensional shift); dark shading EDS (extra-dimensional shift). (a) Behavioural homology: comparison of man, rhesus monkey and marmoset on trials to criterion for the intra- and extra-dimensional shift stages. Note in all three stages the superiority of IDS over EDS performance, indicating selective attention to the different dimensions. (b) Neural homology: similar effects of frontal lesions in marmoset and man selectively to impair EDS, but not IDS, performance (from Roberts *et al.*, 1997, with permission).

clear and simple method of analysing and presenting the main results (see Figure 3.6).

Thus, as mentioned above, the frontal lobe patients were specifically impaired in their ability to shift response set to the previously irrelevant stimulus dimension (i.e. at the EDS stage of learning) but not to shift attention to new exemplars of a previously relevant dimension (i.e. at the IDS stage of learning). This deficit was neurally specific in that a group of patients with temporal lobe excisions were unimpaired in their ability to perform either shift.

Of the three 'frontal lobe' tasks employed, only this test of attentional set-shifting ability revealed significant deficits in *all three* groups of patients with PD, including the never-medicated group. In fact, at the earlier stages of learning prior to the extra-dimensional shift, deficits were, if anything, worst in the non-medicated groups of patients who had relatively mild clinical symptoms (see Figure 3.6).

This test was also particularly sensitive to deficits in the groups of patients with MSA and SRO (Robbins *et al.*, 1994*b*). At the extra-dimensional shift stage of learning, the impairment in the MSA group was approximately equivalent to that seen in the frontal lobe patients (Figure 3.6). The rather more severe deficit at this stage, in the SRO group, resembled that observed in the medicated PD patients with severe clinical symptoms who, in fact, had a similar level of clinical disability. In recent work we have shown that patients early in the course of HD are also susceptible to failure at the EDS stage (Lawrence *et al.*, 1996), although HD patients later in the course fail even at the simple reversal stage, because of a failure to inhibit perseverative responding to the previously reinforced stimulus (see Figure 3.6). The latter deficit was greater than in patients with dementia of the Alzheimer type (DAT) (Lange *et al.*, 1995). Indeed, patients with mild, probable Alzheimer's disease, who exhibit significant memory deficits are no worse than age- and IQ-matched controls at negotiating the ID/ED test (Sahakian *et al.*, 1990 – see Figure 3.6). This is a very significant finding, as it implies that the deficits in attentional set formation and shifting in patients with basal ganglia disorders have some specificity. An obvious hypothesis is that, unlike DAT, these conditions have a profile of cognitive deficits that is reminiscent of frontal lobe dysfunction. By contrast, the deficits present in early DAT resemble those produced by posterior cortical, especially temporal lobe, damage.

However, our own incidental observations, as well as anecdotal reports from the literature, led us to consider once again that the deficit in the ID/ED test following frontal lobe damage and basal ganglia disorders may

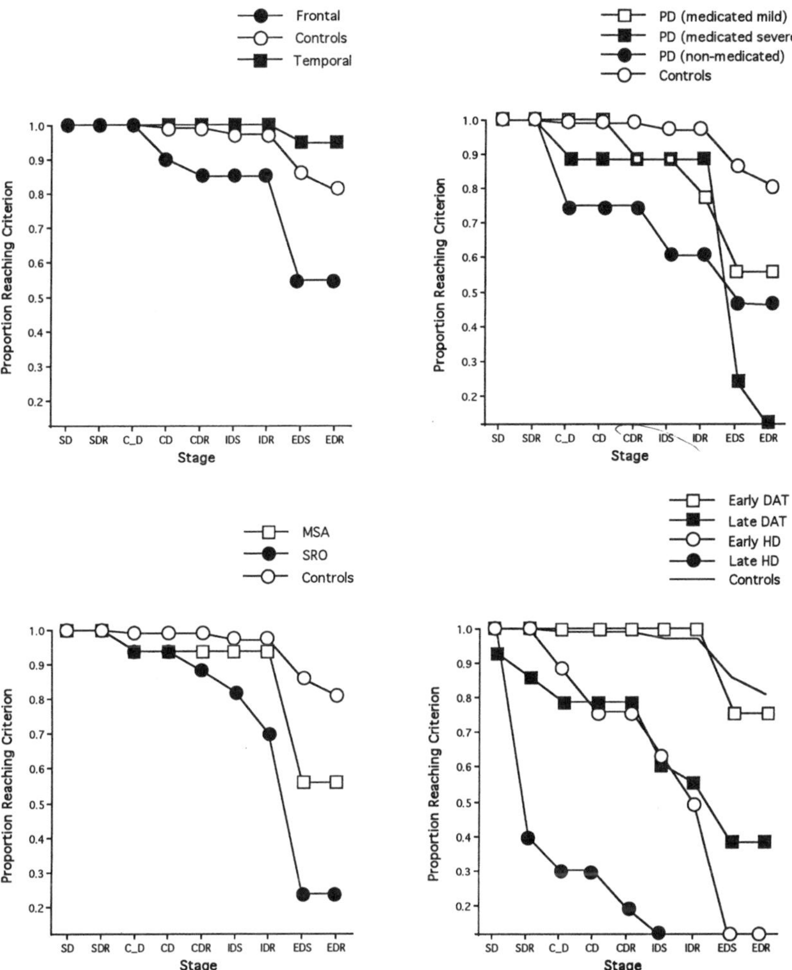

Figure 3.6. Performance on the attentional set-shifting paradigm, assessed in terms of the proportion of subjects reaching each stage of the test. SD, simple discrimination; SDR, simple reversal; C_D, compound discrimination, spatially discontiguous elements; CD, compound discrimination; CDR, compound discrimination reversal; IDS, intra-dimensional shift; IDR, intra-dimensional reversal; EDS, extra-dimensional shift; EDR, extra-dimensional reversal. Other abbreviations as for Figure 3.3. DAT, dementia of Alzheimer type. Data taken from Owen *et al.*, 1991, 1992; Robbins *et al.*, 1992, 1994*b*; Sahakian *et al.*, 1990; Lange *et al.*, 1995.

reflect qualitatively distinct forms of impairment. One possibility is that frontal patients 'perseverate' as described by Milner and others, by failing to disengage their responses from the previously reinforced dimensions, whereas patients with basal ganglia disease fail the shifting task for other reasons. Flowers and Robertson (1985), for example, report how PD patients do not so much perseverate on the WCST as apparently 'lose their way' when a shift is required, by adopting esoteric but inappropriate response strategies. More specifically, we hypothesised that they are impaired because they are reluctant to respond to a stimulus dimension that has never previously been reinforced. An analogous phenomenon in the animal learning literature is called 'learned irrelevance' (Mackintosh, 1983). Therefore, we sought to disconfound these two potential forms of deficit in a novel form of the set-shifting task in which a novel dimension was substituted either for the previously reinforced, or for the previously non-reinforced, dimension at the EDS stage (Owen *et al.*, 1993). In the former case the patient is required to shift to the previously non-reinforced dimension, so any deficit cannot be attributed to perseveration, and must reflect impairments in processing previously non-reinforced stimuli ('learned irrelevance'). In the latter case, it is the non-reinforced dimension that is removed, so any deficit must be attributed to a perseverative tendency, which presumably reflects an inability of the subject to become emancipated from old stimulus-response habits learned on the basis of non-reinforcement. We tested a group of patients with frontal lobe lesions, as well as patients with PD either early in the course and therefore unmedicated, or later in the course and medicated with L-dopa preparations. Each patient received both conditions at different stages in a single test session, in a counterbalanced manner.

The results for frontal patients were clear-cut, with considerable evidence for perseveration, but no deficits in the 'learned irrelevance' condition. Therefore, frontal patients were able to shift when the previously reinforced dimension was removed, even when required to respond to previously irrelevant stimuli. These were, however, unable to shift responses when a previously reinfored dimension was present. It is of interest that a similar, though yet more pronounced perseverative tendency has been demonstrated in a group of chronic schizophrenics (Elliott *et al.*, 1995).

In the group of medicated PD patients completely the opposite pattern of results was obtained. These patients showed no perseverative tendency but made more errors in the 'learned irrelevance' condition, suggesting that the normal reluctance to respond to a never-reinforced dimension had been exacerbated in those patients. However, while these data are consistent with the hypothesis that PD patients exhibit qualitatively distinct problems compared with patients with frontal lobe damage, the interpretation is complicated by the performance of the never-medicated PD patients. These early-in-the-course patients showed *equivalent* deficits in the learned irrelevance and perseveration conditions. Thus, the cross-sectional comparison with the later-in-the-course medicated PD patients would seem to indicate that the effect of medication with L-dopa and related preparations was to reduce perseveration – that aspect of the deficit resembling the effects of frontal lobe damage. However, from these results, it is not possible to say with any confidence what the neural substrates of the 'learned irrelevance' deficit might be. Comparisons with HD might be informative, given the nature of the striatal pathology in this disorder. Preliminary evidence (A. Lawrence, B.J. Sahakian and T.W. Robbins, unpublished observations) suggest that early HD patients have problems in both the learned irrelevance and perseveration components of the task.

Extrapolating from animals to humans (and vice versa)

While the advent of sophisticated neuroimaging techniques provides a way for us to begin to pinpoint the neural underpinnings of some of the deficits described above, and to relate them to the functioning of discrete cortico-striatal loops, it is obvious that studying patients with multiple forms of pathology is not the ideal means of achieving this. An alternative approach is to lesion selectively the brain in experimental animals, but this approach may be limited by the capacity to relate any functional deficits to the cognitive impairments seen in humans. This problem of extrapolation can be circumvented to a degree by employing similar cognitive tests. We have found this most feasible in the case of the attentional set-shifting paradigm described above, which is based on animal learning theory, and where it is possible to use stimuli more or less identical to those employed in the clinic.

Following on from the demonstration that, as in man, damage to the frontal cortex impairs extra-dimensional shift performance, we have also used the neurotoxin 6-OHDA infused into the trajectory of the mesocortical dopamine projections in the marmoset, to test the hypothesis that depletion of frontal cortical DA may be responsible for the set-shifting deficit in patients with PD (Roberts *et al.*, 1994). To our surprise, however, far from being impaired in this task, marmosets with substantial prefrontal DA depletion, actually showed *improved* performance over sham-operated controls. This observation clearly argues against the premise that this particular form of cognitive deficit in PD results from prefrontal DA loss (although it should be noted that there were deficits in performance of the delayed response task in these marmosets). Following a previous hypothesis that there is a reciprocal balance in the regulation of cortical and subcortical DA systems, we also made direct measurements of the functional status of the subcortical DA systems in these monkeys by measuring striatal extracellular DA concentrations following a potassium pulse, and found them to be enhanced. Therefore, it is possible that the improved shifting performance results from an up-regulation of the striatal DA system, consistent with the hypothesis that the deficit in PD reflects striatal DA loss, and its remediation by L-dopa is caused by an up-regulation of striatal dopamine function. This hypothesis can of course be tested efficaciously by producing experimental depletion of striatal DA using 6-OHDA, and this is currently under investigation.

Further convergence of evidence between these studies of the effects of DA depletion in marmosets and patients with PD is provided by a recent study (Leenders, 1993) that has tried to relate the degree of DA loss in the frontal cortex and striatum to the WCST deficit in patients with PD, by determining the extent to which the magnitude of the deficit correlated with the extent of 6-L-[^{18}F]-dopa binding in the striatum and mesial frontal cortex in these patients. In this study a significant inverse relationship between binding in the frontal cortex (as measured by K_i) and perseverative behaviour on the WCST was found. Although this is a counter-intuitive finding, it is in keeping with the results of our animal studies. It is anticipated that future attempts to bridge the gap between clinical and basic studies of cognitive deficits in patients with basal ganglia disorders will be reinforced by this cross-fertilisation of approaches that allows us to determine the nature of the underlying cognitive processes, and how they are normally subserved by defined interactions between the cortex, striatum and their innervation by chemically defined neurotransmitter systems of subcortical origin.

Summary

An approach has been outlined for testing the hypothesis that the cognitive deficits in patients with basal ganglia diseases resemble those executive deficits that follow frontal lobe damage, and are the product of disruptions of functioning of highly organised cortico-striatal anatomical 'loops', which appear to operate in a segregated and parallel manner. This approach makes detailed comparisons of performance following basal ganglia disease, with other informative groups, including DAT, and patients with neurosurgical excisions of the temporal lobe, and most importantly, the frontal lobes themselves. It also allows the possibility of direct comparisons with the effects of selective lesions in monkeys, thus allowing inferences to be made about the causal role of underlying pathology in the human neurodegenerative diseases. The main findings are that certain tests of frontal lobe function are very sensitive to deficits in diseases such as PD, HD, MSA and SRO. In PD, some of these deficits are apparently responsive to L-dopa therapy. However, the nature of the deficits in these conditions often differs qualitatively from those produced by frontal lobe damage, and this suggests that the tests are helping to define the functions of striatal nodes in the cortico-striatal loops, as well as of the prefrontal cortex itself.

Acknowledgements

This work was supported by a Programme grant from the Wellcome Trust. We thank our colleagues for their collaborative contributions.

References

Agid, Y., Javoy-Agid, F. and Ruberg, M. (1987). Biochemistry of neurotransmitters in Parkinson's disease. In *Movement Disorders*, Vol. 2 (ed. C.D. Marsden and S. Fahn), pp. 166–230. London: Butterworth.

Albert, M., Feldman, R.G. and Willis, A.L. (1974). The 'subcortical dementia' of progressive supranuclear palsy. *Journal of Neurology, Neurosurgery and Psychiatry*, **37**, 121–30.

Alexander, G.E., De Long, M.R. and Strick, P.L. (1986). Parallel organisation of functionally segregated circuits linking basal ganglia and cortex. *Annual Review of Neuroscience*, **9**, 357–81.

Arnsten, A.F.T., Cai, J.X. and Goldman-Rakic, P.S. (1988). The alpha-2 adrenergic agonist guanfacine improves memory in aged monkeys without sedative or hypotensive side-effects. *Journal of Neuroscience*, **8**, 4287–98.

Baker, S.C., Rogers, R.D., Owen, A.M. *et al.* (1996). The neural substrates of planning: a PET study with the Tower of London. *Neuropsychologia*, **34**, 515–26.

Bamford, K.A., Caine, E.D., Kido, D.K. *et al.* (1989). Clinical-pathological correlation in Huntington's disease: a neuropsychological and computed tomography study. *Neurology*, **39**, 796–801.

Battig, K., Rosvold, H.E. and Mishkin, M. (1960). Comparison of the effects of frontal and caudate lesions on delayed response and alternation in monkeys. *Journal of Comparative and Physiological Psychology*, **53**, 400–4.

Battig, K., Rosvold, H.E. and Mishkin, M. (1962). Comparison of the effects of frontal and caudate lesions on discrimination learning in monkeys. *Journal of Comparative and Physiological Psychology*, **55**, 458–63

Bowen, F.P. (1976). Behavioural alternations in patients with basal ganglia. In *The Basal Ganglia* (ed. M.D. Yahr), pp. 169–77. New York: Raven Press.

Bowen, F.P., Kamienny, M.A., Burns, M.M. and Yahr, M.D. (1975). Parkinsonism: effects of levodopa treatment on concept formation. *Neurology*, **25**, 701–4.

Brandt, J.A. and Bylsma, F.W. (1993). The dementia of Huntington's disease. In *Neuropsychology of Alzheimer's Disease and other Dementias* (ed. R.W. Parks, R.F. Zec and R.S. Wilson), pp. 265–82. New York: Oxford University Press.

Brown, R.G. (1993). Cognitive function in non-demented patients with Parkinson's disease. In *Mental Dysfunction in Parkinson's Disease* (ed. E.C. Wolters and P. Scheltens), pp. 177–94. Amsterdam: Vrije University Press.

Brown, R.G. and Marsden, C.D. (1988*a*). 'Subcortical dementia': the neuropsychological evidence. *Neuroscience*, **25**, 363–87.

Brown, R.G. & Marsen, C.D. (1988*b*). Internal versus external cues and the control of attention in Parkinson's disease. *Brain*, **111**, 323–45.

Brown, R.G. and Marsden, C.D. (1991). Dual task performance and processing resources in normal subjects and patients with Parkinson's disease. *Brain*, **114**, 215–31.

Canavan, A.G.M., Passingham, R.E., Marsden, C.D. *et al.* (1989). The performance on learning tasks of patients in the early stages of Parkinson's disease. *Neuropsychologia*, **27**, 141–56.

Channon, S.E., Jones, M-C. and Stephenson, S. (1993). Cognitive strategies and hypothesis testing during discrimination learning in Parkinson's disease. *Neuropsychologia*, **31**, 75–82.

Cools, A.R., Van Den Bercken, J.H.L., Horstink, M.W.I. *et al.* (1981). The basal ganglia and the programming of behaviour. *Trends in the Neurosciences*, **4**, 124.

Cools, A.R., Van Den Bercken, J.H.L., Horstink, M.W.I. *et al.* (1984). Cognitive and motor shifting aptitude disorder in Parkinson's disease. *Journal of Neurology, Neurosurgery and Psychiatry*, **47**, 443–53.

Cooper, J.A., Sagar, H., Jordan, N. *et al.* (1991). Cognitive impairment in early, untreated Parkinson's disease and its relationship to motor disability. *Brain*, **114**, 2095–122.

Cronin-Golomb, A., Corkin, S. and Growdon, J.H. (1994). Impaired problem solving in Parkinson's disease: impact of a set-shifting deficit. *Neuropsychologia*, **32**, 579–94.

Cummings, J.L. and Benson, D.F. (1984). Subcortical dementia: neuropsychology, neuropsychiatry and pathophysiology. *Archives of Neurology*, **41**, 874–9.

Dias, R., Roberts, A.C. and Robbins, T.W. (1996). Dissociation in prefrontal cortex of affective and attentional shifts. *Nature*, **380**, 69–72.

Divac, I., Rosvold, H.E. and Szwarcbart, M.R. (1967). Behavioral effects of selective ablation of the caudate nucleus. *Journal of Comparative and Physiological Psychology*, **63**, 184–90.

Downes, J.J., Roberts, A.C., Sahakian, B.J. *et al.* (1989). Impaired extra-dimensional shift performance in medicated and unmedicated Parkinson's disease: evidence for a specific attentional dysfunction. *Neuropsychologia*, **27**, 1329–43.

Downes, J.J., Sharp, H.M., Costall, B.M. *et al.* (1993). Alternating fluency in Parkinson's disease. *Brain*, **16**, 887–902.

Dubois, B., Pillon, B., Legault, F. *et al.* (1988). Slowing of cognitive processing in progressive supranuclear palsy: a comparison with Parkinson's disease. *Archives of Neurology*, **45**, 1194–9.

Elliott, R., McKenna, P.J., Robbins, T.W. and Sahakian, B.J. (1995). Neuropsychological evidence for fronto-striatal dysfunction in schizophrenia. *Psychological Medicine*, **25**, 619–30.
Flowers, K.A. and Robertson, C. (1985). The effects of Parkinson's disease on the ability to maintain a mental set. *Journal of Neurology, Neurosurgery and Psychiatry*, **48**, 517–29.
Goldman-Rakic, P.S. (1990). Cellular and circuit basis of working memory in prefrontal cortex of nonhuman primates. In *Progress in Brain Research* (ed. H.B.M. Uyling, C.G. Van Eden, J.P.C. De Bruin, M.A. Corner and M.G.P. Feenstra), vol. 6, pp. 325–36. Amsterdam: Elsevier.
Goldman-Rakic, P.S. (1992). Dopamine-mediated mechanisms of the prefrontal cortex. *Seminars in the Neurosciences*, **4**, 149–59.
Grafman, J., Litvan, I., Gomez, C. and Chase, T.N. (1990). Frontal lobe function in progressive supranulclear palsy. *Archives of Neurology*, **47**, 553–8.
Hassler, R. (1978). Striatal control of locomotion, intentional actions and of integrating and perceptive activity. *Journal of Neurological Science*, **36**, 187–224.
Lange, K.W., Robbins, T.W., Marsden, C.D. *et al.* (1992). L-dopa withdrawal in Parkinson's disease selectively impairs cognitive performance in tests sensitive to frontal lobe dysfunction. *Psychopharmacology*, **107**, 394–404.
Lange, K.W., Sahakian, B.J., Quinn, N.P. *et al.* (1995). Comparison of executive and visuospatial memory function in Huntington's disease and dementia of Alzheimer-type matched for degree of dementia. *Journal of Neurology, Neurosurgery and Psychiatry*, **58**, 598–606.
Lawrence, A.D., Sahakian, B.J., Hodges, J.R. *et al.* (1996). Executive and mnemonic functions in early Huntington's disease. *Brain*, **119**, 1633–45.
Leenders, K.L. (1993). Mental dysfunction in patients with Parkinson's disease. In *Mental Dysfunction in Parkinson's Disease* (ed. E.C. Wolters and P. Scheltens), pp. 133–139. Amsterdam: Vrije University Press.
Lees, A.J. and Smith, E. (1983). Cognitive deficits in the early stages of Parkinson's disease. *Brain*, **106**, 257–70.
Mackintosh, N.J. (1983). *Conditioning and Associative Learning*. Oxford: The Clarendon Press.
Marsden, C.D. (1980). The enigma of the basal ganglia and movement. *Trends in the Neurosciences*, **3**, 284–7.
Marsden, C.D. (1981). Motor activity and the output of the basal ganglia. *Trends in the Neurosciences*, **4**, 124–5.
McHugh, P.R. and Folstein, M.F. (1975). Psychiatric syndromes in Huntington's disease. In *Psychiatric Aspects of Neurological Disease* (ed. D.F. Benson and D. Blumer), pp. 267–85. New York: Grune & Straton.
Milner, B. (1963). Effects of different brain lesions on card sorting: the role of the frontal lobes. *Archives of Neurology*, **9**, 100–10.
Morris, R.G., Downes, J.J., Evenden, J.L. *et al.* (1988). Planning and spatial working memory in Parkinson's disease. *Journal of Neurology, Neurosurgery and Psychiatry*, **51**, 757–66.
Moss, M., Albert, M.S., Butters, N. and Payne, M. (1986). Differential patterns of memory loss among patients with Alzheimer's disease, Huntington's disease and alcoholic Korsakoff syndrome. *Archives of Neurology*, **43**, 239–46.
Oberg, G.E. and Divac, I. (1981). The basal ganglia and the control of movement. *Trends in the Neurosciences*, **4**, 122–4.

Olton, D.S., Becker, J.T. and Handelman, G.E. (1979). Hippocampus, space and memory. *Behavioural and Brain Sciences*, **2**, 315–65.

Owen, A.M., Downes, J.J., Sahakian, B.J. *et al.* (1990). Planning and spatial working memory following frontal lobe lesions in man. *Neuropsychologia*, **28**, 1021–34.

Owen, A.M., Roberts, A.C., Polkey, C.E. *et al.* (1991). Extra-dimensional versus intra-dimensional set shifting performance following frontal lobe excisions, temporal lobe excisions or amygdalo-hippocampectomy in Man. *Neuropsychologia*, **29**, 993–1006.

Owen, A.M., James, M., Leigh, P.N. *et al.* (1992). Fronto-striatal cognitive deficits at different stages of Parkinson's disease. *Brain*, **115**, 1727–51.

Owen, A.M., Roberts, A.C., Hodges, J.R., Robbins, T.W. (1993*b*). Contrasting mechanisms of impaired attentional set-shifting in patients with frontal lobe damage or Parkinson's disease. *Brain*, **116**, 1159–79.

Owen, A.M., Sahakian, B.J., Semple, J. *et al.* (1995*a*). Visuospatial short term recognition memory and learning after temporal lobe excisions, frontal lobe excisions or amygdala-hippocampectomy in man. *Neuropsychologia*, **33**, 1–24.

Owen, A.M., Sahakian, B.J., Hodges, J.R. *et al.* (1995*b*). Dopamine-dependent fronto-striatal planning deficits in early Parkinson's disease. *Neuropsychology*, **9**, 126–40.

Passingham, R.E. (1985). Memory of monkeys (*Macaca mulatta*) with lesions in prefrontal cortex. *Behavioral Neuroscience*, **99**, 3–21.

Pillon, B., Dubois, B., L'Hermitte, F. and Agid, Y. (1986). Heterogeneity of cognitive impairment in progressive supranuclear palsy, Parkinson's disease, and Alzheimer's disease. *Neurology*, **36**, 1179–85.

Quinn, N.P. (1989). Multiple system atrophy – the nature of the beast. *Journal of Neurology, Neurosurgery and Psychiatry*, Special Supplement, 78–89.

Quinn, N.P. (1993). Dementia and Parkinson's disease. In *Mental Dysfunction in Parkinson's Disease* (ed. E.C. Wolters and P. Scheltens), pp. 113–21. Amsterdam: Frije University Press.

Robbins, T.W., James, M., Lange, K.W. *et al.* (1992). Cognitive performance in multiple system atrophy. *Brain*, **115**, 271–91.

Robbins, T.W., James, M., Owen, A.M. *et al.* (1994*a*). Cambridge Neuropsychological Test Automated Battery (CANTAB): a factor analytic study of a large sample of normal elderly volunteers. *Dementia*, **5**, 266–81.

Robbins, T.W., James, M., Owen, A.M. *et al.* (1994*b*). Cognitive deficits in progressive supranuclear palsy. Parkinson's disease and multiple system atrophy in tests sensitive to frontal lobe dysfunction. *Journal of Neurology, Neurosurgery and Psychiatry*, **57**, 79–88.

Robbins, T.W., James, M., Owen, A.M. *et al.* (1997). A neural systems approach to the cognitive psychology of ageing: using the CANTAB battery. In *Methodology of Frontal and Executive Function* (ed. P. Rabbitt). Psychology Press, London

Roberts, A.C. and Sahakian, B.J. (1993). Comparable tests of cognitive function in monkey and man. In *Behavioural Neuroscience; A Practical Approach* (ed. A. Sahgal), pp. 165–84. Oxford: IRL Press.

Roberts, A.C., Robbins, T.W. and Everitt, B.J. (1988). The effects of intra-dimensional and extra-dimensional shifts on visual discrimination learning in humans and non-human primates. *Quarterly Journal of Experimental Psychology*, **40B**, 321–41.

Roberts, A.C., De Salvia, M.A., Wilkinson, L.S. *et al.* (1994). 6-Hydroxydopamine lesions of the prefrontal cortex in monkeys enhance performance on an analogue of the Wisconsin Card Sorting test: possible interactions with subcortical dopamine. *Journal of Neuroscience*, **14**, 2531–44.

Roberts, A.C., Collins, P. and Robbins, T.W. (1997). The functions of the prefrontal cortex in humans and other animals. In *Modelling the Early Human Mind* (ed. P. Mellars and K. Gibson) Cambridge: McDonald Institute for Archaeological Research.

Sagar, H.J., Sullivan, E.V., Gabrieli, J.D.E. *et al.* (1988). Temporal ordering and short-term memory deficts in Parkinson's disease. *Brain*, **111**, 525–39.

Sahakian, B.J., Downes, J.J., Eagger, S. *et al.* (1990). Sparing of attentional relative to mnemonic function in a subgroup of patients with dementia of the Alzheimer type. *Neuropsychologia*, **28**, 1197–213.

Sahakian, B.J. and Owen, A.M. (1992). Computerised assessment in neuropsychiatry using CANTAB. *Journal of the Royal Society of Medicine*, **85**, 399–402.

Saint-Cyr, J.A., Taylor, A.E. and Lang, A.E. (1988). Procedural learning and neostriatal dysfunction in man. *Brain*, **111**, 941–59.

Schneider, J.S. and Kovelowski, C.J. (1990). Chronic exposure to low doses of MPTP: I Cognitive deficits in motor asymptomatic monkeys. *Brain Research*, **519**, 122–8.

Shallice, T. (1982). Specific impairments in planning. In *The Neuropsychology of Cognitive Function* (ed. D.E. Broadbent and L. Weiskrantz), pp. 199–209. London: The Royal Society.

Starkstein, S.E., Brandt, J., Bylsma, F. *et al.* (1992). Neuropsychological correlates of brain atrophy in Huntington's disease: a magnetic resonance imaging study. *Neuroradiology*, **34**, 487–9.

Talland, G.A. (1962). Cognitive functions in Parkinson's disease. *Journal of Nervous and Mental Disease*, **135**, 196–205.

Taylor, A.E., Saint-Cyr, J.A. and Lang, A.E. (1986). Frontal lobe dysfunction in Parkinson's disease. *Brain*, **109**, 845–83.

Taylor, A.E., Saint-Cyr, J.A. and Lang, A.E. (1990). Memory and learning in early Parkinson's disease: evidence for a 'frontal lobe syndrome'. *Brain and Cognition*, **13**, 211–32.

Wallesch, C-W., Karnath, H.O. and Zimmerman, P. (1992). Is there a frontal lobe dysfunction in Parkinson's disease? A comparison of the effects of Parkinson's disease and circumscribed frontal lobe lesions in a maze learning task. In *Subcortical Disorders Associated With Subcortical Lesions* (ed. G. Vallar, S.F. Cappa and C.-W. Wallesch), pp. 227–41. Oxford: Oxford University Press.

Weingartner, H., Burns, S. and Lewitt, P.A. (1984). Cognitive impairment in Parkinson's disease: distinguishing between effort demanding and automatic cognitive processes. *Psychiatry Research*, **11**, 223–35.

4

The behavioural pharmacology of brain dopamine systems: implications for the cognitive pharmacotherapy of schizophrenia

EILEEN JOYCE & SAM HUTTON

Introduction

Traditionally, the aim of pharmacotherapy in the treatment of neuropsychiatric disorders has been to alleviate any associated movement disorder or emotional manifestation such as depression, anxiety and psychosis. The recognition that cognitive dysfunction in these disorders may also have a specific neurochemical basis ameniable to pharmacotherapy is a relatively recent concept (Stahl, Iversen and Goodman, 1987). To date, the most concerted effort in addressing this possibility has been in the treatment of Alzheimer's disease with compounds thought to enhance acetylcholine neurotransmission. The rationale for the cholinergic hypothesis of dementia was based on two sets of observations. First, a reduction in markers of acetylcholine synthesis was found in the cortex of patients with Alzheimer's disease, which correlated with the severity of the dementia (Davies and Maloney, 1976; Perry *et al.*, 1977, 1978). Second, manipulations of cholinergic systems in animal models and human volunteer studies were found to affect cognitive function (see Hagan and Morris, 1988 and Sahakian, 1988 for reviews). Despite a promising hypothesis, the studies that have investigated the potential of cholinergic enhancement in Alzheimer's disease have been largely disappointing. This is because they have either failed to demonstrate improvement or have shown only modest improvement on a few neuropsychological tests without any demonstrable changes in the performance of activities of daily living (Eagger and Harvey, 1995; Marin *et al.*, 1995). In retrospect, a major reason why this strategy failed is because Alzheimer's disease is a rapidly advancing neurodegenerative disease that progressively destroys cortical and subcortical areas taking many neurotransmitter systems and their target sites in its wake. Therefore, an ideal neuropsychiatric disorder with which to explore the potential of treating cognitive dysfunction should be relatively stable and the abnormality should lie primarily in one neurotransmitter system. Candidate disorders include Parkinson's and Huntington's disease but these are problematic in that they are progressive, although not as rapidly as Alzheimer's disease, and the cognitive dysfunction is usually less significant than the movement disorder.

Although schizophrenia has not been considered a primarily cognitive disorder, there are compelling reasons why this should be so. First, for many years cognitive psychologists have viewed schizophrenic symptoms as a reflection of cognitive dysfunction (e.g. Broen and Storms, 1967). Second, most recent neuropsychological studies of first episode schizophrenia have shown impairment at the beginning of the illness before such factors as institutionalisation or medication effects could have taken hold (e.g. Bilder *et al.*, 1992; Hoff, Riordan *et al.*, 1992; Heaton *et al.*, 1994; Saykin *et al.*, 1994; Holm *et al.*, 1995). Third, neuroimaging and post-mortem research has convincingly demonstrated that schizophrenia involves an abnormality of association cortex (see below for references). However, the fact that the psychotic phenomena can be effectively treated with drugs that specifically inhibit dopamine receptors (Creese, Burt and Snyder, 1976; Seeman *et al.*, 1976) argues for a fundamental role of dopamine in the manifestation of this illness. Indeed this latter observation, together with the finding that long-term ingestion of amphetamine, an indirect dopamine agonist, can mimic the symptoms of schizophrenia (Conell, 1958), led to the dopamine hypothesis of schizophrenia, which postulates that dopaminergic overactivity is the neurobiological basis of the illness (Iversen, 1978). For these reasons, this article will examine whether dopamine has any role to play in the mediation of cognitive dysfunction in schizophrenia and whether schizophrenia is therefore a suitable model for cognitive pharmacotherapy.

Schizophrenia as a model for cognitive pharmacotherapy

There are two problems with the dopamine hypothesis of schizophrenia that make it untenable in its original form. The first reflects the general failure to appreciate both the range of symptoms constituting schizophrenia and the fact that some symptoms are not specific to this illness. For example, the so-called positive symptoms of schizophrenia, hallucinations and delusions, are also seen in other psychiatric disorders such as manic-depressive illness, alcoholic hallucinosis, temporal lobe epilepsy and neurodegenerative disorders. These symptoms are often responsive to dopamine receptor blocking drugs in whatever context they arise. However, the negative symptoms of schizophrenia, such as lack of affect and volition and poverty of movement and thought, tend not to be seen in other psychotic conditions and are not alleviated by conventional antipsychotic drugs. Furthermore, it is the presence of this negative syndrome that has been linked with the presence of cognitive dysfunction and together, these facets of schizophrenia predict a chronic course of illness for which dopamine appears to have no role to play (Crow, 1980). Thus a comprehensive dopamine hypothesis of schizophrenia needs to demonstrate a fundamental role for dopamine in the generation of negative symptoms and cognitive disturbance as well as positive symptoms, otherwise it is only an hypothesis of acute psychosis.

The second problem with the dopamine hypothesis arises because of the lack of consistent evidence to support the view that dopamine function is fundamentally abnormal in patients with schizophrenia. Post-mortem studies measuring tissue concentrations of dopamine and its metabolites or dopamine receptor density have often rendered positive results but the known effect of antipsychotic drugs in inducing increased dopamine turnover and receptor supersensitivity cannot be ruled out as the sole explanation of these data (e.g. Lee *et al.*, 1978; Owen *et al.*, 1978; Bird, Spokes and Iversen, 1979; Crow *et al.*, 1981; Mackay *et al.*, 1982; Reynolds, 1983 and see Kleinman and Nawroz, 1994 for a review). In order to overcome this problem, several studies have used *in vivo* functional imaging techniques, positron emission tomography (PET) or single photon emission tomography (SPET), in antipsychotic drug-naive schizophrenic patients. The initial study by Wong and colleagues (1986), using PET, showed that treatment-naive schizophrenic patients had increased D2 receptor densities in basal ganglia. However Farde and colleagues were unable to repeat this finding using a different kinetic model and tracer (Farde *et al.*, 1987). All subsequent studies have also been non-confirmatory (Martinot *et al.*, 1990; Hietala *et al.*, 1994; Pilowsky *et al.*, 1994). It is possible that extrastriatal dopamine is dysfunctional in schizophrenia and recent attempts at revisiting the dopamine hypothesis have focused on dopamine activity in neocortical and limbic areas (Jaskiw and Weinberger, 1992). However there is as yet no direct evidence from man concerning this because of the difficulty in measuring dopaminergic activity in these less densely innervated areas.

The realisation that cognitive deficits are a major feature of schizophrenia and the lack of evidence to support the dopamine hypothesis instigated a shift in research emphasis away from subcortical dopamine areas to the cortex as the potential site of abnormality. Many studies have now confirmed structural and functional cortical abnormalities, particularly in frontal and temporal areas. Cortical shrinkage and ventricular enlargement have consistently been demonstrated with computed tomography in groups of schizophrenic patients (e.g. Johnstone *et al.*, 1976; Nasrallah *et al.*, 1982 and see Lewis, 1990 for a review) and more detailed magnetic resonance imaging studies have shown both general and focal neuroanatomical abnormalities in cortical areas (e.g. Andreason *et al.*, 1986; DeLisi *et al.*, 1988; Nasrallah *et al.*, 1990; Harvey *et al.*, 1991 and see Chua and McKenna, 1995 for a review). Functional imaging techniques such as positron emission tomography and single photon emission tomography have revealed metabolic abnormalities in frontal and temporal cortices that have been related both to positive and negative schizophrenic symptoms and to cognitive abnormalities (e.g. Buchsbaum *et al.*, 1984; Weinberger *et al.*, 1986; Liddle *et al.*, 1992 and see Joyce, 1992 for a review). Finally, using a variety of neuroanatomical, neurochemical and molecular-genetic techniques, post-mortem studies of schizophrenia have also revealed abnormalities in frontal and temporal cortex. These include both abnormalities of neurotransmitter systems and cytoarchitectural changes (e.g. Kovelman and Scheibel, 1984; Jakob and Beckman, 1986; Hanada *et al.*, 1987; Deakin *et al.*, 1989; Nakai *et al.*, 1991; Benes *et al.*, 1992; Simpson *et al.*, 1992; Akbarian *et al.*, 1993*a*,*b*, 1995).

The lack of evidence concerning an aetiological role for dopamine and the presence of structural abnormalities within cortex must cast doubt both on dopamine as an aetiological variable and the possibility of being able to correct the fundamental schizophrenic abnormality by manipulating dopaminergic activity. However, recent findings concerning the neurobiology and behavioural pharmacology of dopamine systems have caused a resurgence of interest in this neurotransmitter with regard to schizophrenia. For example, evidence suggests that dopamine can modulate cortical processing either directly or via its output at the level of the striatum and that this may affect the type of behaviour that has been shown to be abnormal in schizophrenia. Other studies have shown that there are many more dopamine receptors than originally thought and that these have distinct pharmacological properties and neuroanatomical distributions, thus offering many more abnormal mechanistic possibilities for the mediation of schizophrenia symptoms. Further, studies of the atypical antipsychotic agent clozapine have shown that this drug is not only more effective in alleviating positive symptoms but, apparently, can also improve negative symptoms. Since negative symptoms have been linked to cognitive dysfunction in schizophrenia, it is also possible that this drug may improve cognitive function in this disorder. It is therefore perhaps timely to review these advances and to consider whether pharmacological manipulations of brain dopamine systems have any role to play in treating the manifest cortical abnormalities underlying schizophrenia.

Neuroanatomy of cortico-striatal systems

Much emphasis is currently being placed on the parallel organisation of functionally segregated circuits linking basal ganglia and cortex (Alexander, DeLong and Strick, 1986) because of its power in explaining the symptoms of neurodegenerative diseases such as Parkinson's disease, Huntington's disease and progressive supranuclear palsy. Although extrapyramidal movement disorder is the predominant manifestation of these disorders, reflecting the fact that the basal ganglia are the major site of neuropathology, all three syndromes can also be associated with cognitive dysfunction and psychiatric symptoms. Moreover, the associated cognitive disturbance resembles that seen in patients with frontal lobe lesions despite there being no prominent neuropathology within this area. This observation led to the concept of 'fronto-subcortical dementia' (Albert, 1978) to denote the similarity in expression of basal ganglia disorders and frontal lobe impairment with respect to cognitive dysfunction. Fronto-subcortical dementia can be explained because of the existence of essentially non-overlapping projections from functionally related areas of frontal cortex to discrete areas of striatum as the first step in the output of higher order cortical computations that ultimately result in purposive behaviour and thought. Individual projections are thought to subserve motor, oculomotor, cognitive and motivational/emotive functions. In turn, striatal areas project to segregated areas of the pallidal/substantia nigra pars reticulata complex and thence to segregated areas of thalamus. A partial circuit is then formed by a back projection from thalamus to one of the frontal areas of origin. According to this scheme, basal ganglia pathology, by cutting across and disrupting the normal function of these circuits, can produce various degrees of motor, cognitive and psychological disturbance depending on the severity and distribution of the lesion.

The bearing that this understanding has on schizophrenia is threefold. First, early in the course of Parkinson's disease, when most of the manifestations almost certainly reflect forebrain dopamine depletion, frontal lobe-like cognitive impairments are evident (e.g. Lees and Smith, 1983; Taylor, Saint-Cyr and Lang, 1986; Brown and Marsden, 1988; Owen *et al.*, 1992, 1995). This suggests that manipulation of dopaminergic systems can have a profound influence on cognitive function mediated by frontal cortex in man. Second, there is a body of evidence to suggest that the cognitive dysfunction in schizophrenia is specifically 'frontal' in nature (Shallice, Burgess and Frith 1991; Morrison-Stewart *et al.*, 1992; Elliott *et al.*, 1995) although it should be noted that there is also evidence supporting other specific forms of deficit (McKenna *et al.*, 1990; Saykin *et al.*, 1991; Gold *et al.*, 1992). Third, as well as cognitive dysfunction, there is evidence to suggest that oculomotor and extrapyramidal motor dysfunction is fundamental to the schizophrenic process and is not simply a side-effect of medication (Owens, Johnstone and Frith, 1982; Caligiuri, Lohr and Jeste, 1993; Crawford *et al.*, 1994). Thus schizophrenia can also be viewed in terms of a disruption of the normal processing of frontostriatal circuits (Robbins, 1990; Pantelis, Barnes and Nelson, 1992) perhaps secondary to pathology within the cortex rather than basal ganglia. It remains now to examine whether dopamine can influence the processing within this circuitry.

Functional anatomy of forebrain dopamine systems

The cell bodies of the ascending dopaminergic systems are situated in the ventral mesencephalon and form a mass centred on the substantia nigra pars compacta (A9 group) with a medial extension into the ventral tegmental area of Tsai (A10 group) and a caudal extension into the ventrolateral tegmentum (A8 group) (Dahlstrom and Fuxe, 1965; Ungerstedt, 1971; Lindvall and Bjorklund, 1974, 1978).

The major projection of these cells is to the striatum (caudate-putamen) and this can be separated into two divisions based on neuroanatomical distinctions between the circuitry of the dorsal and ventral aspects of this structure (Heimer and Wilson, 1975). The laterally situated cell bodies (primarily A9) project to dorsal striatum forming the nigrostriatal pathway (Ungerstedt, 1971) also known as the mesostriatal pathway (Lindvall and Bjorklund, 1978). More medial neurones (primarily A10) project to ventral striatum, which now conventionally includes the nucleus accumbens and parts of the olfactory tubercle in addition to the ventral aspect of the striatum proper. This projection forms part of the mesolimbic system (Ungerstedt, 1971).

One distinction between the dorsal and ventral striatum is with respect to their afferent anatomical affiliations (Heimer and Wilson, 1975). Whereas dorsal striatum receives inputs from neocortex, the ventral striatum receives inputs from limbic structures including the amygdala and limbic cortex of the frontal and temporal lobe (hippocampus, anterior cingulate and entorhinal cortex). On this basis, it appears that dorsal striatal dopaminergic afferents are poised to interact with output neuronal systems involved in sensorimotor and cognitive processing whereas ventral striatal dopamine is positioned to influence motivational processing.

An examination of the synaptic arrangement of dopamine terminals appears to confirm this speculation. Most dopaminergic cell bodies project to the matrix of the striatum as opposed to striatal patches (Gerfen *et al.*, 1987) and within the nucleus accumbens, which does not have the patch/matrix organisation, dopamine cells tend to project to the shell rather than the core compartment (Herkenham, Moon Edley and Stuart, 1984; Voorn *et al.*, 1986). In these terminal areas, dopamine neurones synapse with the dendritic shafts or spines of medium-size spiny neurones (Freund, Powell and Smith, 1984), which are the main output cells of the striatum (Kemp and Powell, 1971; Wilson and Groves, 1980). In close proximity to the dopamine synapse is an excitatory synapse derived from neocortex in dorsal striatum and hippocampus in ventral striatum (Bouyer *et al.*, 1984 and see Groenewegen *et al.*, 1991 for a review). Thus synaptic triads are formed consisting of a target dendritic element, an inhibitory dopaminergic terminal and an excitatory, probably glutaminergic, terminal. According to this arrangement, dopamine release is able to exert a modulatory influence on the excitatory drive from neocortical and limbic cortex to striatal output neurones (Kitai *et al.*, 1976).

In addition to this major subcortical projection from mesencephalon to striatum, there are dopamine projections to limbic structures and cortex. Medially situated (mainly A10) cell bodies project to the limbic nuclei, amygdala and septum and form part of the mesolimbic system (Ungerstedt, 1971; Lindvall and Bjorklund, 1978). This cell body area also projects to cortex including, in the rat, prefrontal, anterior cingulate, entorhinal, insular and piriform cortices, thus forming the mesocortical projection (Lindvall and Bjorklund, 1978). Work on human and non-human primates has shown that the cortical dopaminergic innervation is more extensive in these species and additionally includes a dense innervation of the motor, premotor and supplementary motor areas and a light innervation of parietal, temporal and posterior cingulate cortex (Berger, Gaspar and Verney, 1991). The highest density of dopamine innervation appears to be in the anterior cingulate and motor cortex, with ever decreasing density in anterior and posterior directions (Berger *et al.*, 1991).

The synaptic arrangement in cortex appears to be similar to that of striatum (Groenewegen *et al.*, 1991; Goldman-Rakic, 1992). Here, about 60% of dopamine terminals synapse with the dendritic spines of pyramidal cells along with a presumed excitatory synapse, thus forming synaptic triads

(Goldman-Rakic *et al.*, 1989). The cortical pyramidal cells, upon which mesocortical dopamine terminals abut, have different projection sites depending on which layer of cortex they occupy. For example, the main axons of some pyramidal cells of layers 2, 3 and 5 of prefrontal cortex project either to striatal matrix (Gerfen, 1989) or to other cortical regions (Melchitzky *et al.*, 1994). Furthermore, these axons, particularly those of pyramidal cells in layer 3, send collaterals to synapse with the dendrites of more local cortical pyramidal cells (Melchitzky *et al.*, 1994 and see Lewis and Anderson, 1995 for a review). Thus dopamine release in cortex can modulate excitatory activity both within frontal cortex occuring in reverberating circuits, and in output pathways to striatum and other cortical areas.

From these anatomical connections it can be seen that dopamine is in a position to modulate the computational processes occurring within motor, prefrontal and limbic cortex both within the areas of origin of activity and at the level of the striatum where further integration of information takes place.

Multiple dopamine receptors

The original pharmacological classification of dopamine receptors was into D1 and D2 types (Kebabian and Calne, 1979). This was based on the fact that occupation of the D1 receptor by an agonist activates the intracellular adenylate cyclase second messanger system whereas this is inhibited by D2 occupancy. Furthermore, D2 but not D1 receptors were found to be present on dopamine terminals as autoreceptors, which when stimulated cause inhibition of the synthesis and release of dopamine. The clinical importance of being able to differentiate these two receptors became evident when the antipsychotic potency of neuroleptics was shown to correlate strongly with D2 receptor blocking potency (Creese *et al.*, 1976; Seeman *et al.*, 1976).

D1 and D2 receptors are present in all areas innervated by dopamine neurones but are most abundant in dorsal and ventral striatum (Bouthenet *et al.*, 1987; Dawson *et al.*, 1988 and see Sibley and Monsma, 1992 for a review). However the majority of D1 and D2 receptors appear to be present on different populations of striatal neurones (Gerfen *et al.*, 1990). As described above, striatal efferents project to the pallidal/sustantia nigra pars reticulata complex forming part of the cortico–striatal–pallido–thalamic circuitry. There are two routes for this: a direct pathway from cell bodies that express D1 receptors and a polysynaptic pathway from cell bodies that express D2 receptors. Activity in these pathways produces opposite effects at their terminal site, the indirect pathway being ultimately excitatory and the direct pathway being inhibitory. Experiments involving lesions of the ascending dopamine pathways followed by receptor stimulation with specific D1 or D2 agonists have shown that D2 receptor activation causes a decrease in the excitatory output of the indirect pathway whereas stimulation of the D1 receptor cause enhanced activity in the direct inhibitory pathway (Gerfen *et al.*, 1990). Thus dopamine release in striatum can act to decrease the effect of cortical output as it passes through striatum by the dual action of increasing activity in the inhibitory striatal output pathway and decreasing activity in the excitatory output pathway. This ultimately leads to enhanced brainstem outflow and behaviour and enhanced thalamic drive back to cortex. These studies therefore demonstrate that dopamine activity can amplify the output of the cortex at the level of the striatum and that the balance between D1 and D2 receptor activity is of significance to the net behavioural result. Thus the ability to manipulate these receptors independently might have important implications for the pharmacotherapy of neuropsychiatric disorders.

The chances of this being a real possibility have increased since the advent of molecular cloning techniques, which have located the genes and protein sequences for both the D1 and D2 receptors and have consequently led to a greater characterisation of these receptors. Furthermore, other receptors have been identified which are similar, but not identical, to D1 or D2 receptors with respect to their protein sequences. Thus there are two 'families' of dopamine receptors namely the D1-like consisting of D1 and D5 subtypes and the D2-like comprising D2, D3 and D4 subtypes. An important point about these multiple dopamine receptors is that they are pharmacologically distinct and have different neuroanatomical distributions (Schwartz *et al.*, 1992; Sibley and Monsma, 1992; Seeman and Van Tol, 1994) and it is these observations that have revitalised the interest in the putative role of dopamine in schizophrenia.

Because, traditionally, the striatal D2 receptor has been linked to schizophrenia, most studies have focused on the D2-like receptors, D3 and D4, as candidates for mediating psychotic symptoms. For example, the D3 receptor is expressed predominantly in the ventral striatum and hypothalamus (Sokoloff *et al.*, 1992) and antipsychotic drugs that are potent D2 blockers tend also to be potent inhibitors of the D3 receptor (Seeman and Van Tol, 1994). The implication of this finding is significant because it is possible that abnormal D3 mechanisms may be involved in the psychotic response. Thus drugs that specifically manipulate D3 receptors may result in antipsychotic potency without eliciting the debilitating extrapyramidal side-effects thought to be mediated by D2 receptor antagonism in dorsal striatum. A promising link between the D3 receptor and schizophrenia has been found by examining the relationship between populations of schizophrenic patients and the polymorphism that occurs due to a substitution of glycine for serine at amino acid position 9 in some alleles (Ser-9-Gly polymorphism). An initial study of this phenomenon showed an excess of homozygotes for the Gly-9 allele in schizophrenic patients compared to normal controls (Crocq *et al.*, 1992). However many other studies have since failed to replicate this finding but have found other interesting associations between the D3 receptor and schizophrenia (see Shaikh *et al.*, 1996 for a review). Shaikh and colleagues have gone on to clarify this relationship. They have shown, in a group of treatment-resistant schizophrenic patients taking clozapine, that the allele Ser-9 is significantly more common in patients than controls, especially in those patients who are unresponsive to clozapine. Furthermore, in a meta-analysis of all published data in this area, they found a modest association between homozygosity for Ser-9 and schizophrenia. They suggest that either the presence of the Ser-9 allele itself, or a nearby locus in linkage disequilibrium with Ser-9, increases the risk of developing schizophrenia (Shaikh *et al.*, 1996). An alternative possibility is that the presence of this allele may confer some property that makes a schizophrenic illness more difficult to treat.

The D4 receptor (Van Tol, 1991) is also of interest for the pathogenesis of schizophrenia. Highest D4 receptor expression occurs in cortex, hippocampus, amygdala and nucleus accumbens with little in dorsal striatum (Van Tol, 1991; Meadow-Woodruff *et al.*, 1994). This also makes it an ideal candidate for the mediation of psychotic symptoms. Unfortunately population genetic studies have not shown any association between schizophrenia and the D4 receptor by either linkage analysis or allelic association studies (see Kerwin and Collier, 1996 for a review). However a major difficulty with this type of study is that the coding region of the D4 gene is highly variable giving rise to many different D4 receptor proteins (see Seeman and Van Tol, 1994) and one study has shown that only when all of the D4 polymorphisms are taken into account, can an association with schizophrenia be demonstrated and this was only with respect to response to medication (Kennedy *et al.*, 1994).

Post-mortem studies, on the other hand, have implicated the D4 receptor in schizophrenia. Seeman and colleagues (Seeman, Guan and Van Tol, 1993), using tissue homogenate binding, demonstrated that D4 receptors were elevated in post-mortem schizophrenic striatal tissue. However this is a contentious and complex issue because there is no specific ligand for the D4 receptor as yet. Accordingly, in groups of schizophrenic patients and controls (normals, Alzheimer and Huntington patients), they examined the binding of tritiated ritanserin, which binds to D2 and D3 receptors, and subtracted this measure from binding obtained to tritiated emanopride, which has been shown to bind to D2, D3 and D4 receptors. They found a six-fold elevation of D4 receptor binding in striatal tissue compared to only a 10% elevation of combined D2 and D3 receptors. They argue that this is not a medication effect since there was no evidence of such large increases of D4 binding in patients with Alzheimer's and Huntington's diseases who had received moderate doses of neuroleptics prior to death and since chronic haloperidol administration in rats produces only a 2% elevation of striatal D4 receptors. Murray and colleagues, using quantitiative receptor autoradiography, have replicated this finding and extended the observation to include the nucleus accumbens. They found a more modest two-fold increase in striatal D4 receptors (Murray *et al.*, 1995). This was found when compared to normal controls and non-schizophrenic suicides. However, when compared to a non-schizophrenic group that had been taking anti-psychotic drugs for various reasons prior to death (e.g. affective disorder, dementia) the difference in D4 binding failed to reach statistical significance. Thus an elevating effect of neuroleptic drugs on D4 receptor density cannot be strictly ruled out. Further, as pointed out by Kerwin and Collier (1996), 'estimating very low abundance receptors by extracting two estimates of very high abundance receptors is clearly prey to artifact'. Interestingly these findings demonstrated elevated D4 receptors in striatum where this receptor is not thought to be abundant. Whether this is true in other more abundant areas remains to be seen.

Dopamine, behaviour and psychological models of schizophrenia

The role of dopamine in mediating behaviour and cognition is the subject of numerous studies (e.g. Goldman-Rakic, 1992; Koob, 1992; Robbins and Everitt, 1992; Schultz, 1992). Dopamine neurones appear to fire in response to 'salient environmental stimuli which attract the attention of the subject . . . and therefore signal the presence of important stimuli that need to be processed by the subject with high priority without specifying details of the stimulus' (Schultz, 1992). Stress can also increase dopamine neurotransmission (Blanc *et al.*, 1980; Roth *et al.*, 1988) and the exact nature of this depends, in turn, on the nature of the stressor and whether it is transient or chronic (see Robbins and Everitt, 1992 for a discussion). In particular, dopamine release in striatum appears to increase the speed of responding to relevant stimuli by modulating cortical output rather than affecting the precise nature of the response (Robbins and Everitt, 1992). For these reasons dopaminergic mechanisms are important in mediating cognitive behaviour and several of the paradigms employed to measure this have particular relevance for schizophrenia. This is because they suggest that in man, abnormalities of the particular processes subserved by dopaminergic systems might give rise not only to cognitive dysfunction but also to psychotic experiences.

Animal models of striatal dopamine dysfunction

There are several models derived from learning theory that are considered relevant to schizophrenia. Although these are procedurally different, they have in common the fact that the index measure of behaviour – the strength of a certain response – can be modified by a preceding condition so that a subsequent test stimulus fails to fully capture the response. Thus, in these paradigms, *normal* performance in the experimental condition is reflected by a reduction in behaviour compared to that produced by the control condition. The fact that abnormal performance in these paradigms is measured by a failure to inhibit behaviour is important for the interpretation of the performance of schizophrenic patients – if the schizophrenic patient's behavioural output is greater than that of controls, their performance cannot be attributed to poor motivation or nonspecific cognitive dysfunction – a criticism so often levied against neuropsychological studies of schizophrenia.

Blocking

In the blocking paradigm (Kamin, 1968) an animal first learns to associate a simple stimulus (A) with a reinforcer. Next, a compound stimulus is introduced so that the original stimulus plus a new stimulus (AB) is paired with the reinforcer. In the test phase, the strength of conditioning to A and B individually is examined in the absence of the reinforcer. Animals preexposed to A show decreased conditioning to B whereas control animals, which have only been exposed to AB, show a conditioned response to both A and B. Thus normal subjects fail to associate B with reinforcement because B provided no new information about reinforcement during learning (Kamin, 1969; Mackintosh, 1975). Induction of dopamine receptor supersensitivity or chronic amphetamine administration disrupt blocking in animals (Crider, Solomon and McMahon, 1982; Crider, Blocker and Solomon, 1986) and the amphetamine effect can be prevented with simultaneous administration of haloperidol (Crider *et al.*, 1982). Thus dopaminergic systems appear to be involved in this behaviour in that increased dopamine activity causes the animal to fail to ignore an irrelevant aspect of a stimulus. This observation has led to the hypothesis that increased dopamine transmission causes a failure of selective attention, i.e. a failure to ignore irrelevant stimuli, which results in the type of distractability witnessed in schizophrenia (Crider, 1979).

There have been only two studies examining blocking in schizophrenic patients. One found that patients in the acute stages of the disorder exhibited disrupted blocking whereas chronic schizophrenic patients were normal (Jones, Gray and Hemsley, 1992). The second found that blocking was disrupted in non-paranoid psychotic patients but normal in paranoid patients (Oades, Bunk and Eggers, 1992). Therefore, on the basis of these studies, it appears that disrupted blocking is not a general feature of schizophrenia although the paucity of data requires more studies before dismissing this as a model.

Latent inhibition

The paradigm of latent inhibition (LI) is related to blocking in the sense that the normal subject learns to ignore an apparently irrelevant stimulus. Specifically, an animal is exposed to a stimulus that is initially without any consequential reinforcement. The same stimulus is then paired with a reinforcer and the rate of learning the new association is found to be slower in comparison to control animals that have not been pre-exposed to the reinforced stimulus (Lubow, 1973). There are several conditions that need to be satisfied before LI can be demonstrated (Lubow and Gewirtz, 1995) the most important being that the context of the experiment, i.e. the environmental conditions, must be the same during both the pre-exposure and conditioning phases.

The possible link between LI and schizophrenia came about with the observation that amphetamine abolishes LI and that this can be prevented by the concomitant administration of an antipsychotic drug (Solomon *et al.*, 1981; Weiner *et al.*, 1981; Weiner, Lubow and Feldon, 1984). Thus, pre-exposed animals under amphetamine behave during the conditioning phase as if the familiar stimulus were novel. Latent inhibition has been demonstrated in man (Lubow, 1989) and amphetamine is able to disrupt this effect (Gray *et al.*, 1992). In patients with schizophrenia, LI has been shown to be normal in patients who are in the chronic stages of the illness but disrupted in patients tested during the first two weeks of a psychotic episode (Baruch, Hemsley and Gray, 1988*a*; Gray *et al.*, 1992).

There are several existing hypotheses that relate abnormal LI in schizophrenia to a failure of attentional processes. One theory, proposed by Lubow (Lubow and Gewirtz, 1995), is summarised as follows. During preexposure, implicit learning takes place in which the stimulus receives low-level, automatic (i.e. non-resource demanding) attentional processing sufficient to establish a stimulus–no consequence association. This then weakens the associability of the stimulus-reinforcer during the conditioning phase. This weakening occurs because, unlike novel stimuli, the familiar stimulus is not captured by controlled (i.e. effortful, resource demanding) attentional processes that serve to bring the stimulus into working memory and ensure active encoding or learning. The mechanism that prevents the stimulus being treated as novel during the conditioning phase is thought to be provided by the context serving as a cue. Thus, if the individual is in the same context in the conditioning phase as in the preexposure phase, the context itself acts as a cue for the retrieval of the stimulus–no consequence association, which allows continued processing of the stimulus in the automatic mode. It is argued that the utility of this type of learning is to ensure that short-term memory is not flooded with stimuli that are thus experienced as novel but in fact are familiar. Lubow proposes that schizophrenic patients fail to benefit from context as a retrieval cue and therefore short-term memory becomes filled with irrelevant but preoccupying material, which leads to the development of positive symptoms.

Hemsley (1994*a*,*b*) and Gray (Gray *et al.*, 1991; Gray, 1995), in their joint hypothesis, also utilise impaired LI as a demonstration of the type of cognitive failure underpinning positive symptoms but are more specific about the neuroanatomical site of abnormality and the mechanism by which psychotic symptoms are generated.

Hemsley borrows from various cognitive models of normal perception to suggest that the normal influence of past associations or 'regularities' on current sensory input is weakened in schizophrenia. Specifically, he proposes that it is the 'rapid and automatic assessment of the significance of aspects of sensory input (and their implications for action) that is impaired as a result of the weakening of the influence of past associations' (Hemsley, 1994*a*). The failure of past associations to cause an inhibition of irrelevant stimuli causes attention to be captured by them, thereby becoming conscious, and a search for causation to be instigated. This is the basis of delusion formation (Hemsley, 1994*a*). This mechanism, he suggests, also causes a failure to prevent material from long-term memory reaching consciousness, which is then interpreted as hallucinatory (Hemsley, 1994*b*). The parallel between this model, derived from human cognitive psychology, and that of Lubow, derived from animal learning theory, can be seen especially as Hemsley also evokes context as responsible for eliciting stored regularities (Hemsley, 1994*b*). Indeed Hemsley goes on to argue that abnormal LI in schizophrenia supports his cognitive hypothesis because the LI paradigm requires that previously formed associations influence the formation of new associations (Hemsley, 1994*a*,*b*).

Gray elaborated this relationship between LI and schizophrenia by providing a neuroanatomical and neurochemical basis. This centres around his general theory of hippocampal function (Gray, 1982). Here, the limbic forebrain, in particular the hippocampal formation, is thought to perform the role of a comparator, which monitors the outcome of motor programmes executed by the basal ganglia and compares this with the predicted outcome. A declaration of 'match' or 'mismatch' is made by a signal from the hippocampus to the ventral striatum. A mismatch signal causes interruption of the current motor programme in order to give the novel event conscious attention and processing (note the similarity between this and Lubow's account, especially as there is evidence to suggest that the hippocampus encodes context). Gray argued that the neurochemical event caused by a mismatch signal is dopamine release in ventral striatum.

Gray (1995) next postulated that disruption of LI is due to dopamine release in the ventral striatum, on the basis of two experimental observations. First, destruction of dopamine terminals in this area enhances LI in animal models. Second, microdialysis studies in the freely moving rat have shown that pre-exposure to a stimulus attentuates the normal potentiation of dopamine release in the ventral striatum witnessed during the conditioning phase in control animals (Young, Joseph and Gray, 1993). In other words, dopamine release in ventral striatum appears to signal novelty or salience. Since LI is also abolished by lesions of the hippocampus (Weiner, 1990) and this effect is reversed by dopamine receptor blocking drugs (Yee, Feldon and Rawlins, 1995), Gray concluded that hippocampal damage gives rise to a functional state of increased dopamine release in ventral striatum, which disrupts latent inhibition.

For Gray and Hemsley, the phenomenon of latent inhibition and its disruption in schizophrenia adds credence to their more general hypothesis of cognitive dysfunction and schizophrenic symptomology. However, there are several problems with the rleationship between LI and schizophrenia, some of which have been pointed out by Gray himself (1995). First, as explained above, latent inhibition is disrupted in normal volunteers under the influence of amphetamine and in schizophrenic patients who are acutely ill but not when they are in the chronic stages of the illness or indeed after about six or seven weeks of the acute episode have elapsed. The reason why chronic schizophrenic patients do not demonstrate disruption of latent inhibition was initially supposed to be because antipsychotic drugs had normalised the process. However, in a study of medication-free schizophrenic patients, LI was abnormal at the start of the illness but then normalised after about a year in spite of no medication (Gray, 1995). Furthermore, in the study in which LI inhibited in acute but not chronic schizophrenics (Gray *et al.*, 1992), both groups displayed positive symptoms to the same degree.These observations present a problem for their contention that disrupted LI is the basis of the generation of positive symptoms. Gray counters this by suggesting that disrupted LI is a state marker of acute psychosis rather than a trait marker of schizophrenia. There are however problems with interpreting even this modified hypothesis. First, LI is also disrupted in subjects with schizotypy, that is, subjects who are not overtly psychotic and do not have schizophrenia but who have some personality features in common with schizophrenic patients (Baruch, Hemsley and Gray, 1988; Lipp and Vaitl, 1992; Lubow *et al.*, 1992; De la Casa, Ruiz and Lubow, 1993). Second, a recent study comparing drug-treated and drug-naive schizophrenic patients within two weeks of an acute psychotic episode showed that the treated patients had disrupted LI but that LI in the untreated group was normal, suggesting that disrupted LI in earlier studies of schizophrenia is purely a medication effect (Williams *et al.*, 1996). Finally, Swerdlow and colleagues (1996) demonstrated intact LI in both acute and chronic schizophrenic patients. They also found that the schizophrenic patients had elevated learning scores, suggesting that previously observed LI deficits in schizophrenia may be an artifact of performance deficits relating to learning acquisition.

Prepulse inhibition

Prepulse inhibition (PPI), is another animal model that invokes dopaminergic involvement in attentional processes and has therefore been applied to schizophrenia. The phenomenon of PPI occurs at an earlier stage of information processing than LI or blocking and is thought to reflect a sensorimotor gating system that 'screens out the potentially chaotic flow of information or sensory stimuli' (Cadenhead, Geyer and Braff, 1993). Under normal circumstances, animals produce a startle response when a loud burst of white noise is delivered. Startle is significantly diminished if a weaker white noise stimulus is delivered just before the loud stimulus (Graham, 1975). Swerdlow and colleagues (1986, 1994) have shown in the rat that dopamine hyperactivity in ventral striatum, but not dorsal striatum or frontal cortex, also disrupts PPI and that this effect is mediated by the D2 receptor. Thus, like LI and blocking, dopamine release in ventral striatum appears to mediate the disruption of this normal attentional mechanism. PPI can also be demonstrated in man and, like LI and blocking, PPI appears to be disrupted in schizophrenic patients (Braff *et al.*, 1978; Braff, Grillon and Geyer, 1992; Grillon *et al.*, 1992). However, unlike LI and blocking, disrupted PPI occurs in chronic schizophrenic patients on medication (Braff *et al.*, 1992; Perry and Braff, 1994).

The result of failure to screen sensory stimuli at this early stage is thought to result in 'cognitive fragmentation', which in turn is thought to result in thought disorder and other unspecified psychotic symptoms (Braff *et al.*, 1978, 1992; Grillon *et al.*, 1992). Perry and Braff (1994) have examined the relationship between PPI and indices of thought disorder in a group of medicated schizophrenic patients. They found no correlation between PPI and standard measures of thought disorder derived from the Scale for Assessment of Positive and Negative Symptoms but did find an association between PPI and the 'Ego Impairment Index' that was devised by the authors. However this index is based on answers to the Rorscharch inkblot test, which is itself a sensory test and which therefore confounds the interpretation. Cadenhead and colleague (1993) have also demonstrated disrupted PPI in subjects with schizoptypal personality disorder and the deficit was of comparable magnitude to schizophrenic patients. The specificity of PPI as a mechanism explaining schizophrenic symptomology is cast into further doubt by the finding that PPI is also disrupted in obsessive-compulsive disorder (Swerdlow *et al.*, 1993).

Working memory and pre-frontal dopamine dysfunction

The animal models of schizophrenia described above lend themselves to an hypothesis that links abnormal striatal dopamine mechanisms with cognitive impairment and psychotic symptoms in schizophrenia. An alternative animal model postulates a role for abnormal prefrontal-cortical dopamine function in schizophrenia. This work has been carried out by Goldman-Rakic and colleagues using a test of working memory in monkeys. Her studies suggest that dopamine innervation of the principal sulcus, the homologue of the human dorsolateral prefrontal cortex, plays a crucial role in this cognitive function. Extrapolations have been made from this work to suggest that abnormalities in the dopaminergic control of cognitive processing within the cortex have relevance for the symptomology of schizophrenia, especially thought disorder (Goldman-Rakic, 1992).

The concept of working memory (WM) was developed several years ago by cognitive psychologists and, in its current form, is conceived of as a transient and active memory system that encompasses many different cognitive processes including covert verbal rehearsal, active short-term storage of phonological information, and the manipulation of images (Baddeley, 1986). Other properties of WM are assumed to be mediated by a 'central executive' component which, among other things, is involved in bringing information to mind from long-term memory, updating the current contents of working memory, problem solving, planning future behaviour and coordinating ongoing behaviour (Shallice, 1988). A common factor linking these processes is that they are effortful and under voluntary, conscious control (Desimone, 1995). Within the human cognitive psychology literature this model has proved to be extremely influential because of its capacity to explain a wide variety of cognitive functions (Baddeley, 1992).

The concept of working memory that Goldman-Rakic and colleagues have developed is somewhat more focused than that employed in human cognitive neuropsychology. They have argued that the cardinal properties of WM are 'to access and hold information in mind and then to use that information to guide responses in the absence of external cues' (Goldman-Rakic, 1992). These properties are thought to be essential for the successful performance of delayed response tasks in which macaque monkeys are required to remember a spatial location over a short delay. Using this paradigm and a variety of experimental approaches, Goldman-Rakic and colleagues have detailed the neuroanatomical, neuropharmacological and neuropsychological properties of working memory in this species.

Initial research established that ablation of the principal sulcus causes a specific impairment in delayed response performance (Goldman and Rosvold, 1970; Goldman, 1971). Later studies concentrated on the role of dopamine in mediating this behaviour. Using intracerebral injections of the selective catecholamine neurotoxin 6-OHDA into the principal sulcus, in combination with a noradrenaline uptake blocker to maximise dopamine depletion, Brozoski and colleagues found that those monkeys with the lowest levels of dopamine exhibited the largest deficits in delayed response performance (Brozoski *et al.*, 1979). Peripheral injections of apomorphine or levodopa reversed the deficits in several monkeys. Further, the monkeys with severe dopamine depletion did not differ from control animals that had intracerebral injections of the vehicle solution only, in performance on a pattern discrimination task presumed to depend on associative rather than working memory.

It has been well established that some prefrontal neurones become active during the delay phase of the delayed response task, suggesting that these are involved in maintaining an active memory for the stimulus (Kubota and Niki, 1971; Fuster, 1973). More recently, single unit recordings from the principal sulcus of monkeys have revealed three types of neurone involved in a prefrontal circuit during performance of an oculomotor delayed response task. Here monkeys are required to fixate a central stimulus for 0.5 seconds after which a target stimulus appears for 0.5 seconds in one of eight surrounding spatial locations. The animal is then required to maintain central fixation for a further 3 second delay period, after which the central stimulus is removed and the monkey must make a saccade to the location in which the target stimulus appeared. Neurones have been identified that appear to be responsible for stimulus registration (Funahashi, Bruce and Goldman-Rakic, 1990), maintaining the information in mind during the delay period (Funahashi, Bruce and Goldman-Rakic, 1989) and guiding the timing and direction of appropriate responses (Funahashi, Bruce and Goldman-Rakic, 1991). Importantly, principal sulcus lesions have been shown not to affect the accuracy or timing of eye movements of the same direction and amplitude made to external cues which remain present.

Recently, the availability of selective dopamine antagonists has allowed the contributions of different dopamine receptors to be assessed. Sawaguchi and Goldman-Rakic (1991) found that performance on the oculomotor delayed response task was impaired in a dose-dependent manner by injections into the principal sulcus of SCH23390 and SCH39166, both selective D1 antagonists. Performance was unimpaired by injections of raclopride, a selective D2 antagonist. Again it was found that performance was normal when the targets remained visible throughout the task. Thus D1, but not D2, antagonists impair performance specifically when the accuracy of the behavioural response is governed by remembered information. The importance of the involvement of D1 but not D2 in cortically mediated cognitive processes tallies with the finding that, in contradistinction to the striatum, D1 receptors are ten times more abundant than D2 receptors (Lidow *et al.*, 1991).

In a recent iontophoretic study, Williams and Goldman-Rakic (1995) examined the effect of the selective D1 antagonist SCH39166 on single cells that responded maximally during the delay period for targets in one location, i.e. cells with 'memory fields'. When the D1 antagonist was applied, the activity of the cell during the delay was actually enhanced for those cues presented within the memory field of the cell and this enhancement was reversed by the selective D1 agonist SKF38393. The discrepancy between this and previous results, which demonstrated that D1 antagonists impair behavioural performance of the delayed response task (Sawaguchi and Goldman-Rakic, 1991), was resolved when the concentrations of the drug were manipulated. Thus, whereas low concentrations of SCH39166 enhanced the signal-to-noise ratio of cells with memory fields, higher concentrations nonspecifically inhibited the firing of these cells throughout all periods of the task. Control studies demonstrated that the concentration of SCH39166 that caused enhanced activity in memory cells did not increase activity in cells that were active during either the cue presentation or response initiation phases of the delayed response task. Furthermore, the selective D2 antagonist, raclopride, produced a general inhibition of memory cell activity during all phases of the task.

These results suggest that dopaminergic activity in the prefrontal cortex modulates, in a highly specific manner, cognitive processing via its action on D1 receptors. Whether this is the D1 or D5 subtype of the D1 family is unresolved. The D1 receptors appear to be concentrated on cells involved in the active maintenance of memory for a relevant stimulus and Williams and Goldman-Rakic have proposed that the normal action of dopamine is to dampen the excitatory input to these memory cells responsible for generating the sustained activity during the delay period and that this action is feasible because of the synaptic triad arrangement previously described. Moreover, they argue that the ultimate effect of this modulatory activity will depend on the amount of endogenous ligand present. In their study, they presume that the stress of performance of the delayed response task was enough to cause an increased release of cortical dopamine. Since they found that low concentrations of D1 blockers improved memory cell activity, they suggest that the high levels of intrinsic dopamine in their study were suboptimal for memory cell performance. This conclusion is supported by behavioural studies of working memory. In the monkey, stress induced by either white noise or the administration of an anxiogenic benzodiazepine inverse agonist has been shown to disrupt delayed response performance and this is ameliorated by pretreatment with the specific D1 blocker SCH 23390 and by antipsychotics that have activity at the D1 site (Arnsten and Goldman-Rakic, 1990; Murphy *et al.*, 1995).

While high levels of intrinsic dopamine are detrimental to optimal cognitive performance, low levels of intrinsic ligand are equally detrimental, as shown by the studies of dopaminergic lesions described above and by the effect of ageing in monkeys, which reduces dopaminergic activity and delayed response performance (Arnsten *et al.*, 1994). Thus it appears that there is an optimal level of dopamine receptor occupation for the performance of working memory tasks with too much or too little being disruptive (Arnsten and Goldman-Rakic, 1990; Williams and Goldman-Rakic, 1995).

The work described above represents a substantial body of converging evidence that extends the role of dopamine in controlling behaviour from the subcortical regulation of motor acts to the cortical regulation of behaviour guided by internal representations. Does this role of dopamine in mediating this type of working memory have relevance for schizophrenia? Park and Holzman (1992) have used a modified version of the oculomotor and manual delayed response tasks used by Goldman-Rakic and colleagues to examine performance in 12 schizophrenic patients. They found that the schizophrenic subjects were impaired on the memory-guided conditions of both oculomotor and manual paradigms but were not impaired on any of the sensory-guided conditions. These results are therefore directly comparable to those found by Goldman-Rakic in monkeys with sulcus principalis lesions. In a more recent study, Park and Holzman (1993) replicated this deficit in a larger group of schizophrenic patients and showed that it correlated with another measure of frontal dysfunction, namely impaired smooth pursuit eye tracking performance.

Neuropsychological studies of schizophrenia have found wide-ranging cognitive deficits and it is possible that the findings of Park and Holtzman are non-specific. However, Fleming, Goldberg and Gold (1994) have argued that several important aspects of the generalised cognitive dysfunction of schizophrenia can be reduced to a deficit in working memory. By contrast, the model of working memory they used is that of Baddeley, which is generated from human cognitive psychology and is more elaborate than the model of working memory proposed by Goldman-Rakic for the monkey as explained above. Fleming and colleagues suggested that a common theme in the cognitive failure of schizophrenic patients is a dysfunction of the central executive component of Baddeley's working memory model, which controls the inflow of information into short-term store and allocates processing resources to priority functions, among other things (Shallice, 1988; Baddeley, 1992). Whether this can be reduced to the system in the monkey, which holds information 'on line' until it can be acted upon remains to be seen.

Another problem is that other tests of working memory akin to that of the delayed response task have been shown to be normal in schizophrenia.

For example, in the human cognitive psychology literature the standard measure of working memory capacity is digit span – essentially the number of digits a person can maintain 'on line'. Goldman-Rakic has argued that the ability of a monkey to perform the delayed response task is akin to this function in man (Goldman-Rakic, 1994). However digit span is one of the few neuropsychological tests on which schizophrenic patients consistently perform as well as controls (Park and Holzman, 1992; Ganzelves and Haenen, 1995; Morice and Delahunty, 1996). Corsi's block tapping task is a spatial equivalent of the digit span test, and is probably even more comparable in terms of cognitive processing to spatial delayed response tasks. Again, schizophrenic patients tend to perform this task as well as controls (Elliott, *et al.*, 1995). A more demanding test of spatial working memory has been developed by Robbins, Sahakian and colleagues (Sahakian and Owen, 1992). Although schizophrenic patients perform poorly on this test (Pantelis *et al.*, 1993), it has been shown that this poor performance does not represent a deficit in spatial working memory per se, but rather appears to reflect inefficient use of a search strategy. Thus it is clear that the cognitive deficits present in schizophrenia are considerably more complex than an inability to retain spatial locations on line. Yet another difficulty with reducing the cognitive failure of schizophrenia to a dopamine-mediated dysfunction of working memory, is that dopamine is not the only neurotransmitter implicated in modulating this function. Within the human psychopharmacology literature it is the cholinergic system that has received most research attention with respect to working memory (Rusted, 1988; Warburton and Rusted, 1993).

In addition to providing a link between dopaminergic dysfunction and schizophrenic cognitive dysfunction, Goldman-Rakic (1994) has suggested that schizophrenic thought disorder is 'reducible to an impairment of the operational mechanisms by which symbolic representations are both accessed from long-term memory, and held "in mind" to guide behaviour in the absence of instructive stimuli in the outside world' and cited evidence such as the studies described above as support this proposition. There is clearly a large conceptual leap from the type of working memory system responsible for performance on a delayed response task in which internal representations of spatial locations are kept on line for a few seconds to a working memory system in which the items held in short-term memory are symbolic representations called from long-term memory as this might suggest that single cells would fire only when the memorandum (symbolic representation) is an abstract concept rather than a childhood memory or a high rather than low imagery word. Further, as with the other animal models described above, there is also a problem in relating the dopamine mediated disruption of a simple learning paradigm to the complex phenomenology witnessed in schizophrenia. Nevertheless the hypothesis of Goldman-Rakic is thematically similar to those described in the preceding section in that these all suggest that difficulties in the cognitive processes that relate events in long-term memory to current perceptions in consciousness or working memory give rise to the disruption of normal patterns of thinking, resulting perhaps in such phenomena as hallucinations, delusions and thought disorder and all invoke a central role of dopamine. It therefore remains to be seen if drugs that correct positive schizophrenic symptoms also normalise these cognitive functions.

Do antipsychotic drugs treat cognitive dysfunction in schizophrenia?

Traditional antipsychotic drugs are ineffective in treating the positive symptoms in approximately one-third of patients and can produce debilitating side-effects in many more. It is unsurprising therefore that the effect of these compounds on neuropsychological performance in schizophrenia is very variable, with improvement and deterioration both having been reported (see Lee, Thompson and Meltzer, 1994 for a review). In this respect it is worth examining the effect of clozapine on the cognitive disorder in schizophrenia as this drug is superior to all other compounds in treating the positive symptoms of schizophrenia (Claghorn *et al.*, 1987; Kane, Honigfeld and Singer, 1988; Lindstrom, 1988; Pickar *et al.*, 1992; Breier *et al.*, 1994) and is said also to improve negative features (Kane *et al.*, 1988; Meltzer *et al.*, 1989, 1992; Miller *et al.*, 1994 but see also Carpenter *et al.*, 1995 and Meltzer, 1995 for a discussion). Further it has a different profile of action to the more traditional drugs in that clozapine is a relatively weak blocker of the D2 (and D3) receptor *in vitro* (see Seeman and Van Tol, 1994 for a discussion) and *in vivo* (Brucke *et al.*, 1992; Farde *et al.*, 1992; Pilowsky, 1992) and exerts its main effect in ventral striatum and cortex (Deutch, 1994; Fibiger, 1994; Knable and Weinberger, 1994).

There have been five peer-reviewed publications to date. The first study compared three groups of patients receiving haloperidol, flupenthixol and clozapine and found no differences on a variety of tests of psychomotor speed and general cognition (Classen and Laux, 1988). A study by Goldberg and colleagues used a superior within-subjects design and also found no effect of clozapine treatment. They examined IQ, memory and executive function in 15 treatment-resistant psychotic patients first on haloperidol and then on clozapine (Goldberg *et al.*, 1993). The baseline performance on haloperidol showed impairments of psychomotor function, long-term memory and executive function. Following a mean of 15 months on clozapine, performance on these tests had not changed and performance on a test of visual memory had actually deteriorated. Importantly, although these patients failed to improve with respect to cognition, symptom scores on the Brief Psychiatric Rating Scale (BPRS) fell by a mean of 19 points (haloperidol score 51, clozapine score 32) with a distinct improvement in both positive (paranoia, thought disturbance) and negative (anergia) symptoms.

Several studies have claimed to have demonstrated improvement in cognitive function following clozapine treatment. Hagger and colleagues (1993) tested 36 treatment-resistant psychotic patients, the majority of whom (27) had been drug free for a mean of nine days before baseline testing. They were initially impaired on a variety of executive and memory tests compared to an age- and education-matched group of controls. They were then tested after six weeks and six months of clozapine treatment with most improvement being evident at the latter time point when they had improved on five of the nine tests administered. Psychopathology, as measured by the BPRS, improved on positive but not on negative symptom scores and a regression analysis showed that a change in psychopathology predicted a change in cognitive function. However, the improvement of symptoms in this study, although significant, was small with a mean fall of 3.4 BPRS points and no change between the six week and six month ratings (baseline score 41.9, six week score 38.5, six month score 38.4). Most cognitive improvement occurred in treatment responders, defined as a fall of 20% or more in BPRS score. However the improvement in verbal fluency occurred in both responders and non-responders. There was no change in symptoms between six weeks and six months despite an improvement in cognitive function over that period. Further, because the majority of patients had been drug free at the time of initial testing, it is possible that these results could be explained in terms of decreased distractability due to the reduction of positive symptoms rather than a direct effect of clozapine on cognitive function.

In a parallel study by the same group, Lee and colleagues (1994) found similar results after six weeks and six months of clozapine treatment in 24 schizophrenic patients who were not considered to be treatment resistant. In this study, the clozapine group was compared to a group of patients, matched for IQ and BPRS score, receiving a range of traditional antipsychotic drugs and an additional test session occurred after 12 months of treatment. At six months, the traditional group showed improvement in only one of the nine tests administered, compared to seven in the clozapine group. After 12 months of treatment, the profile of performance had changed for both groups. Improved performance of the clozapine group was sustained on four of the seven tests: category and letter fluency, digit symbol substitution and perseverative error score on the Wisconsin Card Sorting Test. For the traditional group, performance had shifted so that they were better than at baseline on two different tests. Taking this changing profile over the four test sessions into consideration, the authors concluded that the main difference between the two drug groups was that the clozapine group showed a sustained improvement over time on tests of digit symbol substitution and letter fluency. There were no differences in change of psychopathology between the two drug groups. In this study, the criticism that changes in cognitive function may be secondary to improvement in positive symptoms is overcome by demonstrating the superiority of clozapine over other antipsychotics that produced the same degree of improvement in positive symptoms. However, other explanations of the results can be considered that do not invoke a direct action of clozapine on the cognitive abnormalities fundamental to schizophrenia. For example, one of the two most striking effects was on digit symbol substitution. This is a test of psychomotor speed where subjects have to draw an appropriate symbol under a series of numbers in a given amount of time. Slowness on this test might be expected in the traditional group compared to the clozapine group purely on the grounds that clozapine rarely produces extrapyramidal effects whereas these are common with other compounds. The authors prescribed anticholinergic drugs when clinically indicated but this does not preclude a subclinical effect of these drugs on psychomotor speed. The other major effect was found with verbal fluency. This finding may also be nonspecific and attributable to the potent anticholinergic action of clozapine, as there are reports of improved verbal fluency following administration of scopolamine in volunteers (Lines *et al.*, 1991; Dunne *et al.*, 1993).

Buchanan, Holstein and Breir (1994) have also found improvement in cognitive function after treatment with clozapine in a tightly controlled study. They examined 39 schizophrenic patients with residual positive and negative symptoms following traditional treatment with two antipsychotic drugs as measured by the BPRS and Scale for Assessment of Negative Symptoms (SANS). Nineteen patients were randomised to take 400 mg clozapine and 20 patients were given 20 mg haloperidol for ten weeks. At baseline, all patients were taking fluphenazine and were tested for measures of visuospatial function, memory and executive function. There were no differences between the groups. After 10 weeks, there were also no differences in performance that could be attributable to a superior action of clozapine. All patients were then given clozapine for one year. Improvements were subsequently found, compared to baseline, on letter fluency, the Mooney faces test and the block design test from the Wechsler Adult Intelligence Scale. There was a trend for improvement on tests of category fluency and story recall and on the Stroop test. There were positive associations between changes in psychiatric symptoms and changes in neuropsychological performance. Again, all of these tests but one were timed tests and therefore the differences could again be attributable to extrapyramidal side-effects slowing performance at baseline and in the haloperidol group.

In a preliminary report, Dye, Mortimer and Lock (1996) compared patients remaining on their usual treatment with matched patients who changed to clozapine. They showed that there was a significant improvement in positive symptoms by six months but improvement in cognitive function did not emerge until 12 months in the clozapine group.

The evidence as to whether clozapine improves cognition in schizophrenia is currently inconclusive and open to criticism. The fact that cognitive function appears not to bear any relation to change in symptoms in most studies has been taken to show that positive symptoms are not a by-product of neuropsychological disturbance. This is an erroneous conclusion. First, theories postulating a neuropsychological basis for symptoms have invoked sophisticated cognitive models that have not been tested in these studies. Second, the kinds of function tested in these studies have been more linked to the presence of negative than positive symptoms. Whether clozapine improves negative symptoms is also currently under debate (Carpenter *et al.*, 1995), there being evidence for and against – like the effect on cognition. Thus the question of whether antipsychotic drugs can improve neuropsychological function in relation to improvement in symptoms will not be answered until more rigorous and sophisticated studies are performed.

Conclusions

The main positive conclusion that can be made from these studies is that dopamine neurotransmission plays a significant role in cognitive function. The question remains as to whether this has anything to do with schizophrenia. Several animal models have demonstrated a role for dopamine in working memory and selective attentional processes and these results have been extrapolated to provide appealing explanations of the development of schizophrenic phenomenology. Unfortunately when some of these paradigms have been applied to patient groups, the results fail to show clear deficits that can be firmly linked to the patient's mental state. Other approaches that explore whether antipsychotic treatment can concommitantly change both positive symptoms and cognition are flawed because the neuropsychological tests used have no theoretical basis in relation to symptom generation. Thus there is clearly a need for more rigorous exploration of phenomenology in relation to cognition. This is difficult to achieve however because schizophrenic patients can be difficult to work with because of fluctuations in both motivation and phenomenology. Furthermore, if Goldman-Rakic is correct and cognitive performance can be disrupted by both high and low levels of intrinsic dopamine, then dopamine function would need to be finely modulated in patients to obtain meaningful results. This is currently impossible with the current range of drugs available.

It is important to appreciate that cognition is not the only type of higher function involving dopamine. Research over many years has established without doubt that this neurotransmitter is also important for motor activity and motivational behaviour (Koob, 1992; Robbins and Everitt, 1992). Although the precise nature of the information carried in dopaminergic pathways has not been fully elucidated, it appears that striatal dopamine acts to enhance responding, in the form of action (or thought?), to significant external and internal events. Ventral striatal dopamine appears to mediate the behavioural excitement witnessed in animals when they receive a reward and the possible human analogue of this is the experience of pleasure. Dorsal striatal dopamine appears to be important for superior cognitive performance and skilled motor acts, as animal studies have shown that dopamine release here enhances sensori-motor coordination. In the cortex, the role of dopamine is less clear although the work of Goldman-Rakic (1994) on cognition and others on motivation (e.g. McGregor, Baker and Roberts, 1996) suggest that dopamine is also involved in cortical computational processes themselves. Thus, given that in schizophrenia there are disturbances of motivation, cognition and movement, there continues to be a theoretical appeal in invoking a fundamental abnormality of dopamine systems in schizophrenia. Equally, however, there continues to be a lack of direct evidence to support this. Further, the fact that other research, outlined above, provides direct evidence that a disturbance of neuronal cytoarchitecture in temporal and frontal cortex underlies schizophrenia and presumably involves many neurotransmitter systems, makes it foolish to continue to plead for a single neurotransmitter defect in this illness. Given the fact that these changes are structural, it also suggests that the ability to treat established schizophrenia over and above the relief of some symptoms might be unrealistic. Nevertheless as long as the mainstay of treatment of schizophrenia is dopamine receptor blockade, a form of the dopamine hypothesis will persist and the important work for the future is to put it in the context of these other findings. For example, the knowledge that dopamine in the cortex can modulate intrinsic activity and that cortical dopamine receptor types are different in distribution from striatum suggest that pharmacotherapy might be able to ameliorate intrinsic aberrant function when more precise details are available about the function of cortical dopamine from animal studies. Further, the current knowledge that the dopamine receptor types are differentially distributed within striatum and have different functions also gives rise to the hope that more specific drugs may be used to modulate the outflow of aberrant cortical processing in a way that can provide more effective relief of symptoms.

References

Akbarian, S., Bunney, W.E., Potkin, S.G. *et al.* (1993*a*). Altered distribution of nicotinamide-adenine dinucleotide phosphate-diaphorase cells in frontal lobe of schizophrenics implies disturbances of cortical development. *Archives of General Psychiatry*, **50**, 169–77.

Akbarian, S., Vinuela, A., Kim, J.J. *et al.* (1993*b*). Distorted distribution of nicotinamide-adenine dinucleotide phosphate-diaphorase neurones in temporal lobe of schizophrenics implies anomolous cortical development. *Archives of General Psychiatry*, **50**, 178–87.

Akbarian, S., Kim, J.J., Potkin, S.G. *et al.* (1995). Gene expression for glutamic acid decarboxylase is reduced without loss of neurons in prefrontal cortex of schizophrenics. *Archives of General Psychiatry*. **52**, 258–66.

Albert, M.L. (1978). Subcortal dementia. In *Alzheimer's Disease: Senile Dementia and Related Disorders* (ed. R. Katzman, R.D. Terry and K. Beck), pp. 173–80. New York: Raven Press.

Alexander, G., DeLong, M. and Strick, P. (1986). Parallel organization of functionally segregated circuits linking basal ganglia and cortex. *Annual Review of Neuroscience*, **9**, 357–81.

Andreason, N.C., Nasrallah, H.A., Dunn, V. *et al.* (1986). Structural abnormalities in the frontal system in schizophrenia. A magnetic resonance imaging study. *Archives of General Psychiatry*, **43**, 136–144.

Arnsten, A.F.T. and Goldman-Rakic, P.S. (1990). Stress impairs prefrontal cortex cognitive function in monkeys: role of dopamine. *Society for Neurosciences Abstracts*, **16**, 7475.

Arnsten, A.F.T., Cai, J.X., Murphy, B.L. *et al.* (1994). Dopamine D-Sub.1 receptor mechanisms in the cognitive performance of young adult and aged monkeys. *Psychopharmacology*, **116**, 143–51.

Baddeley, A.D. (1986). *Working Memory*. Oxford: Clarendon Press.

Baddeley, A.D. (1992). Is working memory working? *Quarterly Journal of Experimental Psychology. Human Experimental Psychology*, **44A**, 1–31.

Baruch, I., Hemsley, D.R. and Gray, J.A. (1988*a*). Differential performance of acute and chronic schizophrenics in a latent inhibition task. *Journal of Nervous and Mental Diseases*, **176**, 598–606.

Baruch, I., Hemsley, D.R. and Gray, J.A. (1988*b*). Latent inhibition and psychotic proneness. *Personality and Individual Differences*, **9**, 777–83.

Benes, F.M., Vincent, S.L., Alsterberg, G. *et al.* (1992). Increased GABA-A receptor binding in superficial layers of cingulate cortex in schizophrenics. *Journal of Neuroscience*, **12**, 924–9.

Berger, B., Gaspar, P. and Verney, C. (1991). Dopaminergic innervation of the cerebral cortex: unexpected differences between rodents and primates. *Trends in Neurosciences*, **14**, 21–7.

Bilder, R.M., Lipschutz-Broch, L., Reiter, G. *et al.* (1992). Intellectual deficits in first episode schizophrenia: evidence for progressive deterioration. *Schizophrenia Bulletin*, **18**, 437–48.

Bird, E.D., Spokes, E.G.S. and Iversen, L.L. (1979). Increased dopamine concentrations in limbic areas of brain from patients dying with schizophrenia. *Brain*, **102**, 347–60.

Blanc, G., Herve, D., Simon, H. *et al.* (1980). Response to stress of mesocortical frontal neurones in rats after long term isolation. *Nature*, **284**, 265–7.

Bouthenet, M.L., Martres,M.P., Sales, N. *et al.* (1987). A detailed mapping of dopamine D2 receptors in the rat central nervous system by autoradiography with [^{125}I] iodosulpiride. *Neuroscience*, **20**, 117–55.

Bouyer, J.J., Park, D.H., Joh, T.H. *et al.* (1984). Chemical and structural analysis of the relation between cortical inputs and tyrosine hydroxylase containing terminals in rat neostriatum. *Brain Research*, **302**, 267–75.

Braff, D.L., Stone, C., Callaway, E. *et al.* (1978). Prestimulus effects on human startle reflex in normals and schizophrenics. *Psychophysiology*, **14**, 339–43.

Braff, D.L., Grillon, C. and Geyer, M.A. (1992). Gating and habituation of the startle reflex in schizophrenic patients. *Archives of General Psychiatry*, **49**, 206–15.

Breier, A., Buchanan, R.W., Kirkpatrick, B. *et al.* (1994). Effects of clozapine on positive and negative symptoms in outpatients with schizophrenia. *American Journal of Psychiatry*, **151**, 20–6.

Broen, W.E. and Storms, L.H. (1967). A theory of response interference in schizophrenia. In *Progress in Experimental Personality Research*, 4 (ed. L. Maher). New York: Academic Press.

Brown, R.G. and Marsden, C.D. (1988). 'Subcortical dementia': the neuropsychological evidence. *Neuroscience*, **25**, 363–87.

Brozoski, T., Brown, R.M., Rosvold, H.E. *et al.* (1979). Cognitive deficit caused by depletion of dopamine in prefrontal cortex. *Science*, **205**, 929–31.

Brucke, T., Roth, J., Podrecka, I. *et al.* (1992). Striatal D2 dopamine blockade by typical and atypical neuroleptics. *Lancet*, **339**, 497.

Buchanan, R.W., Holstein, C. and Breier, A. (1994). The comparative efficacy and long-term effect of clozapine treatment on neuropsychological test performance. *Biological Psychiatry*, **36**, 717–25.

Buchsbaum, M., DeLisi, L. and Holcomb, H. (1984). Anteroposterior gradients in cerebral glucose use in schizophrenia. *Archives of General Psychiatry*, **41**, 1159–66.

Cadenhead, K.S., Geyer, M.A. and Braff, D.L. (1993). Impaired startle prepulse inhibition and habituation in patients with schizotypal personality disorder. *American Journal of Psychiatry*, **150**, 1862–7.

Caligiuri, M., Lohr, J. and Jeste, D. (1993). Parkinsonism in neuroleptic naive schizophrenic patients. *American Journal of Psychiatry*, **150**, 1343–8.

Carpenter, W.T., Conley, R.R., Buchanan, R.W. *et al.* (1995). Patient response and resource management: another view of clozapine treatment of schizophrenia. *American Journal of Psychiatry*, **152**, 827–32.

Chua, S.E. and McKenna, P.J. (1995). Schizophrenia – a brain disease? A critical review of structural and functional cerebral abnormality in the disorder. *British Journal of Psychiatry*, **166**, 563–82.

Claghorn, J., Honigfeld, G., Abuzzahab, F.S. *et al.* (1987). The risks and benefits of clozapine versus chlorpromazine. *Journal of Clinical Psychopharmacology*, **7**, 377–84.

Classen, W. and Laux, G. (1988). Sensorimotor and cognitive performance of schizophrenic impatients treated with haloperidol, flupenthixol or haloperidol. *Pharmacopsychiatry*, **21**, 295–7.

Connell, P.H. (1958). *Amphetamine Psychosis*. London: Chapman & Hall.

Crawford, T., Haeger, B., Kennard, C. *et al.* (1995). Saccaotic abnormalities in psychotic patients. II. The role of neuroleptic treatment. *Psychological Medicine*, **25**, 473–83.

Creese, I., Burt, D.R. and Snyder, S.H. (1976). Dopamine receptor binding predicts clinical and pharmacological potencies of antischizophrenic drugs. *Science*, **192**: 481–3.

Crider, A. (1979). *Schizophrenia: A Biopsychological Perspective*. Hillsdale: Erlbaum.

Crider, A., Solomon, P.R. and McMahon, M. (1982). Disruption of selective attention in the rat following chronic d-amphetamine administration: possible relationship to schizophrenic attention disorder. *Biological Psychiatry*, **17**, 351–61.

Crider, A., Blockel, L. and Solomon, P.R. (1986). A selective attention deficit in the rat following induced dopamine receptor supersensitivity. *Behavioural Neuroscience*, **100**, 315–19.

Crocq, P.R., Mant, R., Asherson, P. *et al.* (1992). Association between schizophrenia and homozygosity at the dopmaine D3 receptor gene. *Journal of Medical Genetics*, **29**, 858–60.

Crow, T. (1980). Molecular pathology of schizophrenia: more than one disease process? *British Medical Journal*, **280**, 1–9.

Crow, T.J., Owen, F., Cross, A.J. *et al.* (1981). Neurotransmitter enzymes and receptors in post-mortem brains in schizophrenia; evidence that an increase in D2 receptors is associated with the type 1 syndrome. In *Transmitter Biochemistry of Human Brain Tissue* (ed. P. Riederer and E. Usdin). London: Macmillan.

Dahlstrom, A. and Fuxe, K. (1965). Evidence for the existence of monoamine containing neurones in central nervous system. I: Demonstration of monoamines in the cell bodies of brainstem neurones. *Acta Physiologica Scandinavica*, **62**, Suppl. 232, 1–55.

Davies, P. and Maloney, A.F.J. (1976). Selective loss of cerebral cholinergic neurones in Alzheimer's disease. *Lancet*, **ii**, 1403.

Dawson, T.M., Barone, P., Sidhu, A. *et al.* (1988). The D1 dopamine receptor in the rat brain: quantitative autoradiographic localisation using iodinated ligand. *Neuroscience*, **26**, 83–100.

Deakin, J.F.W., Simpson, M.D.C., Gilchrist, A.C. *et al.* (1989). Frontal cortical and left temporal glutamatergic dysfunction in schizophrenia. *Journal of Neurochemistry*, **52**, 1781–6.

De la Casa, L.G., Ruiz, G. and Lubow, R.E. (1993). Latent inhibition and recall/recognition of irrelevant stimuli as a function of pre-exposure duration in high and low psychotic prone normals. *British Journal of Psychology*, **33**, 119–32.

DeLisi, L.E., Dauphinais, I.D. and Gershon, E.S. (1988). Perinatal complications and reduced size of brain limbic structures in familial schizophrenia. *Schizophrenia Bulletin*, **14**, 185–91.

Desimone, R. (1995). Is dopamine a missing link? *Science*, **376**, 549–50.

Deutch, A.Y. (1994). Identification of the neural systems subserving the actions of clozapine: clues from immediate-early gene expression. *Journal of Clinical Psychiatry*, **55** Suppl B, 37–42.

Dunne, M.E., Stathan, D., Raphael, B. *et al.* (1993). Further evidence that scopolamine can improve verbal fluency. *Journal of Psychopharmacology*, **7**, 159–63.

Dye, S.M., Mortimer, A.M. and Lock, M. (1996). Clozapine versus treatment as usual in schizophrenia. *Schizophrenia Research*, **18**, 126.

Eagger, S.A. and Harvey, R.J. (1995). Tacrine and other anticholinesterase drugs in dementia. *Current Opinion in Psychiatry*, **8**, 264–7.

Elliott, R., McKenna, P.J., Robbins, T.W. *et al.* (1995). Neuropsychological evidence for frontostriatal dysfunction in schizophrenia. *Psychological Medicine*, **25**, 619–30.

Farde, L., Wiesel, F.-A., Hall, H., *et al.* (1987). No D2 receptor increase in PET study of schizophrenia. *Archives of General Psychiatry*, **44**, 671–2.

Farde, L., Nordstrom, A.-L., Wiesel, F.-A. *et al.* (1992). Positron emission tomography of central D1 and D2 receptor occupancy in patients treated with classical neuroleptics and clozapine. *Archives of General Psychiatry*, **49**, 538–44.

Fibiger, H.C. (1994). Neuroanatomical targets of neuroleptic drugs as revealed by fos immunochemistry. *Journal of Clinical Psychiatry*, **55** Suppl B, 33–6.

Fleming, K., Goldberg, T.E. and Gold, J.M. (1994). Applying working memory constructs to schizophrenic cognitive impairment. In *The Neuropsychology of Schizophrenia*, (ed. A.S. Dvid and J.C. Cutting, pp. 197–213. Hove: Lawrence Erlbaum Associates.

Freund, T.F., Powell, J.F. and Smith, A.D. (1984). Tyrosine hydroxylase-immunoreative boutons in synaptic contact with identified striatonigral neurones, with particular reference to dendritic spines. *Neuroscience*, **13**, 1189–215.

Funahashi, S., Bruce, C.J. and Goldman-Rakic, P.S. (1989). Mnemonic coding of visual space in the monkey's dorsolateral prefrontal cortex. *Journal of Neurophysiology*, **61**, 331–49.

Funahashi, S., Bruce, C.J. and Goldman-Rakic, P.S. (1990). Visuospatial coding in primate prefrontal neurons revealed by oculomotor paradigms. *Journal of Neurophysiology*, **63**, 814–31.

Funahashi, S., Bruce, C.J. and Goldman-Rakic, P.S. (1991). Neuronal activity related to saccadic eye-movements in the monkey's prefrontal cortex. *Journal of Neurophysiology*, **65**, 1464–83.

Fuster, J.M. (1973). Unit activity in prefrontal cortex during delayed response performance: neuronal correlates of transient memory. *Journal of Neurophysiology*, **36**, 61–78.

Ganzelves, P.G.J. and Haenen, M.-A. (1995). A preliminary study of externally and self-ordered task performance in schizophrenia. *Schizophrenia Research*, **16**, 67–71.

Gerfen, C.R. (1989). The neostriatal mosaic: striatal patch-matrix organisation is related to cortical lamination. *Science*, **246**, 385–8.

Gerfen, C.R., Herkenham, M. and Thibault, J. (1987). The neostraital mosaic: II. Patch and matrix-directed mesostriatal dopaminergic and non-dopaminergic systems. *Journal of Neuroscience*, **7**, 3935–44.

Gerfen, C.R., Engber, T.M., Mahan, L.C. *et al.* (1990). D1 and D2 dopamine receptor-regulated gene expression of striatonigral and striatopallidal neurones. *Science*, **250**, 1429–32.

Gold, J., Randolph, C., Carpenter, C. *et al.* (1992). Forms of memory failure in schizophrenia. *Journal of Abnormal Psychology*, **101**, 487–94.

Goldberg, T.E., Greenberg, R.D., Griffin, S.J. *et al.* (1993). The effect of clozapine on cognition and psychiatric symptoms on patients with schizophrenia. *British Journal of Psychiatiatry*, **162**, 43–8.

Goldman, P.S. (1971). Funcational development of the prefrontal cortex in early life and the problem of neuronal plasticity. *Experimental Neurology*, **32**, 366–87.

Goldman, P.S. and Rosvold, H.E. (1970). Localisation of function within the dorsolateral prefrontal cortex of the rhesus monkey. *Experimental Neurology*, **27**, 291–304.

Goldman-Rakic, P.S. (1992). Dopamine-mediated mechanisms of the prefrontal cortex. *Seminars in the Neurosciences. Milestones in Dopamine Research*, **4**, (ed. T.W. Robbins), pp. 149–160. London: Saunders Scientific Publications, Academic Press Ltd.

Goldman-Rakic, P.S. (1994). Working memory dysfunction in schizophrenia. *Journal of Neuropsychiatry and Clinical Neurosciences*, **6**, 348–57.

Goldman-Rakic, P.S., Leranth, C., Williams, M.S. *et al.* (1989). Dopamine synaptic complex with pyramidal neurones in primate cerebral cortex. *Proceedings of the National Academy of Science USA*, **86**, 9015–19.

Graham, F. (1975). The more or less startling effects of weak prestimuli. *Psychophysiology*, **12**, 238–48.

Gray, J.A. (1982). *The Nueropsychology of Anxiety: An Enquiry into the Functions of the Septohippocampal System*. Oxford: Oxford University Press.

Gray, J.A. (1995). Dopamine release in the nucleus accumbens: the perspective from aberrations of consciousness in schizophrenia. *Neuropsychologia*, **33**, 1143–53.

Gray, J.A., Feldon, J., Rawlins, J.N.P. *et al.* (1991). The neuropsychology of schizophrenia. *Behavioural Brain Sciences*, **14**, 56–84.

Gray, N.S., Hemsley, D.R. and Gray, J.A. (1992*a*). Abolition of latent inhibition in acute but not chronic schizophrenics. *Neurology and Psychiatry Brain Research*, **1**, 83–9.

Gray, N.S., Pickering, A.D., Hemsley, D. *et al.* (1992*b*). Abolition of latent inhibition by a single 5 mg dose of d-amphetamine in man. *Psychopharmacology*, **107**, 425–30.

Grillon, C., Ameli, R., Charney, D.S. *et al.* (1992). Startle gating deficts occur across prepulse intensities in schizophrenic patients. *Biological Psychiatry*, **32**, 939–43.

Groenewegen, H.J., Berendse, G.E., Meredith, G.E. *et al.* (1991). Functional anatomy of the ventral, limbic system-innervated striatum. In *The Mesolimbic Dopamine System: From Motivation to Action* (ed. P. Willner and J. Scheel-Kruger), pp. 19–59. Chichester: John Wiley and Sons Ltd.

Hagan, J.J. and Morris, R.G.M. (1988). The cholinergic hypothesis of memory: a review of animal experiments. In *Handbook of Psychopharmacology* (ed. L.L. Iversen, S.D. Iversen and S.H. Snyder), pp. 237–323. New York: Plenum Press.

Hagger, C., Buckley, P., Kenny, J.T. *et al.* (1993). Improvement in cognitive functions and psychiatric symptoms in treatment refractory schizophrenic patients receiving clozapine. *Biological Psychiatry*, **34**, 702–12.

Hanada, S., Mita, T., Nishinok, N. *et al.* (1987). ^{3}H -Muscimol binding sites increased in autopsied brains of chronic schizophrenics. *Life Sciences*, **40**, 259–66.

Harvey, I., Ron, M., DuBoulay, G., *et al.* (1993). Reduction in cortical volume in schizophrenia on magnetic resonance imaging. *Psychological Medicine*, **23**, 591–604.

Heaton, R., Paulsen, J.S., McAdams, L.A. *et al.* (1994). Neuropsychological deficits in schizophrenia. *Archives of General Psychiatry*, **51**, 469–76.

Heimer, L. and Wilson, R.D. (1975). The subcortical projections of the allocortex: similarities in the neural connections of the hippocampus, the pyriform cortex and the neocortex. In *Golgi Centennial Symposium: Perspectives in Neurobiology* (ed. M. Santini), pp. 177–93. New York: Raven Press.

Hemsley, D.R. (1994). Cognitive disturbances as a link between schizophrenic symptoms and their biological bases. *Neurology, Psychiatry and Brain Research*, **2**, 163–79.

Hemsley, D.R. (1994*b*). Perceptual and cognitive abnormalities as the bases for schizophrenic symptoms. In *The Neuropsychology of Schizophrenia* (ed. A.S. David and J.C. Cutting), pp. 97–118. Hove: Lawrence Erlbaum Associates.

Herkenham, M., Moon Edley, S. and Stuart, J. (1984). Cell clusters in the nucleus accumbens of the rat, and the mosaic relationship of opiate receptors, acetylcholinesterase and subcortical afferent terminations. *Neuroscience*, **11**, 561–93.

Hietala, J., Syvalahti, E., Vuorio, K. *et al.* (1994). Striatal D2 dopamine receptor characteristics in neuroleptic-naive schizophrenic patients studied with positron emission tomography. *Acrhives of General Psychiatry*, **51**, 116–23.

Hoff, A.L., Riordan, H., O'Donnell, D.W. *et al.* (1992). Neuropsychological functioning of first-episode schizophreniform psychosis. *American Journal of Psychiatry*, **149**, 898–903.

Holm, R.P., Moller-Madsen, A., Videbech, S. *et al.* (1995). Neuropsychological deficit in newly diagnosed patients with schizophrenia or schizophreniform disorder. *Acta Psychiatrica Scandinavica*, **92**, 35–43.

Iversen, L.L. (1978). Biochemical and pharmacological studies: the dopamine hypothesis. In *Schizophrenia: Towards a New Synthesis* (ed. J.K. Wing), pp. 89–286. London: Academic Press.

Jakob, H. and Beckman, H. (1986). Prenatal developmental disturbances in the limbic allocortex of schizophrenics. *Journal of Neural Transmission*, **65**, 303–26.

Jaskiw, G.E. and Weinberger, D.R. (1992). Dopamine and schizophrenia – a cortically corrective perspective. In *Seminars in the Neurosciences. Milestones in Dopamine Research* (ed. T.W. Robbins), pp. 179–188. London: Saunders Scientific Publications, Academic Press.

Johnstone, E.C., Crow, T.J., Frith, C.D. *et al.* (1976). Cerebral ventricular size and cognitive impairment in chronic schizophrenia. *Lancet*, **ii**, 924–7.

Jones, S.H., Gray, J.A. and Hemsley, D.R. (1992). Loss of the Kamin blocking effect in acute but not chronic schizophrenics. *Biological Psychiatry*, **32**, 739–55.

Joyce, E.M. (1992). The significance of functional imaging for psychiatry. *Journal of Neurology, Neurosurgery and Psychiatry*, **55**, 427–30.

Kamin, L.J. (1968). 'Attention-like' processes in classical conditioning. In *Miami Symposium on the Prediction of Behaviour* (ed. E. Jones). Miami: University of Miami Press.

Kamin, L.J. (1969). Predictability, surprise, attention and conditioning. In *Punishment and Aversive Behaviour* (ed. Campbell and Church). New York: Appleton Century Crofts.

Kane, J., Honigfeld, G. and Singer, J. (1988). Clozapine for the treatment of resistant schizophrenia. *Archives of General Psychiatry*, **45**, 789–96.

Kebabian, J.W. and Calne, D.B. (1979). *Nature*, **277**, 93–6.

Kemp, J.M. and Powell, T.P.S. (1971). The structure of the caudate nucleus of the cat: light and electron microscopic study. *Philosophical Transactions of the Royal Society of London (Biology)*, **262**, 383–401.

Kennedy, J.L., Petronis, A., Gao, J. *et al.* (1994). Genetic studies of DRD4 and clinical response to neuroleptic medications. *American Journal of Human Genetics*, **55**, 3.

Kerwin, R.W. and Collier, D. (1996). The dopamine D4 receptor inschizophrenia: an update. *Psychological Medicine*, **26**, 221–8.

Kitai, S.T., Koscis, J.D., Preston, R.J. *et al.* (1976). Monosynaptic inputs to caudate neurones identified by intracellular injections of horseradish peroxidase. *Brain Research*, **109**, 601–6.

Kleinman, J.E. and Nawroz, S. (1994). Schizophrenia: post mortem studies. In *Biology of Schizophrenia and Affective Disease* (ed. S.J. Watson). New York: Raven Press.

Knable, M.B. and Weinberger, D.R. (1994). Limbic-prefrontal connectivity and clozapine. *Journal of Clinical Psychiatry*, **55** Suppl B, 70–3.

Koob, G.F. (1992). Dopamine, addiction and reward. In *Seminars in the Neurosciences*, 4 (ed. T.W. Robbins), pp. 139–48. London: Saunders Scientific Publishers.

Kovelman, J.A. and Scheibel, A.B. (1984). A neurohistological correlate of schizophrenia. *Biological Psychiatry*, **19**, 1601–21.

Kubota, K. and Niki, H. (1971). Prefrontal cortical unit activity and delayed cortical unit activity and delayed alternation performance in monkeys. *Journal of Neurophysiology*, **34**, 337–47.

Lee, M.A., Thompson, P.A. and Meltzer, H.Y. (1994). Effects of clozapine on cognitive function in schizophrenia. *Journal of Clinical Psychiatry*, **55** Suppl B, 82–7.

Lee, T., Seeman, P., Tourtelotte, V.W. *et al.* (1978). Binding of ^{3}H-neuroleptics and ^{3}H-apomorphine in schizophrenic patients. *Nature*, **274**, 897–900.

Lees, A.J. and Smith, E. (1983). Cognitive deficits in the early stages of Parkinson's disease. *Brain*, **106**, 257–70.

Lewis, D.A. and Anderson, S.A. (1995). The functional architecture of the prefrontal cortex and schizophrenia. Editorial. *Psychological Medicine*, **25**, 887–94.

Lewis, S. (1990). Computerised tomography in schizophrenia 15 years on. *British Journal of Psychiatry*, **157** (suppl 9), 160–25.

Liddle, P., Friston, K.J., Frith, C.D. *et al.* (1992). Patterns of cerebral blood flow in schizophrenia. *British Journal of Psychiatry*, **160**, 179–86.

Lidow, M.S., Goldman-Rakic, P.S., Gallager, D.W. *et al.* (1991). Distribution of dopaminergic receptors in the primate cerebral cortex. *Neuroscience*, **40**, 657–71.

Lindstrom, L.H. (1988). The effect of long term treatment with clozapine in schizophrenia: a retrospective study in 96 patients treated with clozapine for up to 13 years. *Acta Psychiatrica Scandinavica*, **77**, S24–29.

Lindvall, O. and Bjorklund, A. (1974). The organisation of the ascending catecholamine neurone system in rat brain. *Acta Physiologica Scandinavica*, Suppl 412.

Lindvall, O. and Bjorklund, A. (1978). Organisation of the catecholamine neurones in the rat central nervous system. In *Handbook of Psychopharmacology*, **9**, (ed. L.L. Iversen, S.D. Iversen and S.H. Snyder). New York: Plenum Press.

Lines, C.R., Preston, G.C., Brocks, P. *et al.* (1991). The effects of scopolamine on retrieval from semantic memory. *Journal of Psychopharmacology*, **5**, 234–7.

Lipp, O.V. and Vaitl, D. (1992). Latent inhibition in human Pavlovian differential conditioning: effect of additional stimulation after preexposure and relation to schizotypal traits. *Personality and Individual Differences*, **13**, 1003–12.

Lubow, R.E. (1973). Latent inhibition. *Psychological Bulletin*, **79**, 398–407.

Lubow, R.E. (1989). *Latent Information and Conditioned Attention Theory*. Cambridge: Cambridge University Press.

Lubow, R.E. and Gewirtz, J.C. (1995). Latent inhibition in humans: data, theory, and implications for schizophrenia. *Psychological Bulletin*, **117**, 87–103.

Lubow, R.E., Ingberg-Sachs, Y., Zalstein-Orda, N. *et al.* (1992). Latent inhibition in low and high psychotic prone normal subjects. *Personality and Individual Differences*, **13**, 563–72.

Mackay, A.V.P., Iversen, L.L., Rossor, M. *et al.* (1982). Increased brain dopamine and dopamine receptors in schizophrenia. *Archives of General Psychiatry*, **39**, 991–7.

Mackintosh, N.J. (1975). A theory of attention: variations in the associability of stimuli with reinforcement. *Psychological Review*, **82**, 276–98.

Marin, D.B., Bierer, C.M., Lawlor, B.A. *et al.* (1995). L-Deprenyl and physostigmine for the treatment of Alzheimer's disease. *Psychiatry Research*, **58**, 181–9.

Martinot, J.-L., Peron-Magnan, P., Huret, J.-D. *et al.* (1990). Striatal D2 dopaminergic receptors assessed with positron emission tomography and [^{76}Br] Bromospiperone in untreated schizophrenic patients. *American Journal of Psychiatry*, **147**, 44–50.

McGregor, A., Baker, A.G. and Roberts, D.C.S. (1996). The effect of 6-hydroxy-dopamine lesions of the medial frontal cortex on intravenous cocaine self administration under a progressive ratio of reinforcement. *Pharmacology, Biochemistry and Behaviour*, **53**, 5–10.

McKenna, P., Tamlyn, D., Lund, C. *et al.* (1990). Amnesic syndrome in schizophrenia. *Psychological Medicine*, **20**, 967–72.

Meadow-Woodruff, J.H., Mansour, A., Saul, J. *et al.* (1994). Neuroanatomical distribution of dopamine receptor messenger RNAs. In *Domamine Receptors and Transporters: Pharmacology, Structure and Function* (ed. H.B. Niznik), pp. 403–15. New York: Dekker.

Melchitzky, D.S. Pucak, M.L., Dammerman, R.S. *et al.* (1994). Morphology and extrisic targets of pyramidal neurones furnishing intra-renal connections in monkey prefrontal cortex. *Society for Neuroscience Abstracts*, **20**, 1416.

Meltzer, H.Y. (1992). Clozapine: pattern of efficacy in treatment-resistant schizophrenia. In *Novel Antipsychotic Drugs* (ed. H.Y.Meltzer). New York: Raven Press.

Meltzer, H.Y. (1995). Clozapine: is another view valid? *American Journal of Psychiatry*, **152**, 821–5.

Meltzer, H.Y., Bastani, B., Kwon, K.Y. *et al.* (1989). A prospective study of clozapine in treatment-resistant schizophrenic patients, I: preliminary report. *Psychopharmacology*, **99**, S68–S72.

Miller, D.D., Perry, P.J., Cadoret, R.J. *et al.* (1994). Clozapine effects on negative symptoms in treatment-refractory schizophrenia. *Comprehensive Psychiatry*, **35**, 8–15.

Morice, R. and Delahunty, A. (1996). Frontal/executive impairments in schizophrenia. *Schizophrenia Bulletin*, **22**, 125–37.

Morrison-Stewart, S., Williamson, P., Corning, W. *et al.* (1992). Frontal and non-frontal neuropsychological test performance and clinical symptomatology in schizophrenia. *Psychological Medicine*, **22**, 353–9.

Murphy, B.L., Arnsten, A.F.T., Goldman-Rakic, P.S. *et al.* (1996). Increased dopamine turnover in the prefrontal cortex impairs spatial working memory performance in rats and monkeys. *Proceedings of the National Academy of Sciences USA*, **93**, 1325–9.

Murray, A.M., Hyde, T.M., Knable, M.B. *et al.* (1995). Distribution of putative D4 dopamine receptors in post mortem striatum from patients with schizophrenia. *Journal of Neuroscience*, **15**, 2186–91.

Nakai, T., Kitamura, N., Hashimoto, T. *et al.* (1991). Decreased histamine H1 receptors in the frontal cortex of brains from patients with schizophrenia. *Biological Psychiatry*, **30**, 349–56.

Nasrallah, H.A., Jacoby, C.G., McCalley-Whitters, M. *et al.* (1982). Cerebral ventricula enlargement in subtypes of chronic schizophrenia. *Archives of General Psychiatry*, **39**, 774–7.

Nasrallah, H.A., Caffman, J.A., Schwarzkopf, S.B. *et al.* (1990). Reduced cerebral volume in schizophrenia. *Schizophrenia Research*, **3**, 17.

Oades, R.D., Bunk, D. and Eggers, C. (1992). Paranoid schizophrenics may not use irrelevant signals. The use of measures of blocking and urinary dopamine. *Acta Paedopsychiatrica*, **55**, 183–4.

Owen, A., James, M., Leigh, P. *et al.* (1992). Fronto-striatal cognitive deficits at different stages of Parkinson's disease. *Brain*, **115**, 1727–51.

Owen, A.M., Sahakian, B.J., Hodges, J.R. *et al.* (1995). Dopamine-dependent fronto-striatal planning deficits in early Parkinson's disease. *Neuropsychology*, **9**, 126–40.

Owen, F., Crow, T.J., Poulter, M. *et al.* (1978). Increased dopamine receptor sensitivity in schizophrenia. *Lancet*, **ii**, 223–5.

Owens, D., Johnstone, E. and Frith, C. (1982). Spontaneous involuntary disorders of movement: their prevelance, severity and distribution in chronic schizophrenics with and without treatment with neuroleptics. *Archives of General Psychiatry*, **39**, 452–61.

Pantelis, C., Barnes, T. and Nelson, H. (1992). Is the concept of subcortical dementia relevant to schizophrenia? *British Journal of Psychiatry*, **160**, 442–60.

Pantelios, C., Barnes, T., Nelson, H. *et al.* (1993). The nature of dementia in schizophrenia. *Schizophrenia Research*, **9**, 184.

Park, S. and Holzman, P.S. (1992). Schizophrenics show spatial working memory deficts. *Archives of General Psychiatry*, **49**, 975–82.

Park, S. and Holzman, P.S. (1993). Association of working memory deficit and eye tracking dysfunction in schizophrenia. *Schizophrenia Research*, **11**, 55–61.

Perry, E.K., Perry, R.H., Blessed, G. *et al.* (1977). Necropsy evidence of cerebral cholinergic deficits in senile dementia. *Lancet*, **ii**, 1–89.

Perry, E.K., Tomlinson, B.E., Blessed, G. *et al.* (1978). Correlation of cholinergic abnormalities with senile plaques and mental test scores in senile dementia. *British Medical Journal*, **2**, 1457–9.

Perry, W. and Braff, D.L. (1994). Information-processing deficits and thought disorder in schizophrenia. *American Journal of Psychiatry*, **151**, 363–7.

Pickar, D., Owen, R.R., Litman, R.E. *et al.* (1992). Clinical and biologic responses to clozapine in patients with schizophrenia: crossover comparison with fluphenazine. *Archives of General Psychiatry*, **49**, 345–53.

Pilowsky, L. (1992). Clozapine, single photon emission tomography and the D2 dopamine receptor blockage hypothesis of schizophrenia. *Lancet*, **340**, 199–202.

Pilowsky, L.S., Costa, D.C., Ell, P.J. *et al.* (1994). D2 dopamine receptor binding in the basal ganglia of antipsychotic-free schizophrenic patients. *British Journal of Psychiatry*, **164**, 16–26.

Reynolds, G.P. (1983). Increased concentrations and lateral assymetry of amygdala dopamine in schizophrenia. *Nature*, **305**, 527–9.

Robbins, T. (1990). The case for frontostriatal dysfunction in schizophrenia. *Schizophrenia Bulletin*, **16**, 391–401.

Robbins, T.W. and Everitt, B.J. (1992). Functions of dopamine in the dorsal and ventral striatum. In *Seminars in the Neurosciences*, **4**, (ed. T.W. Robbins), pp. 119–28. London: Saunders Scientific Publishers.

Roth, R.H., Tam, S.Y., Ida, Y. *et al.* (1988). *Annals of the New York Academy of Sciences*, **537**, 138–47.

Rusted, J.M. (1988). Dissociative effects of scopolamine on working memory in healthy young volunteers. *Psychopharmcology*, **96**, 487–92.

Sahakian, B.J. (1988). Cholinergic drugs and human cognitive performance. In *Handbook of Psychopharmacology* (ed. L.L. Iversen, S.D. Iversen and S.H. Snyder), pp. 393–424. New York: Plenum Press.

Sahakian, B.J. and Owen, A.M. (1992). Computerised assessment in neuropsychiatry using CANTAB: discussion paper. *Journal of the Royal Society of Medicine*, **85**, 399–402.

Sawaguchi, T. and Goldman-Rakic, P.S. (1991). D1 dopamine receptors in prefrontal cortex: involvement in working memory. *Science*, **251**, 947–50.

Saykin, A., Gur, R., Gur, R. *et al.* (1991). Neuropsychological function in schizophrenia. *Archives of General Psychiatry*, **48**, 618–24.

Saykin, A., Shtasel, D.L., Gur, R.E. *et al.* (1994). Neuropsychological deficts in neuroleptic naive patients with first-episode schizophrenia. *Archives of General Psychiatry*, **51**, 124–31.

Schultz, W. (1992). Activity of dopamine neurones in the behaving primate. In *Seminars in the Neurosciences*, **4**, (ed. T.W. Robbins), pp. 129–38. London: Saunders Scientific Publishers.

Schwartz, J.C., Giros, B., Martres, M.-P. *et al.* (1992). The dopamine receptor family: molecular biology and pharmacology. In *Milestones in Dopamine Research* (ed. T.W. Robbins), pp. 99–108. London: Saunders Scientific Publishers.

Seeman, P. and Van Tol, H.M. (1994). Dopamine receptor pharmacology. *Trends in Pharmacological Sciences*, **15**, 264–70.

Seeman, P., Guan, H.-C. and Van Tol, H.H.M. (1993). Dopamine D4 receptors elevated in schizophrenia. *Nature*, **365**, 441–5.

Seeman, P., Lee, T., Chan-Wong, M. *et al.* (1976). Antipsychotic drug doses and neuroleptic/dopamine receptors. *Nature*, **261**, 717–19.

Shaikh, S., Collier, D.A., Sham, P.C. *et al.* (1996). Allelic association between a Ser-9-Gly polymorphism in the dopamine D3 receptor gene and schizophrenia. *Human Genetics*, **97**, 714–19.

Shallice, T. (1988). *From Neuropsychology to Mental Structure*. Cambridge: Cambridge University Press.

Shallice, T., Burgess, P. and Frith, C. (1991). Can the neuropsychological case study approach be applied to schizophrenia? *Psychological Medicine*, **21**, 661–73.

Sibley, D.R. and Monsma, F.J. (1992). Molecular biology of dopamine receptors. *Trends in Pharmacological Sciences*, **13**, 61–9.

Simpson, M.D.C., Slater, P., Royston, M.C. *et al.* (1992). Regionally selective deficits in uptake sites for glutamate and gamma aminobutyric acid in the basal ganglia in schizophrenia. *Psychiatry Research*, **42**, 273–82.

Sokoloff, P., Lannfelt, L., Martres, M.P. *et al.* (1992). The third dopamine receptor (D3) as a novel target for antipsychotics. *Biochemistry and Pharmacology*, **43**, 659–66.

Solomon, P.R., Crider, A., Winkelman, J.W. *et al.* (1981). Disrupted latent inhibition in the rat with chronic amphetamine or haloperidol-induced supersensitivity:relationship to schizophrenic attention disorder. *Biological Psychiatry*, **16**, 519–37.

Stahl, S.M., Iversen, S.D. and Goodman, E.C. (1987). *Cognitive Neurochemistry*. Oxford: Oxford University Press.

Swerdlow, N., Braff, D., Geyer, M. *et al.* (1986). Central dopamine hyperactivity in rats mimics abnormal acoustic startle response in schizophrenics. *Biological Psychiatry*, **21**, 23–33.

Swerdlow, N.R., Benbow, C.H., Zisook, S. *et al.* (1993). A preliminary assessment of sensorimotor gating in patients with obsessive compulsive disorder. *Biological Psychiatry*, **33**, 298–301.

Swerdlow, N.R., Braff, D.L., Taaid, N. *et al.* (1994). Assessing the validity of an animal model of sensorimotor gating in schizophrenic patients. *Archives of General Psychiatry*, **51**, 139–54.

Swerdlow, N.R., Braff, D.L., Hartston, H. *et al.* (1996). Latent inhibition in schizophrenia. *Schizophrenia Research*, **20**, 91–103.

Taylor, A.E., Saint-Cyr, J.A. and Lang, A.E. (1986). Frontal lobe dysfunction in Parkinson's disease – the cortical focus of neostriatal outflow. *Brain*, **109**, 845–83.

Ungerstedt, U. (1971). Stereotaxic mapping of the monoamine pathaways in the rat brain. *Acta Physiologica Scandinavica*, Suppl 367, 49–68.

Van Tol, H.H.M. (1991). Cloning of the gene for human D4 receptor with high affinity for the antipsychotic clozapine. *Nature*, **350**, 616–19.

Voorn, P., Jorritsma-Byham, B., Van Dijk, C. *et al.* (1986). The dopaminergic innervation of the ventral striatum in the rat; a light and electron-microscopal study with antibodies against dopamine. *Journal of Comparative Neurology*, **251**, 507–21.

Warburton, D.M. and Rusted, J.M. (1993). Cholinergic control of cognitive resources. *Neuropsychobiology*, **28**, 43–6.

Weinberger, D.R., Berman, K.F. and Zec, R.F. (1986). Physiological dysfunction of the dorsolateral prefrontal cortex in schizophrenia. I. Regional cerebral blood flow (rCBF) evidence. *Archives of General Psychiatry*, **43**, 114–25.

Weiner, I. (1990). Neural substrates of latent inhibition: the switching model. *Psychological Bulletin*, **108**, 442–61.

Weiner, I., Lubow, R.E. and Feldon, J. (1981). Chronic amphetamine and latent inhibition. *Behavioural Brain Research*, **2**, 285–6.

Weiner, I., Lubow, R.E. and Feldon, J. (1984). Abolition of the expression but not the acquisition of latent inhibition by chronic amphetamine in rats. *Psychopharmacology*, **83**, 194–9.

Williams, G.V. and Goldman-Rakic, P.S. (1995). Modulation of memory fields by dopamine D1 receptors in prefrontal cortex. *Nature*, **376**, 572–5.

Williams, J.H., Wellman, N.A., Geaney, D.P. *et al.* (1996). Latent inhibition is not reduced in drug free patients with schizophrenia. *Schizophrenia Research*, **18**, 205.

Wilson, C.J. and Groves, P.M. (1980). Fine structure and synaptic connections of the common spiny neurone of the rat neostriatum: a study employing intracellular injection of horseradish peroxidase. *Journal of Comparative Neurology*, **194**, 599–615.

Wong, D.F., Wagner, H.N., Tune, L.E. *et al.* (1986). Positron emission tomography reveals elevated D2 dopamine receptors in drug-naive schizophrenics. *Science*, **234**, 1558–63.

Yee, B.K., Feldon, J. and Rawlins, J.N. (1995). Latent inhibition in rats is abolished by NMDA-induced neuronal loss in the retrohippocampal region, but this lesion effect can be prevented by systemic haloperidol treatment. *Behavioural Neuroscience*, **109**, 227–40.

Young, A.M., Joseph, M.H. and Gray, J.A. (1993). Latent inhibition of conditioned dopamine release in rat nucleus accumbens. *Neuroscience*, **54**, 5–9.

Section III

Memory and its disorders

5

Neuropsychology of memory and amnesia

ANDREW R. MAYES

Introduction

The amnesia syndrome is only one of the memory disorders that can be caused by brain damage, Lesions in different brain regions can, in fact, cause memory to break down in several distinct ways. The resultant memory syndromes can be divided into the following groups: (a) disorders of immediate memory, (b) disorders of previously well-established, primarily semantic memory, (c) memory disorders caused by damage to the prefrontal association neocortex, (d) the amnesic syndrome, (e) disorders of skill learning and memory, (f) disorders of classical conditioning, and (g) disorders of non-associative kinds of memory, (f) disorders of classical conditioning, and (g) disorders of non-associative kinds of memory, such as habituation (see Mayes, 1988). This categorisation of the kinds of memory disorder assumes that the disorders within each group have more in common with each other than they do with disorders in other groups. For example, there is evidence to suggest that dissociable deficits in immediate memory for different types of information are caused by lesions to adjacent association neocortical regions that share similar neural architecture and this architecture differs radically from that of the basal ganglia and cerebellum where differently located lesions are believed to cause deficits in various forms of skill learning and memory.

Organic amnesia is a syndrome with four major features. First, patients show anterograde amnesia in which there is impaired recall and recognition of post-morbidly experienced facts and personal episodes. Second, they show retrograde amnesia in which there is impaired recall and recognition for pre-morbidly experienced facts and personal episodes. Third, they may show preservation of intelligence. Fourth, they may show preservation of short-term or immediate memory as assessed by the digit span or Corsi blocks tests. These features can be found following lesions to any one of several interconnected brain regions including the medial temporal lobes, the midline diencephalon, and the basal forebrain (see Mayes, 1988). The syndrome has a variety of aetiologies including not only infarctions that affect the blood vessels supplying these regions, but also anoxia, viral infections of the brain (such as that caused by herpes simplex), chronic alcoholism and other conditions associated with thiamine deficiency, invasive tumours within the critical structures, and the rupture and repair of aneurysms of certain cerebral arteries (and possibly the anterior communicating artery in particular, although recent evidence does not support this specific association). Anterograde and retrograde amnesia also typically occur after severe closed head injury and early in Alzheimer's disease although this dementing condition disrupts intelligence and immediate memory as well. Amnesia is, in fact, a common result of brain damage although in 'pure' form (in which intelligence and immediate memory are preserved) it is much rarer.

When information is recalled or recognised, rememberers are aware that they have encountered it in one or more situations in the past. For this reason, such forms of remembering are referred to as explicit or declarative memory. Explicit memory is contrasted with implicit memory in which rememberers are unaware that the remembered information was encountered in one or more situations in the past, but display signs of memory through changes in the way they process or behave towards the remembered information. Amnesia is, therefore, defined as a particular kind of explicit memory disorder for pre- and post-morbidly experienced facts and events. Research aims to resolve whether (a) the syndrome comprises one or several functional deficits, (b) what the exact characteristics of this or these deficits is or are, and (c) what lesions cause the deficit or deficits. It remains unresolved, however, whether the deficits characteristic of amnesia are dissociable and, therefore, whether one or more than one kind of functional deficit underlies the syndrome. The precise characterisation of this or these functional deficits also remains unresolved. Relevant to the resolution of these issues is the neuroanatomy of amnesia because the precise location of the lesions within the medial temporal lobes, midline diencephalon and basal forebrain may help determine whether one or more deficits underlie amnesia, and perhaps even what their characteristics are likely to be.

The neuroanatomy of amnesia

The detailed characterisation of the anatomy of amnesia is still controversal. Although it is believed that the syndrome is caused by lesions to the medial temporal lobes, the midline diencephalon, or the basal forebrain, it is uncertain to which structures within these regions the critical damage occurs. Work with humans has been hampered because brain lesions are adventitious and rarely selectively damage one structure. Relatively few patients have been described in whom there was fairly selective brain damage, detailed neuropsychological assessment, and post-mortem assessment of the brain damage. This situation has, however, been improved in recent years by the advent of much more sophisticated means of imaging the structure and function of living brains. Given the problems with human patients, the use of monkey and other animal models of amnesia has provided an important avenue for exploring the neuroanatomy of the syndrome in recent years (see Zola-Morgan and Squire, 1993). Such models have the advantage of enabling specific lesions to be made, but face the difficulty of establishing that the same memory processes have been affected in the animal models as are disrupted in human amnesics. Indeed, Horel (1994) has questioned whether many of the lesion effects are mnemonic at all. He challenges the widely believed view that lesioned animals are more impaired after a delay of 30 seconds or longer than they are after a minimal delay of between zero and few seconds when appropriate control procedures are used. Such an interaction is essential otherwise the deficit might be simply the result of a processing problem.

Within the medial temporal lobes, it has been claimed by Squire (1992) that amnesia can be caused by hippocampal, but not by amygdala lesions. In addition, he has claimed that parahippocampal and perirhinal cortex lesions cause severe amnesia. These claims have been largely based on work with a monkey model of amnesia that focuses on recognition tasks (see Zola-Morgan and Squire, 1993) and have been challenged by Horel (1994). They have been insufficiently explored in humans although Zola-Morgan, Squire, and Amaral (1986) have described a patient, who suffered bilateral damage to the CA1 field of the hippocampus following an ischemic episode that caused an anterograde amnesia of moderate severity, but no measurable retrograde amnesia. It is, however, impossible to exclude the possibility that the patient also suffered undetected cortical damage from the anoxia that damaged his hippocampus (see Horel,1994). Post-encephalitic amnesics with damage to hippocampus, amygdala, parahippocampal and perirhinal cortices, which may also extend to other cortical structures, show a far more severe anterograde amnesia and often a devastatingly severe retrograde amnesia. Finally, although evidence from monkeys shows that selective amygdala damage does not contribute to an impairment on delayed nonmatching to sample performance, the few extant case studies of humans with selective amygdala damage suggest that damage to this structure causes recall and recognition deficits for non-verbal material (for example, see Tranel and Hyman, 1990). Amygdala damage and damage to its downstream diencephalic connections might, therefore, exacerbate at least the non-verbal amnesia shown by patients with medial temporal lobe lesions.

The parahippocampal and perirhinal polysensory association cortices provide about two-thirds of the input to the hippocampus, which itself sends projections back to them as well as to other polysensory cortices that feed it with processed sensory information. Amnesia might, therefore, result from damage to any part of this system. This is most unlikely to be a complete account of amnesia, however, because it not only ignores the role of the diencephalic and basal forebrain structures believed to be implicated in amnesia as well as the possible contributory role of the amygdala in non-verbal amnesia, but also ignores the strong evidence that suggests that damage to the parahippocampal and perirhinal cortices produces a far more severe amnesia than does hippocampal damage. Damage to these cortices may cause a more severe amnesia than hippocampal lesions for one or both of two reasons. First, as they also send backprojections to earlier stages of sensory processing, a lesion to them is likely to cause a much more severe disruption of the backprojected information than would a lesion further downstream in the hippocampus. Provided the backprojected information is involved in memory processing, as seems likely, then a more severe amnesia should result from parahippocampal and perirhinal cortex lesions than from hippocampal lesions. Second, these cortices may project to midline thalamic nuclei, involved in memory processing, that do not form part of the hippocampal circuit.

If the amnesic syndrome can be caused by lesions to a polysensory cortex–hippocampal loop and separately by lesions to a polysensory cortex–non-hippocampal–midline diencephalic loop, the older view that it can also be caused by damage to a downstream hippocampal circuit should not be ignored. This third circuit, damage to which may cause amnesia, is the downstream projection path from the hippocampus to the midline diencephalon. It runs from the hippocampus via the fornix directly to the mammillary bodies and the anterior thalamus (which also receives an indirect projection via the mammillothalamic tract). There is evidence that links damage to each of these structures with memory disturbances that have at least some of the features of organic amnesia. Thus, Hodges and Carpenter (1991) found that fornix damage following removal of a third ventricle colloid cyst was associated with an anterograde amnesia primarily comprising a recall deficit. Gaffan (1992) has argued, however, that fornix lesions in monkeys and humans disrupt recognition for previously encountered complex scenes, a form of recognition that centrally involves spatial memory. Dusoir *et al.* (1990) studied a patient with a penetrating paranasal injury, which magnetic resonance imaging (MRI) showed had primarily damaged the mammillary bodies, and found similar effects to those that have been described following fornix lesions. Their patient was impaired on tests of free recall, but relatively normal on recognition tests, and gave no indication of having a severe retrograde amnesia. Some evidence also links lesions of the anterior thalamic nucleus to amnesia although it is unlikely that any lesion is completely specific to this structure. Daum and Ackerman (1994) have formally assessed a woman with bilateral ischemic damage affecting the blood supply of the paramedian thalamic artery. The damage was shown by MRI to have primarily affected the anterior thalamic region of the patient, who showed recognition as well as recall deficits. One of the issues that requires much more detailed study is the extent to which hippocampal, fornix, mammillary body and anterior thalamic lesions cause recognition as well as recall deficits. Midline thalamic lesions to structures that do not form part of the hippocampal circuit may also cause memory deficits (for example, see Mennemeier *et al.*, 1992), although it remains to be shown whether or not these deficits are amnesic in kind. If they are, it would be of interest to determine whether the lesions responsible are to structures that receive projections from the parahippocampal and/or perirhinal cortices.

It remains uncertain how the downstream hippocampal and non-hippocampal circuits through the midline diencephalon are routed back to the medial temporal lobe (if indeed they are). The midline thalamic nuclei do, of course, have projections to the prefrontal association cortex, and the anterior thalamus is known to project back to the medial temporal lobe area. It has reciprocal connections to the posterior cingulate and retrosplenial cortices, both of which are densely interconnected with the hippocampus. A case study has shown that retrosplenial cortex lesions may cause a mild memory deficit that has some of the features of the full amnesia syndrome, although the fornix may also have been damaged in the patient described (Valenstein *et al.*, 1987) and Cramon and Schuri (1992) have argued that retrosplenial lesions may not cause a permanent amnesia.

There has also been very little research on the effects on memory of basal forebrain lesions in humans. Some evidence exists that implicates septal lesions in the production of an amnesic-like memory deficit. Thus, Berti, Arienta and Papagno (1990) have described a patient who suffered a lesion that damaged the upper part of the septum, but may have spared the diagonal band of Broca following the removal of a tumour. This patient displayed a moderate degree of anterograde amnesia that persisted for at least four months after surgery. Rupture and repair of anterior communicating artery aneurysms can also damage the septum as well as other structures within the basal forebrain, and is known to cause amnesia sometimes. For example, Phillips, Sangalang and Sterns (1992) reported anterograde amnesia in a case who, at post-mortem, was shown to have suffered damage to the septum, the diagonal band of Broca, and the nucleus accumbens, but not the nucleus basalis of Meynert. Cramon and Schuri (1992) have argued that lesions to basal forebrain structures such as the septum may cause an amnesic-like disturbance because they disrupt the modulation of the hippocampus that these structures normally perform. There is evidence that disruption of such modulation can cause functional disruptions that are just as severe as lesions to the structures of which the activity is being modulated (T.W. Robbins, personal communication). If so, basal forebrain lesions may sometimes cause quite severe amnesia.

The current picture of the neuroanatomy of amnesia is, therefore, unclear. It needs to be determined by systematic study whether lesions to the structures discussed above really cause a complete amnesic syndrome, a partial amnesic syndrome, or a different kind of memory deficit. Only when this has been decided will it be possible to say whether amnesia is caused by damage to one or more circuits, and hence whether it is likely to be underlain by more than one kind of functional deficit. At present, it remains an open possibility that separate damage to a polysensory cortex–hippocampal circuit, to the hippocampal–fornix–midline diencephalic circuit, and to a polysensory cortex–non-hippocampal midline diencephalic circuit could each cause distinct memory deficits, some or all of which are found in most amnesics.

If identifying the structural lesions that cause amnesia has the potential to throw light on the functional deficits that underlie the syndrome, so has the ability to demonstrate metabolic changes in neural systems that are structurally intact in patients. For example, in one study by Levasseur *et al.* (1992) of patients with midline thalamic lesions and varying degrees of amnesia following paramedian thalamic infarcts, a reduced level of oxygen metabolism in the cerebral cortex was shown in a Positron Emission Tomography (PET) study. A similar study of Korsakoff patients, who also have midline diencephalic lesions, by Paller *et al.* (1993) found that these patients also show a widespread reduction in metabolic activity in the neocortex. One interpretation of these results is that one cause of the memory deficits produced by at least some midline diencephalic lesions is a reduction of efficiency in the cortical systems that process and store much, if not all, episodic and semantic information. This reduction may be sufficient to impair memory processing of such information without significantly disrupting its initial encoding. PET studies may also be useful in identifying the regions where structural damage may cause amnesia. For example, in a PET study of cerebral glucose metabolism in a mixed group of amnesics, Perani *et al.* (1993) showed that the patients revealed hypometabolism in the hippocampus, thalamus, cingulate, and frontal basal cortex. This study failed to find clear evidence of a global reduction in neocortical metabolism and, therefore, differs from the studies by Levasseur *et al.* (1992) and Paller *et al.* (1993). Clearly, more work with this promising approach needs to be done before unequivocal conclusions can be drawn, but it should be possible to determine whether lesions in the hypothetically distinct neural systems implicated in amnesia are associated with different regional patterns of hypometabolism, and hence whether several functional deficits may underlie the syndrome.

Theories of the functional deficit(s) and what they predict

It remains uncertain, therefore, whether the amnesic syndrome comprises one or more functional deficits. Functional deficit theories have nearly all assumed that there is only one underlying deficit so if it turns out that the symptoms of the syndrome can be dissociated, these theories will have to be modified. However, all hypotheses about the functional deficit that underlies amnesia must postulate a disruption of the encoding, storage, and/or retrieval of some or all components of information about facts and personally experienced episodes. Although encoding deficits may contribute to the memory deficits of amnesics with additional cognitive impairments (such as Alzheimer disease patients), there is little reason to believe that encoding deficits are a feature of amnesia *per se*. Not only is poor encoding hard to reconcile with patients' preserved intelligence, but their memory also improves to the same degree as does that of normal subjects when they are encouraged to process information semantically (see Mayes, 1988). When amnesics are asked unpredictable questions about briefly displayed complex pictures immediately after the pictures are removed, it has been shown that they are able to answer questions about the pictures' meaning and about items' spatial location, colour and size as well as their control subjects (Mayes *et al.* 1993). Normal performance was found in amnesic patients with probable lesions in the medial temporal lobes, the midline diencephalon, and the basal forebrain. It therefore seems likely that amnesics encode information at the same rate as and in the same manner as normal people unless they have additional brain damage that affects the ability to represent incoming sensory information in a rich manner. Amnesia must then be caused by a failure to store and/or a failure to retrieve some or all aspects of fact and event information.

At present, storage deficit accounts of amnesia seem to be dominant (for example, see Squire, 1992). Such accounts can differ from each other in several ways (see Mayes, 1988). One way relates to the nature of the storage deficit. Damage to some or all of the structures implicated in amnesia is postulated on one account to disrupt the modulation of storage processes that take place in the association neocortex. (This account might be derived from some of the PET data described at the end of the last section.) The effect of this disruption is that storage is very deficient. An alternative and more widely held view is that key aspects of fact and event information are held initially in the hippocampus, but that, with the passage of time, these memories are transferred to the association neocortex (for example, see Squire, 1992). The work of Zola-Morgan and Squire (1990) has suggested that, in monkeys, medial temporal cortex lesions only disrupt memories that were acquired up to around four weeks before the lesions. This work requires replication but, if correct, it would be consistent with transfer of storage to neocortex in a fairly short period of time. Unless the temporal characteristics of transfer are different in humans, there would be a severe problem in explaining retrograde amnesias that extend back 20 or 30 years before the occurrence of brain damage, as is found with many human amnesics.

Another way in which storage deficit hypotheses about amnesia differ is with respect to what aspects of fact and event information they postulate are not stored properly. Many accounts are not at all clear on this issue so that it is plausible to suppose that the accounts intend to claim that all aspects of fact and event information are inadequately stored. To deny this would be to claim that these accounts postulate that some aspects of fact and event information are stored normally. One hypothesis that does make exactly this assumption is the context-memory deficit hypothesis (CMDH) of amnesia (see Mayes, Meudell and Pickering, 1985). This hypothesis makes a distinction between target information that lies at the focus of attention during a learning experience and the background context of this target information that typically receives far less attention. Exactly what kinds of information constitute context has never been clearly worked out, but it is usual to distinguish between spatiotemporal features that do not affect the meaningful interpretation of targets (independent context) and features that do influence the meaningful interpretation of targets (interactive context). Some versions of the CMDH postulate a selective storage deficit in some or all aspects of independent context (for example, see Gaffan, 1992), others concentrate more on interactive context (Warrington and Weiskrantz, 1982), whereas yet others postulate that storage of both kinds of context is impaired in amnesics. The CMDH postulates that amnesics are impaired at storing some or all aspects of a target item's context or the associations between the target and those contextual features, and as a result are impaired at recalling or recognising the target, which has been stored normally.

Recently, Eichenbaum, Otto and Cohen (1994) advanced another hypothesis that has many of the features of a storage deficit account that applies to specific components of fact and event information. They proposed that hippocampal lesions disrupt the ability to store particular kinds of flexible relational information that presumably incorporates certain complex contextual–target associations. Hippocampal–neocortical interactions are necessary to establish lasting memories of these relationships. It was also postulated that parahippocampal and perirhinal cortex lesions disrupt the workings of an intermediate memory store for specific items (presumably targets in the terminology of the CMDH). Such lesions would also prevent the ability of an intact hippocampus to store relational information because, of course, these polysensory cortices not only provide the major input of processed sensory information to the hippocampus, but also intermediate memory is necessary to help form many complex relational memories.

Although retrieval deficit accounts of amnesia used to be widely held (see, for example, Warrington and Weiskrantz, 1982, and Mayes, 1988 for discussions), they are currently far less influential than storage deficit hypotheses. Nevertheless, there has been little discussion of the evidence that is relevant for discriminating between these broad groups of hypotheses. Any hypothesis about the functional deficit underlying amnesia must be able to explain the pattern of memory performance shown by patients with the amnesic syndrome. Two aspects of memory performance found in patients offer a powerful means of discriminating between storage and retrieval deficit hypotheses. The first concerns areas of preserved memory in amnesia and the second concerns forgetting rate patterns in amnesia.

It is well known that amnesics show preservation of learning and memory for skills and classical conditioning (see Mayes, 1988). It is probable, however, that all this reveals is that classical conditioning and skill memory are radically different from recall and recognition of facts and events and are mediated by brain regions, such as the basal ganglia and cerebellum, that are organised in a very different way from the regions implicated in amnesia and are not involved in any way with the storage of facts and events. But it has also been claimed that amnesics show preservation of what might be referred to as item-specific implicit memory (ISIM). This is supposed to be a form of memory revealed by a change in the way that the rememberer processes repeated items or components of repeated items. This item-specific processing change does not involve the kind of awareness of pastness that is the central feature of explicit forms of memory such as recall and recognition. Also, unlike explicit memory, which involves effortful retrieval processes, implicit memory retrieval is believed to be automatic. But the key point is that implicit and explicit memory can be of apparently the same information. If amnesics show preservation of ISIM for information that was novel prior to learning, then it becomes plausible to argue that they must have stored this information normally even though they show very impaired explicit memory for it. In other words, to the extent that amnesics show preserved ISIM for novel information, they cannot be said to have a storage deficit, and, therefore, they must have a kind of retrieval deficit that prevents normal explicit memory being shown.

The only way to avoid this conclusion is to argue that the same information is held in different stores, one for implicit and one for explicit memory, with amnesics having a storage deficit that is selective for explicit memory. No one seems to hold this view. The recent reports that two patients showed a selective impairment of ISIM for perceptual information in the face of apparently normal recognition for the same verbal items (Gabrieli *et al.*, 1995; Keane *et al.*, 1995) does not prove that explicit and implicit memory for the same information is stored in different brain regions. Much more probably, it means that ISIM for verbal, perceptual items involves retrieving different information (such as perceptual features) from word recognition memory (which involves retrieval of more semantic information retrieval), or even if they do (contrary to majority opinion) involve retrieving the same information, the double dissociation arises because Gabrieli *et al.*'s and Keane *et al.*'s patients' lesions selectively disrupted the automatic retrieval route used by ISIM, whereas the lesions underlying amnesia disrupt the effortful retrieval route used by explicit memory. Only if a double dissociation between explicit memory and ISIM could be shown to result from two *storage* deficits would it be necessary to postulate a dual storage system. Nevertheless, it is difficult to avoid the conclusion that preservation of ISIM for previously novel information in amnesics shows that they can store fact and event information normally. If their ISIM is normal for all fact/event information (including perceptual, semantic and contextual features), all storage accounts of amnesia would be refuted, but if they only show impaired ISIM for novel contextual associations or complex relations, then the CMDH and Eichenbaum's hypothesis (at least of the hippocampus) would be respectively supported. It is, therefore, critical to determine whether amnesics show preservation of ISIM for some or all aspects of novel fact and event information.

Amnesics seem to encode facts and events normally and hold the encoded information normally in immediate memory, but, following distraction, an impairment in the ability to recall and recognise the same information becomes apparent. If this impairment is caused by a deficit in an explicit memory retrieval process, there is no clear reason to expect it to worsen as the learning–test delay is increased, that is, to expect amnesics to show accelerated forgetting. This would only be expected if amnesics show increased susceptibility to interference during the delay. For example, retroactive interference might build up in the delay to cause forgetting, the degree of which would depend on how much interference there was and how susceptible to it one was. It has been claimed that amnesics are more susceptible to interference. The claim rests on the use of a paradigm that depends on the learning of related paired associate words like 'soldier–rifle'. Subjects first learn an A–B list comprising items like 'soldier–rifle', and then learn an A–C list comprising items like 'soldier–army'. When tested on the A–B list using the first word as a cue for the second, it has been claimed that amnesics perform normally. But when tested on the A–C list, it has been claimed that they are abnormally sensitive to interference because they are grossly impaired and make many intrusion errors from the A–B list.

We examined this effect further under two conditions (Mayes, Pickering and Fairbain, 1987). In the first condition, at test subjects were shown the first words from the pairs one at a time and asked to do their best to *recall* which word had been presented with it in the earlier learning phase. In the second condition, at test subjects were again shown the first words from the pairs one at a time and asked to produce the first related associate word that came to mind. In the first condition, the amnesics showed worse cued recall of the A–C list and made more intrusion errors than did their control subjects just as had previously been reported. But, unlike in some of the earlier work, their memory was also worse for the A–B list. In the second condition, there was no difference between the two groups and they both performed on the A–C list like the amnesics had in the first condition. We interpreted this as showing that the amnesics had worse explicit memory on the A–B list and that their sensitivity to proactive interference arose because their performance depended on ISIM, which does not use contextual information, and so is very susceptible to proactive interference. When normal people also rely on ISIM, then they show a similar level of sensitivity to interference. There is, therefore, no direct evidence that amnesic explicit memory is any more sensitive to proactive and retroactive interference than is normal people's explicit memory. Given this, it is highly probable that a retrieval deficit account of amnesia should predict a normal rate of forgetting in patients following the initial distraction that reveals their explicit memory deficit.

If amnesia is caused by a deficit in the storage processes that lead to long-term memory, then it is plausible to argue that their explicit memory deficit should become more severe as consolidation into long-term memory progresses in normal people in the period after learning, that is, they should show accelerated forgetting. This would be the case whether amnesics fail to modulate consolidation processes in an optimal manner or whether their fact and event memories are initially maintained in a structure damaged in patients so as to impair the development of their long-term memories. The time scale over which forgetting might be expected to be accelerated is uncertain because this depends on the time course of the affected consolidation processes. This prediction leaves a major problem, which has been inadequately addressed in the literature. The problem concerns what supports memory whilst consolidation into long-term memory is occurring. However, although this problem is unsolved, its solution should not undermine the validity of the prediction of accelerated amnesic forgetting by storage deficit accounts. Which kinds of explicit memory should be lost at an accelerated rate should be a function of the storage deficit account. For example, if all aspects of fact and event information are deficiently stored, then forgetting should be accelerated for recall and recognition of any aspect of this information. If, on the other hand, the CMDH is correct, then forgetting should only be accelerated when it depends on explicitly retrieving contextual associations.

Item-specific implicit memory in amnesia

It is widely agreed that amnesics, regardless of aetiology (and, therefore, probable lesion location) show preserved item-specific implicit memory for verbal, non-verbal, and contextual information that was familiar prior to learning (for example, see Mayes, 1988; Priestley and Mayes, 1992). One popular way of explaining this pattern of results is to postulate that the learning experience activates an extant long-term memory, that the memory remains active for some time or is modified in some relatively long-lasting manner, so as to influence how items whose memories have been activated are processed at test. This does not require one to postulate that amnesics have stored new fact/event memories normally. Other accounts of familiar item implicit memory are, of course, possible, but it is very improbable that the creation of new memories of any kind is required although the strengthening of old memories is perhaps more likely to be involved than is continued activation of an otherwise unchanged memory trace as discussed above (because activation would have to persist for a very long time in many cases). It is, therefore, unwise to view the preservation of familiar item implicit memory in amnesia as support for their having preserved storage of new fact and event information.

The same cannot be said for ISIM for information that was novel prior to learning because memory for such information must depend on the creation of new memories. There is, however, greater doubt about whether amnesics show preserved implicit memory for all kinds of novel items. Some workers now believe that amnesics show impaired implicit memory for novel associations, particularly if these are semantic in nature (see Graf and Masson, 1993; Mayes and Downes, 1997 *passim*). For example, we and others have failed to find normal (indeed any) enhanced word-stem completion priming in amnesics (Mayes and Gooding, 1989). Performance on this test is likely to depend on memory for semantic associations between previously unassociated or weakly associated words so it might be argued that amnesics fail to store such associations whereas normal people do.

There is, however, a major interpretative problem which relates to how ISIM and explicit memory are measured. Implicit memory is tapped by indirect memory tasks in which no reference is made to memory or the learning experience and subjects' memories are revealed by how they process repeated items or components/associates of repeated items. In contrast, explicit memory is tapped by direct memory tasks in which reference is made to the learning experience and subjects are overtly asked to remember information encoded during that experience. It has been argued, however, that performance on both direct and indirect memory tasks may often (if not always) depend on both explicit and implicit memory to varying degrees, and explicit memory could be used to either enhance or inhibit performance on indirect memory tasks (Jacoby and Kelley, 1992). For example, amnesics have been reported to show a normal tendency to complete dot templates with previously shown patterns (Gabrieli *et al.*

1990). Although we have replicated this indirect memory test result at least with some measures of pattern completion (Gooding *et al.*, 1993), we have more recently found strong evidence that normal subjects' performance on this task seems to rely almost entirely on explicit memory (P.A. Gooding, A.R. Mayes and P.R. Meudell, submitted). We found this evidence of explicit memory mediation of task performance using a modified version of the task which provides a better method of measuring baseline effects. In order to try to explain the puzzle about why amnesics' performance on the original version of this indirect memory task seemed to be preserved, we are currently retesting a group of amnesics using the modified version of the task from which we derived evidence that normals' performance is based almost entirely on explicit memory. Although the experiment is not yet complete, the results to date strongly suggest that amnesics' performance is impaired.

If the impurity of item-specific indirect memory tests is to be taken seriously, then much current work on amnesia is hard to interpret. If amnesics' performance is normal, this could be because they have preservation of ISIM or because their controls are inhibiting their performance by using their superior explicit memory. Conversely, if patients' performance is impaired, this could be because their ISIM is deficient or because normal subjects are enhancing their performance by using their superior explicit memory.

To resolve the question of whether amnesic novel ISIM is preserved, it will be necessary to adopt a convergent operations approach in which similar results must be obtained using several procedures designed to minimise or control for the contribution of explicit memory to memory performance. These procedures could include: (a) tasks where implicit memory is indicated by a reduction in reaction time to repeated items so as to reduce the chances of explicit memory contributing to performance; (b) tasks where implicit memory is indicated by changed autonomic responses to repeated items; (c) tasks where attention is divided at test so as to prevent a significant contribution from explicit memory; (d) the use of a modified form of Jacoby's process dissociation procedure (see Jacoby and Kelley, 1992) to estimate the strengths of both explicit and implicit memory from task performance. All these procedures make different assumptions so one can only be confident about conclusions reached by using them when these conclusions are reasonably congruent.

We have developed a modified form of Jacoby's process dissociation procedure (Jacoby and Kelley, 1992) to examine explicit memory (recollection) and implicit-like memory (familiarity) in a recognition task. By using an inclusion condition in which scores comprise both explicitly and implicitly remembered items, and an exclusion condition in which scores comprise only items that are implicitly, but not explicitly remembered items, it is possible to calculate the explicit and implicit memory contributions provided one assumes the two kinds of memory are stochastically independent. Whereas Jacoby only corrects for familiarity false alarms, we also correct for recognition false alarms by using multidimensional signal detection theory (van Eijk, Mayes and Meudell, 1997).

Recently, we (R. van Eijk, D. Dewhurst and A.R. Mayes, in preparation) have applied this procedure to two versions of the famous names task (Jacoby, Woloshyn and Kelley, 1989) in one of which names were used and in the other of which faces were used. The central feature of this task is that subjects falsely attribute fame to studied previously unknown items because these items are familiar, but not recollected from the study episode. We found that an amnesic group with patients of several aetiologies showed very impaired recollection for both studied names and faces, but also a slight, but significant degree of impairment of familiarity memory. Other unpublished work with the modified procedure had previously shown familiarity (see van Eijk *et al.*, 1997), as is expected for implicit memory, is unaffected by dividing attention at test. It is likely that the information encoded at study was novel and required some new intra-item associations to be formed at least for the face stimuli. So our finding suggests that amnesics have mildly impaired implicit memory for some forms of novel item information that may require the storage of new intra-item associations between the components of novel items.

Before one can be confident about this conclusion, however, it would be desirable to assess implicit memory for the novel faces using procedures which rely on different assumptions from Jacoby's modified procedure. One might, for example, examine whether amnesics also show a preserved ability to discriminate autonomically between unknown faces that have been studied and similar ones that have not been. Diamond, Mayer and Mendell (1996) have found that amnesics are able to discriminate autonomically between repeated and non-repeated words as well as normal people, but this has not been shown for items that were entirely novel prior to study. The convergent operations approach needs to be applied to determine whether amnesics fail to show preservation of ISIM for novel complex associations. At present, our results weakly suggest that amnesics may have mildly impaired ISIM for some kinds of novel information, and perhaps more severe ISIM deficits for complex associations across different items (see Mayes and Downes, 1997 *passim*).

Forgetting rate in amnesia

Nearly all work on amnesic forgetting rates has investigated rate of loss of recognition at delays beyond ten minutes with the intention of determining whether patients with medial temporal lobe lesions show a different pattern of memory breakdown than do patients with midline diencephalic lesions. In order to compare amnesic and normal forgetting rates, it was necessary to avoid floor and ceiling effects and possible scaling effects by matching patient and control recognition at the shortest delay used. This was achieved by allowing amnesics longer to learn the target material. So, for example, amnesics might receive eight-second exposures to each of 120 targets whereas their controls would be given only one-second exposures. A ten minute delay would then typically be given before testing recognition for a proportion of the items. This procedure gives rise to an artefact in which amnesic forgetting rates tend to be underestimated because the initial mean item presentation-to-test delay is actually longer for them than it is for their controls and forgetting rate tyically slows as a function of delay (see Mayes, 1988). So results of studies using the procedure are difficult to interpret with confidence. Nevertheless, it has to be said that there is little good evidence suggesting that patients with medial temporal lobe lesions lose the ability to recognise recently perceived items over delays between ten minutes and one week faster than do patients with midline diencephalic lesions. Indeed, there is little evidence to suggest that any amnesics lose the ability to recognise pictures and simple verbal material over these delays faster than do normal people.

There has been hardly any research that has looked at forgetting over shorter delays in amnesics and examined their rate of loss of free and cued recall as well as recognition. Recently, we have done this using short story material similar to that found in the Logical Memory subtest of the Wechsler Memory Scale (Isaac and Mayes, 1997*a*). A large number of these stories were matched for difficulty in a pilot study with student subjects. Recognition tests were constructed with a subset of the stories. These tests comprised test items that tapped memory for specific components of the stories. Amnesic free recall of the stories was matched to that of their controls after a filled delay of 15 seconds by giving the patients up to five presentations of each story compared to the controls' single presentation. Free recall of equivalent stories was tested after the same exposures at delays of one minute, two minutes, five minutes and ten minutes. Recognition was tested in the same way except that the delays used were 15 seconds, ten minutes and one hour because recognition was lost more slowly. During all of the longer delays for both recall and recognition tests, subjects were occupied with other tasks to minimise rehearsal. At the shortest delay, amnesics and their controls were matched on free recall and recognition performance, which suggests that these forms of explicit memory are equally impaired at this delay. After ten minutes, however, the amnesics had lost free recall, but not recognition, pathologically fast so that at this delay they were more impaired at free-recalling the stories than they were at recognising them.

One possible explanation of these results is that the normal subjects surreptitiously rehearsed during the longer delays despite having to perform the filler activities, and this specifically enhanced their free recall ability. The amnesics might have been less likely to try to do this because they would not remember that their memory would shortly be tested. To check this we tested an equivalent group of controls on the same stories at the ten minute delay when they had no expectation of a memory test and hence no motivation to rehearse. These subjects recalled no worse than the controls in the first experiment. Another possibility was that long-term memory free recall is lost at a normal rate in amnesics, but that at 15 seconds delay their free recall performance depends not only on long-term memory, but also on their residual, but normal, short-term memory. At the ten minute delay, performance might be mediated solely by long-term memory, which is impaired in the patients, and this would give the illusion that they have lost long-term memory pathologically fast. All the patients included in the experiment had suffered from amnesia of mild to moderate severity in order to be able to achieve a match at the short delay on recall. To test the other possibility, therefore, we presented the stories five times to three severely amnesic patients with normal short-term memories, and found that their story recall at the 15 seconds delay was either zero or negligible. This makes it unlikely that residual short-term memory could have been significantly assisting free recall at that delay.

We confirmed the main results in a second experiment in which we matched at a short filled delay of 20 seconds and tested free recall, cued recall, and recognition at ten minutes. When the cues provided some of the information that needed to be recalled, we found that cued recall, like recognition, was lost at a normal rate by the amnesics although free recall was lost pathologically fast. In a third experiment, we examined the effects of proactive interference on free recall at 15 second and one minute delays, and of retroactive interference on recognition at delays of ten minutes and one hour. In all cases, interference was produced by presentation of three stories that were very similar to the target story. Both amnesic and control memory was disrupted to a small and closely similar degree by the interference, which makes it hard to argue that the amnesic accelerated loss of free recall resulted from increased sensitivity to interference. The effects, found in the three experiments, occurred in amnesics of several aetiologies, who probably had lesions respectively in the medial temporal lobes, the midline diencephalon, and the basal forebrain. Lesion location, therefore did not seem to influence the degree to which loss of free recall was accelerated.

In order to determine whether this pattern of accelerated loss of free recall in amnesics also occurs with other kinds of material, Isaac and Mayes (1997*b*) repeated the story forgetting rate procedure with three kinds of word list: (a) unrelated word lists; (b) lists of semantically related words that are randomly arranged; (c) lists of related words that are arranged so as to facilitate the organization of their semantic encoding. The results with the two kinds of related word list were similar to those that we had already obtained with the stories, but with the unrelated word lists we found no evidence of accelerated loss of free or cued recall, or of recognition, in the amnesics. This result agrees with that of Haist, Shimamura and Squire (1992), who found that amnesic recall and recognition of unrelated word lists decays at a normal rate between delays of 15 seconds and up to two weeks.

Free recall of related word lists (and stories), but not of unrelated word lists, probably depends on forming complex associations between semantically related words and their encoding context whereas recognition of individual words does not depend on retrieving these complex associations. The most likely explanation of our results is that amnesics, regardless of lesion location, have a storage deficit for complex target-contextual associations that involve two or more targets. If this is correct, then recognition that depends on retrieving such complex associations should also decline at an accelerated rate in amnesics in the first ten minutes after learning. For example, if the pairs 'horse–chisel' and 'train–mountain' appeared in a list, amnesics should show accelerated loss of the ability to decide whether 'horse–chisel', 'horse–mountain' or 'horse–train' appeared in the list. This prediction remains to be tested.

Conclusion

It is clear that no consensus currently exists about the neuroanatomy of amnesia, the syndrome's possible functional heterogeneity, and the detailed characterisation of the functional deficit or deficits. A plausible speculative characterisation of the syndrome might, however, be as follows. First, damage to any part of the Papez circuit that includes the hippocampus, fornix, mammillary body, anterior thalamus, and possibly the cingulate and retrosplenial cortices disrupts the storage of complex associations between two or more attended items and their background context. This deficit only begins to become apparent around one minute following encoding, prior to which explicit memory is relatively normal. Explicit memory for simple associations and single items should be relatively normal. Some evidence to support this hypothesis can be gleaned from temporal lobe epilepsy. These patients can show relatively selective lateralised hippocampal sclerosis and Lencz *et al.* (1992) have shown a significant correlation between the volume of the left hippocampus and the rate at which stories are forgotten. Similar results relating left-sided hippocampal sclerosis to delayed, but not immediate story recall were reported by Miller, Munoz and Finmore (1993), who also reported normal word recognition memory. Further work needs to be done to confirm the relative normality of explicit memory tested shortly after encoding and the specificity of the delayed explicit memory deficit.

If the hippocampal circuit hypothesis is correct, then one would also predict that lesions to the circuit will impair ISIM for complex associations, which remains to be shown convincingly by finding convergent results from several sources of evidence. There is also a need to explain why all the amnesics in the Isaac and Mayes study showed impaired explicit memory for all fact and event material after filled delays of 15 seconds or less. To explain this one can propose a second kind of functional deficit. The proposal is that most or all amnesics also have damage to another circuit involving the parahippocampal and perirhinal cortices and their midline thalamic projections. Damage to this circuit disrupts retrieval from what Eichenbaum *et al.* (1994) have referred to as intermediate memory. Intermediate memory could hold information about single items and simple associations, reach its maximum strength within a few seconds and fade within a few minutes or less. Damage to such a memory system would be associated with an impairment in global explicit memory that would become apparent immediately following distraction, but not worsen as time passes. Such a deficit would be compatible with preservation of ISIM for simple forms of novel information and might also explain some aspects of retrograde amnesia.

Third, damage to parts of temporal association neocortex might affect the storage of memories acquired up to decades prior to the onset of brain damage and hence produce a retrograde amnesia. This is compatible with reports of selective retrograde amnesia following temporal association neocortex lesions (see Kapur, 1993). It may even be that differently located lesions cause retrograde amnesia for different kinds of memories as patients have been reported with selective retrograde amnesias. For example, McCarthy and Warrington (1992) described a patient whose memory for famous people and family friends was far better than for the specific episodes in which those people had appeared.

Coda

Since this chapter was written, there have been some important developments related to the heterogeneity of the amnesia syndrome. First, Aggleton and Shaw (1996) have conducted a meta-analysis in which they argued that selective lesions to the hippocampus, fornix, mammillary bodies or the anterior nucleus of the thalamus ('Papez circuit') minimally affect item-forced choice recognition, but disrupt free recall to about the same extent as is found in more globally impaired amnesics. Consistent with this argument, Baxendaele (1997) has shown that selective hippocampal sclerosis in epileptics impaired free recall, but not item recognition and, in unpublished work, my group has found similar results in a patient with selective hippocampal damage. Second, there is animal evidence that a double dissociation exists between the mnemonic effects of perirhinal cortex and 'Papez circuit' lesions, which suggests that the former is concerned with single items and perhaps simple associative memory whereas the latter is concerned with spatial and other kinds of associative memory. For example, Ennaceur *et al.* (1996) found that rats with fornix lesions showed spatial memory, but not object recognition, deficits whereas the reverse pattern was found following perirhinal cortex lesions. Third, there is some evidence that lesions to the temporal pole and prefrontal cortex can cause relatively selective retrograde amnesia (for example, see Kroll *et al.*, 1997) although, in my view, the underlying deficit remains to be elucidated.

References

Aggleton, J.P. and Shaw, C. (1996). Amnesia and recognition memory: a reanalysis of psychometric data. *Neuropsychologia*, **34**, 51–62.

Baxendaele, S.A. (1997). The role of the hippocampus in recognition memory. *Neuropsychologia*, **35**, 591–8.

Berti, A., Arienta, C. and Papagno, C. (1990). A case of amnesia after excision of the septum pellucidum. *Journal of Neurology, Neurosurgery and Psychiatry*, **53**, 922–4.

Cramon, D.Y. von and Schuri, U. (1992). The septo-hippocampal pathways and their relevance to human memory: A case report. *Cortex*, **28**, 411–22.

Daum, I. and Ackerman, H. (1994). Dissociation of declarative and nondeclarative memory after bilateral thalamic lesions: A case study. *International Journal of Neuroscience*, **75**, 153–65.

Diamond, B.J., Mayes, A.R. and Mendell, P.R. (1996). Autonomic and recognition indices of memory in amnesic and healthy control subjects. *Cortex*, **32**, 439–59.

Dusoir, H., Kapur, N., Byrnes, D. *et al.* (1990). The role of diencephalic pathology in human memory disorder: evidence from a penetrating paranasal brain injury. *Brain*, **113**, 1695–706.

Eichenbaum, H., Otto, T. and Cohen, N.J. (1994). Two component functions of the hippocampal memory system. *Behavioral and Brain Sciences*, **17**, 449–517.

Ennaceur, A., Neave, N. and Aggleton, J.P. (1996). Neurotoxic lesions of the perirhinal cortex do not mimic the behavioural effects of fornix transection in the rat. *Behavoural Brain Research*, **80**, 9–25.

Gabrieli, J.D.E., Milberg, W., Keane, M.M. and Corkin, S. (1990). Intact priming of patterns despite impaired memory. *Neuropsychologia*, **28**, 417–27.

Gabrieli, J.D.E., Fleischman, D.A., Keane, M.M. *et al.* (1995). Double dissociation between memory systems underlying explicit and implicit memory in the human brain. *Psychological Science*, **6**, 76–82.

Gaffan, D. (1992). The role of the hippocampal-fornix-mammillary system in episodic memory. In *Neuropsychology of Memory*, second edition (ed. L.R. Squire and N. Butters), pp. 336–46.

Gooding, P.A., Eijk, R. van, Mayes, A.R. and Meudell, P.R. (1993). Preserved pattern completion priming for novel abstract geometric shapes in amnesics of several aetiologies. *Neuropsychologia*, **31**, 789–810.

Graf, P. and Masson, M.E.J. (1993). *Implicit Memory*. Hove: Lawrence Erlbaum Associates.

Haist, F., Shimamura, A.P. and Squire, L.R. (1992). On the relationship between recall and recognition memory. *Journal of Experimental Psychology: Learning, Memory and Cognition*, **18**, 691–702.

Hodges, J.R. and Carpenter, K. (1991). Anterograde amnesia with fornix damage following removal of a third ventricle colloid cyst. *Journal of Neurology, Neurosurgery and Psychiatry*, **54**, 633–8.

Horel, J.A. (1994). Some comments on the special cognitive functions claimed for the hippocampus. *Cortex*, **30**, 269–80.

Isaac, C. and Mayes, A.R. (1997*a*). Rate of forgetting in amnesia. 1: Recall and recognition of prose, submitted.

Isaac, C. and Mayes, A.R. (1997*b*). Rate of forgetting in amnesia. 2: Recall and recognition of word lists with different levels of organization, submitted.

Jacoby, L.L. and Kelley, C. (1992). Unconscious influences of memory: dissociations and automaticity. In *The Neuropsychology of Consciousness* (ed. A.D. Milner and M.D. Rugg), pp. 201–33. London: Academic Press.

Jacoby, L.L., Woloshyn, V. and Kelley, C. (1989). Becoming famous without being recognized: unconscious influences of memory produced by dividing attention. *Journal of Experimental Psychology: General*, **118**, 115–25.

Kapur, N. (1993). Focal retrograde amnesia in neurological disease: a review. *Cortex*, **29**, 217–34.

Kroll, N.E.A., Markowitsch, H.J., Knight, R.T. and von Cramon, D.Y. (1997). Retrieval of old memories: the temporopolar hypothesis. *Brain*, **120**, 1377–99.

Keane, M.M., Gabrieli, J.D.E., Mapstone, H.C. *et al.* (1995). Double dissociation of memory capacities after bilateral occipital-lobe or medial temporal-lobe lesions. *Brain*, **118**, 1129–48.

Lencz, T., McCarthy, G., Bronen, R.A. *et al.* (1992). Quantitative magnetic resonance imaging in temporal lobe epilepsy: relationship to neuropathology and neuropsychological function. *Annals of Neurology*, **31**, 629–37.

Levasseur, M., Baron, J.C., Sette, G. *et al.* (1992). Brain energy metabolism in bilateral paramedian thalamic infarcts. *Brain*, **115**, 795–807.

McCarthy, R.A. and Warrington, E.K. (1992). Actors not scripts: the dissociation of people and events in retrograde amnesia. *Neuropsychologia*, **7**, 633–44.

Mayes, A.R. (1988). *Human Organic Memory Disorders*. Cambridge: Cambridge University Press.

Mayes, A.R. and Downes, J.J. (eds) (1997). Theories of organic amnesia. *Memory*, **5**, 1–315.

Mayes, A.R. and Gooding, P. (1989). Enhancement of word completion priming in amnesics by cueing with previously novel associates. *Neuropsychologia*, **27**, 1057–72.

Mayes, A.R., Meudell, P.R. and Pickering, A. (1985). Is organic amnesia caused by a selective deficit in remembering contextual information? *Cortex*, **21**, 167–202.

Mayes, A.R., Pickering, A. and Fairbairn, A. (1987). Amnesic sensitivity to proactive interference: its relationship to priming and the causes of amnesia. *Neuropsychologia*, **25**, 211–20.

Mayes, A.R., Downes, J.J., Shoqeirat, M. *et al.* (1993). Encoding ability is preserved in amnesia: evidence from a direct test of encoding. *Neuropsychologia*, **31**, 745–59.

Mennemeier, M., Fennell, E., Valenstein, E. and Valenstein, K.M. (1992). Contributions of the left intralaminar and medial thalamic nuclei to memory: comparisons and report of a case. *Archives of Neurology*, **49**, 1050–8.

Miller, L.A., Munoz, D.G. and Finmore, M. (1993). Hippocampal sclerosis and human memory. *Archives of Neurology*, **50**, 391–4.

Paller, K.A., Richardson, B.C., Shimamura, A.P. *et al.* (1993). Neurophysiological substrates of human memory impairments: altered regional cerebral glucose utilization in alcoholic Korsakoff's syndrome and Alzheimer's disease, as measured by positron emission tomography (PET). *Society for Neuroscience Abstracts*, **19**, 1078.

Perani, D., Bressi, S., Cappa, S.F. *et al.* (1993). Evidence of multiple memory systems in the human brain. *Brain*, **116**, 903–19.

Phillips, S., Sangalang, V. and Sterns, G. (1992). Basal forebrain infarction. *Achives of Neurology*, **44**, 1134–8.

Priestley, N.M. and Mayes, A.R. (1992). Preservation of priming for interactive context. *Cortex*, **28**, 555–74.

Squire, L.R. (1992). Memory and the hippocampus: a synthesis from findings with rats, monkeys, and humans. *Psychological Review*, **99**, 195–231.

Tranel, D. and Hyman, B.T. (1990). Neuropsychological correlates of bilateral amygdala damage. *Archives of Neurology*, **47**, 349–55.

Valenstein, E., Bowers, D., Verfaellie, M. *et al.* (1987). Retrosplenial amnesia. *Brain*, **110**, 1631–46.

van Eijk, R., Mayes, A.R. and Meudell, P.R. (1997). Measures of the contributions of recollection and familiarity to recognition memory.

Warrington, E.K. and Weiskrantz, L. (1982). A disconnection syndrome? *Neuropsychologia*, **20**, 233–48.

Zola-Morgan, S. and Squire, L.R. (1990). The primate hippocampal formation: evidence for a time-limited role in memory storage. *Science*, **250**, 288–90.

Zola-Morgan, S. and Squire, L.R. (1993). The neuroanatomy of amnesia. *Annual Review of Neuroscience*, **16**, 547–63.

Zola-Morgan, S., Squire, L.R. and Amaral, D.G. (1986). Human amnesia and the medial temporal region: enduring memory impairment following a bilateral lesion limited to field CA1 of the hippocampus. *Journal of Neuroscience*, **10**, 2950–67.

6

Clinical and neuropsychological studies of patients with amnesic disorders

MICHAEL D. KOPELMAN

Introduction

Amnesic states arise in the context of (i) the organic amnesic syndrome, such as the alcoholic Korsakoff syndrome; (ii) a more global dementia, such as Alzheimer's disease; (iii) as a transient or 'discrete' episode of amnesia; and (iv) in psychogenic amnesia. Examples of each of these will be considered in turn, and then inferences and broad conclusions will be drawn at the end of the chapter.

Korsakoff syndrome

Clinical features

This is probably the best described, and most intensively investigated, amnesic syndrome (Kopelman, 1995*a*), although in certain ways it is not entirely typical – for example, there is commonly concurrent frontal lobe involvement.

Korsakoff (1889*a,b*) described a characteristic memory disturbance, which occurred in a setting of clear consciousness: 'At first, during conversation with such a patient . . . (he or she) gives the impression of a person in complete possession of his (or her) faculties; he (she) reasons about everything perfectly well, draws correct deductions from given premises, makes witty remarks, plays chess or a game of cards, in a word comports himself (herself) as a mentally sound person'. However, 'the patient constantly asks the same questions and repeats the same stories . . . may read the same page over and again sometimes for hours . . . is unable to remember those persons whom he (she) met only during the illness, for example, the attending physician or nurse'. Characteristically, 'the memory of recent events . . . is chiefly disturbed . . . everything that happened during the illness and a short time before'. However, in some cases 'not only memory of recent events is lost, but also that of the long past', in which case the impairment may involve memories of up to 30 years earlier. Korsakoff also emphasised the variability in the severity of the disorder. In mild cases, recent memories are 'remembered vaguely . . . (without) complete abrogation . . . the forgetfulness chiefly affects the patients' own thought processes . . . (and) facts are remembered' although their retrieval requires 'specially favourable conditions'. In some instances, events may be remembered 'but not the time when they occurred'. In more severe cases, 'the amnesia is much more profound . . . the memory of facts is completely lost'.

As is widely known, Korsakoff mentioned that 'such patients invent some fiction and constantly repeat it . . . (for example) of conversations which have never occurred . . . so that a peculiar delirium develops, rooted in false recollections (pseudo-reminiscences)'. However, he tended to place greater emphasis upon the confusion of 'old recollections with present impressions', and he gave several examples of this: 'In telling of something about the past, the patient would suddenly confuse events and would introduce the events related to one period into the story about another period . . . Telling of a trip she had made to Finland before her illness and describing her voyage in fair detail, the patient mixed into the story her recollections of Crimea, and so it turned out that in Finland people always eat lamb and the inhabitants are Tartars'.

Korsakoff (1887, 1889*a,b*) described the syndrome occurring in 30 or more cases of chronic alcohol abuse, as well as in 16 patients in whom alcohol had not been implicated. De Wardener and Lennox (1947) also gave an excellent clinical description of the onset of Wernicke-type symptoms, followed by severe memory impairment, in thiamine-deprived prisoners of war. Moreover, there is a substantial literature indicating that Wernicke features and pathology can follow various aetiologies such as hyperemesis gravidarum and malignancies. However, 'pure' cases of the Korsakoff syndrome from non-alcoholic aetiologies have been harder to demonstrate in modern times, presumably because of a higher standard of underlying nutrition (see Kopelman, 1995*a*).

Critical lesion site

Although there is now a general agreement about the overlapping distribution of the lesions in Wernicke's encephalopathy and Korsakoff's syndrome, debate has ensued regarding the critical lesion(s) for the development of an amnesic syndrome, the thalamus and the mammillary bodies being the sites most commonly implicated. Victor, Adams and Collins (1971) pointed out that all 24 of their cases, in whom the medial–dorsal nucleus of the thalamus was affected, had a clinical history of persistent memory impairment (Korsakoff's syndrome), whereas five cases, in whom it was unaffected, had a history of Wernicke features without any recorded clinical history of subsequent memory disorder. By contrast, the mammillary bodies were implicated in all the Wernicke cases examined, whether or not there was subsequent memory impairment. Amnesia in association with unilateral or bilateral involvement of the thalamic nuclei, with apparent sparing of the mammillary bodies, has also been described in cases of tumour or infarction (McEntee *et al.*, 1976; Speedie and Heilman, 1982; Guberman and Stuss, 1983; Winocur *et al.*, 1984; Graff-Radford *et al.*, 1985, 1990; Katz, Alexander and Mandell, 1987; Parkin *et al.*, 1994).

However, Mair, Warrington and Weiskrantz (1979) provided a careful pathological and neuropsychological description of two Korsakoff patients, whose autopsies showed lesions in the mammillary bodies and the midline and anterior portion of the thalamus, but *not* in the medial dorsal nuclei. Mair *et al.* suggested that the lesions they described might 'disconnect' a critical circuit running between the temporal lobes and the frontal cortex, and Warrington and Weiskrantz (1982) put forward an hypothesis concerning the functional significance of this circuit. Mayes *et al.* (1988) provided findings in two further patients, who had had careful neuropsychological and autopsy investigations, which closely replicated the findings in the Mair *et al.* (1979) study. Von Cramon, Hebel and Schuri (1985) reviewed findings in a personal series of six cases of thalamic infarction (four of whom were amnesic and two of whom were not), together with a further five cases from the literature. These authors found that the region of the thalamus always implicated in the amnesic cases (and not implicated in the non-amnesic patients) lay in the anterior thalamus, involving the mammillo–thalamic tract, ventral to the medial dorsal nucleus (see Graff-Radford *et al.*, 1990).

Role of thiamine

Alexander and colleagues (1938, 1940) demonstrated: (1) the lesions of Wernicke's encephalopathy could be produced in pigeons following thiamine deprivation; (2) these lesions were not produced on deprivation of all other vitamins, when doses of thiamine were adequate; (3) the histology and topography of these lesions were identical to those obtained in a series of sixteen Wernicke patients. Thereafter, Jolliffe, Wortis and Fein (1941) reported clinical evidence of thiamine deficiency in 27 Wernicke patients, amongst whom 12 survivors manifested a Korsakoff syndrome.

Subsequently, De Wardener and Lennox (1947) reported their observations in malnourished prisoners-of-war. The onset of symptoms generally occurred 6 to 14 weeks after captivity, i.e. at the same time as symptoms of beriberi but before the symptoms of other vitamin deficiencies. De Wardener and Lennox showed that there was a very favourable response to thiamine treatment by injection, when it was available.

A genetic factor has been postulated to explain why only a minority of heavy drinkers develop the syndrome, which is far less common than the hepatic or gastro-intestinal complications of alcohol abuse. Transketolase is an enzyme that requires thiamine pyrophosphate (TPP) as a co-factor, and Blass and Gibson (1977) postulated that a hereditary abnormality of transketolase metabolism predisposed some alcoholics to the Korsakoff syndrome. More recently, McCool *et al.* (1993) have identified the transketolase gene, but found that no particular allelic variants could account for the biochemical properties of the enzyme, when cultures from two Wernicke–Korsakoff patients with extremely low affinity (K_m) for the TPP co-enzyme were compared with cultures from two non-alcoholic controls with extremely high affinity. Hence, McCool *et al.* (1993) argued that (extragenic) variation in post-translational processing and modifcation of the tranketolase polypeptide, rather than allelic variation, might underlie differential susceptibility to the development of the syndrome amongst alcoholics. Witt (1985) has pointed out that six neurotransmitter systems are affected by thiamine depletion, either by reduction of TPP-dependent enzyme activity or by direct structural damage, and four of these neurotransmitters (acetylcholine, glutamate, aspartate, GABA) are directly related to glucose metabolism.

Neuropsychology: general cognitive impairments

Jacobson and Lishman (1987) showed a variable degree of general cognitive impairment on standard IQ tests in this disorder. Their findings suggested a continuum between those patients who showed a disproportionate impairment of anterograde memory, and those patients with a fairly severe, general cognitive decline, suggestive of 'alcoholic dementia' – even though alcoholic patients with clear clinical evidence of generalised dementia had been excluded from their study. However, these authors had employed the original version of the Wechsler Memory Scale, which is confounded by the inclusion of digit span and mental control as determinants of the Memory Quotient. The revised Wechsler Memory Scale (WMS-R) avoids this problem, and tends to give substantially lower quotients to Korsakoff and other amnesic patients (Butters *et al.*, 1988). It seems quite likely that, had Jacobson and Lishman been able to use the WMS-R (which was not available at the time of their study) or some other relatively 'pure' measure of anterograde memory, their patients would all have shown a disproportionate impairment of anterograde memory, although the degree of general cognitive impairment would still have varied considerably between individual patients.

There is also considerable evidence of frontal or 'executive' dysfunction in Korsakoff patients (Shimamura, Jernigan and Squire, 1988; Leng and Parkin, 1988; Janowsky *et al.*, 1989; Kopelman, 1989, 1991*a*; Jacobson, Acker and Lishman 1990; Shoqeirat *et al.*, 1990; Joyce and Robbins, 1991). Various aspects of the memory deficits found in Korsakoff's patients have been attributed to frontal dysfunction (e.g. Moscovitch, 1982; Squire, 1982; Schacter, Harbluk and McLachlan, 1984; Mayes, Mendell and Pickering, 1985; Janowsky *et al.*, 1989; Shimamura, Janowsky and Squire, 1990; Kopelman, 1991*a*).

Neuropsychology: memory deficits

By definition, episodic or 'explicit' memory is severely impaired in Korsakoff patients. It is plausible that this deficit results from an underlying dysfunction in the process of physiological 'consolidation', and this may have neurochemical or electrophysiological correlates (Meudell and Mayes, 1982; Kopelman, 1986). In addition, various psychological deficits have also been postulated, including an impairment in the encoding of semantic or meaningful information (Cutting, 1978; Butters and Cermak, 1980) or in the encoding of contextual information (Huppert and Piercy, 1976, 1978*a*; Hirst, 1982; Mayes *et al.*, 1985; Mayes, 1992; Parkin, 1992). However, for various reasons, it seems unlikely that either a semantic or a contextual memory deficit accounts for the severity of the memory disorder in the Korsakoff syndrome (see Kopelman, 1995*a*).

Another possibility would be that information is forgotten faster by Korsakoff patients, once it has been learned. This possibility was tested by Huppert and Piercy (1978*b*), who 'matched' the initial learning of Korsakoff patients to that of healthy controls by prolonging the exposure time to stimulus material (pictures from magazines) to the amnesic patients. They found that the rate of long-term forgetting was normal, once the target information had been learned to an adequate degree for as long as 10 minutes, and various other researchers have replicated this result in Korsakoff patients (Squire, 1981; Kopelman, 1985; Martone, Butters and Trauner, 1986; McKee and Squire, 1992). However, all these studies involved recognition memory, as 'matching' is extremely difficult to achieve on recall tests; and forgetting was assessed only after intervals longer than 10 minutes. A recent study by Kopelman and Stanhope (1997) suggests that there is accelerated forgetting of pictorial material, when tested by recall, between 1 minute and 10 minutes delays.

In addition, there is an extensive retrograde memory loss in the Korsakoff syndrome, extending back several decades, as Korsakoff (1889*a*) himself noted. Modern neuropsychological studies have confirmed that this retrograde memory loss extends back at least 25 to 30 years (Albert *et al.*, 1979; Cohen and Squire, 1981; Squire, Haist and Shimamura, 1989; Kopelman, 1989; Parkin *et al.*, 1990). This extensive retrograde loss includes memory for remote public or 'semantic' information, facts about a patient's own life ('personal semantic memory'), and 'autobiographical' memory for incidents or events from the patient's past (Kopelman, 1989). All these aspects of retrograde memory show a 'temporal gradient' with relative sparing of the most distant memories, and the gradient is significantly steeper than that seen in dementing disorders such as Alzheimer's disease (Kopelman, 1989). The relative sparing of early memories may result from their greater salience and rehearsal, such that they have become assimilated within semantic memory (Cermak, 1984; Weiskrantz, 1985).

Particularly interesting are those aspects of memory which are preserved in Korsakoff patients. These include simple conditioning (Weiskrantz and Warrington, 1979), procedural learning of perceptuo-motor skills (Claparede, 1911; Brooks and Baddeley, 1976; Martone *et al.*, 1984), and various measures of the response to 'priming' (Warrington and Weiskrantz, 1970; Graf, Squire and Mandler, 1984; Shimamura and Squire, 1984; Graf and Schcter, 1985; Schacter and Graf, 1986; Tulving and Schacter, 1990). Korsakoff patients also show preserved affective or evaluative memory responses (Johnson, Kim and Risse, 1985; Frith *et al.*, 1992); and, in general, they show relative preservation of semantic memory compared with dementing patients (Weingartner *et al.*, 1983; Perani *et al.*, 1993).

Degenerative dementia

We will discuss Alzheimer dementia, as there is an extensive literature discussing the nature of the memory deficits in this disorder. In many respects, the memory disorder of Alzheimer dementia resembles that seen in the Korsakoff syndrome except: (i) primary or 'working' memory is more severely affected; (ii) semantic memory is much more affected than in the Korsakoff syndrome; (iii) there is a more severe loss of early, 'retrograde' memories; and (iv) there is controversy over the extent to which priming is affected.

Explicit memory

An example of the similarity of the explicit memory deficit to that in the Korsakoff syndrome comes from studies of forgetting rates. Kopelman (1985) took the opportunity to use the Huppert–Piercy test to investigate 'long-term' forgetting in Alzheimer (and Korsakoff) patients. Alzheimer patients show extensive pathology within the hippocampi and the temporal lobes, implying that these patients would show accelerated forgetting according to Huppert and Piercy's (1979) hypothesis, which was that temporal lobe lesions produce faster forgetting. Using exposure times that were approximately 14 times as long in Alzheimer (and Korsakoff patients) than in healthy controls, the Alzheimer group's recognition memory performance at 10 minutes was matched to that of the Korsakoff group, and was only a little below that of the healthy control subjects. The rate of forgetting over 24 hours and a week (indicated by the slopes of the curves) was the same in the Alzheimer group as in the other two groups. This was true whether scoring was in terms of per cent correct scores, recognition scores as a proportion of scores at 10 minutes, or d prime. However, using a *recall* task, Christensen *et al.* (1997) have found accelerated forgetting of pictures of objects between 1 minute and 10 minutes delay, similar to that obtained on the same task by Kopelman and Stanhope (see above) in Korsakoff and other amnesic patients.

Working memory

On the other hand, there is a much more extensive involvement of working memory in Alzheimer dementia than in the amnesic syndrome (see Kopelman, 1994 for a review; also Morris, 1994). For example, studies of the (verbal) Brown–Peterson test uniformly demonstrate severe impairment in Alzheimer patients (Corkin, 1982; Kopelman, 1985; Morris, 1986; Dannenbaum, Parkinson and Inman, 1988). Non-verbal analogues of this task, using Corsi block retention, also reveal a severe impairment in Alzheimer patients (Sullivan, Corkin and Growdon, 1986; Kopelman,

1991*a*). In two studies, Kopelman (1985, 1991*b*) demonstrated that this deficit in Alzheimer patients was much more severe than the relatively mild impairment in Korsakoff patients, and that the Alzheimer patients exhibited significantly more omission errors on the verbal task than either Korsakoff patients or healthy controls. Moreover, the clinical validity of the verbal test was demonstrated by the fact that, whereas younger healthy subjects of high IQ performed best at this test, younger Alzheimer patients performed particularly poorly, consistent with the greater severity of their expected neuropathological and neurochemical abnormalities.

Becker (1988) postulated that, although Alzheimer patients generally show deficits in both working memory and secondary memory, sub-groups of patients might show disproportionate impairment on measures of either 'executive' (working memory) or secondary memory function, just as Martin *et al.* (1986) had demonstrated that particular individuals and sub-groups of Alzheimer patients exhibited disproportionate impairment on either verbal or visuo-spatial tasks. Becker and colleagues (Becker, 1988; Becker, Bajulaiye and Smith, 1992) examined Alzheimer patients using several measures of 'executive' function (verbal similarities, letter cancellation, word generation, card-sorting) and several measures of anterograde memory (paired-associate learning, story and complex figure recall). From a sample of 191 patients, these authors did indeed find that relatively small sub-groups of patients could be identified, who had either disproportionate impairment on the measures of executive function (a dysexecutive syndrome, N=8) or on the memory tasks (an amnesic syndrome, N=43).

Similarly, Baddeley *et al.* (1986) examined dual task performance in Alzheimer patients, demonstrating that concurrent performance of a digit-span task and a tracking task produced a significant decrement in the performance of each task, even though the difficulty of the tasks had been manipulated such that Alzheimer patients' performance at the *individual* tasks was matched to that of controls. In a follow-up study, Baddeley *et al.* (1991) showed that the deterioration in Alzheimer patients' performance was far greater for dual-task performance than it was for the individual tasks alone.

Semantic memory

There is general agreement that semantic memory is much more severely implicated in Alzheimer dementia than in the Korsakoff syndrome, or indeed other patients with an amnesic syndrome (Weingartner *et al.*, 1983; Huff, Corkin and Growdon, 1986). Various authors have documented that

Alzheimer patients show deficits on (for example) verbal fluency and object naming (Huff *et al.*, 1986; Nebes and Brady, 1989; Nebers, 1992). Martin and Fedio (1983; Martin, 1990) argued that a degradation of semantic representations occurs in this disease, which becomes more severe as it advances. Martin (1992*a,b*) pointed out that the disparity between Alzheimer patients' *ability* to demonstrate knowledge about *superordinate* categories and their *failure* to identify *specific attributes* of objects indicates that the loss of knowledge proceeds from the more particular to the more general level (see Huff *et al.*, 1986). Similarly, Hodges *et al.* (1992) reported a consistency in the individual items to which dementing patients produce errors across a variety of naming, matching, or sorting tasks; and they also argued for an explanation in terms of degraded storage.

Retrograde memory

There has been only one direct comparison of the retrograde memory loss in Alzheimer and Korsakoff patients (Kopelman, 1989), which showed a 'flatter' temporal gradient in the Alzheimer patients, i.e. a more severe loss of early (childhood and young adult) memories. However, there was some relative sparing of the earlier memories (compared with more recent memories) even in this group. The findings in other recent studies of Alzheimer patients are broadly consistent with these observations (Beatty *et al.*, 1988; Sagar *et al.*, 1988; Hodges, Salmon and Butters, 1993).

Implicit memory

There is more controversy concerning aspects of 'priming'. In the most widely cited study (Shimamura *et al.*, 1987) Alzheimer patients failed to show priming on a word-stem completion task, for which priming had clearly been demonstrated in amnesic patients in earlier studies (Graf *et al.*, 1984; Shimamura and Squire, 1984). However, widely conflicting results have been obtained since that time. It appears that word-completion priming may be intact where the Alzheimer patient has had *longer* to encode the original material, or has been encouraged to encode the material to a 'deeper' level (Patridge, Knight and Feehan, 1990; Christensen and Birrell, 1991; Christensen *et al.*, 1992; Ostergaard, 1994). Moreover, semantic priming appears to be intact (Nebes, Martin and Horn, 1984), and there is even evidence that Alzheimer patients may show 'hyper-priming' in certain circumstances (Chertkow *et al.*, 1994). Reviewing this literature, Ober and Shenaut (1994) have recently argued that hyper-priming, when it occurs, results from a specific slowing in 'controlled' or 'explicit' processing in Alzheimer patients, which allows 'automatic' or 'implicit' mechanisms to be facilitated.

Transient amnesia

Transient amnesia refers to a 'discrete episode' of memory loss, which subsequently recovers, characteristically leaving an 'amnesic gap' for the period of the acute memory loss. Transient organic amnesias have been reviewed in more detail elsewhere (Kopelman, 1996), and in the present chapter we will consider (i) the transient global amnesia (TGA) syndrome, (ii) head injury, and (iii) ECT.

TGA syndrome

Hodges and Ward (1989) recently defined transient global amnesia (TGA) as 'a witnessed amnesia, occurring in clear consciousness, without focal signs or other signs of epilepsy, resolving within 24 hours'. In a combined retrospective and prospective study, these authors obtained 114 cases, aged between 39 and 82, of whom 61% were male. The duration of the amnesia ranged between 15 minutes and 12 hours (mean=4.2 hours), and 15% of the sample reported multiple episodes. In the preceding 24 hours, 10% had experienced either headache or nausea, and 14% a stressful life event, whilst in others the attack was preceded by a medical procedure or severe exercise. Repetitive questioning was a characteristic feature, as others had previously described (e.g. Whitty, Stores and Lishman, 1977), and no patients reported a loss of personal identity. In 25% of the sample, there was a past history of migraine, which was considered to have a possible aetiological role. In a further 7%, the episode was subsequently attributed to previously undiagnosed epilepsy (see below). However, there was *no* association with *either* a history or clinical signs of *or* known risk factors for vascular disease: this pattern was quite different from that obtained in a sample of patients who had had transient ischaemic attacks (TIAs). Moreover, the underlying aetiology of the TGA attacks remained unclear in 60 to 70% of the sample. In general, these findings are consistent with those obtained in other large-scale studies of TGA (Heathfield, Croft and Swash, 1973; Fisher, 1982; Miller *et al.*, 1987).

Hodges and Ward (1989) administered neuropsychological tests to five patients during their acute episode of memory loss. As expected, all these patients showed a profound anterograde amnesia on tests of both verbal and non-verbal memory. Performance on retrograde memory tests was variable. Three out of five patients showed impairments on a test requiring the recognition of famous faces from earlier decades; the other two patients performed within the 'normal' range for this test. Similarly, on a test requiring the subjects to produce autobiographical memories to specific cue-words, one out of the three patients administered this task performed normally. In short, whilst anterograde memory is always severely impaired, the effect of a TGA episode upon retrograde memory is very variable. In addition, Hodges and Oxbury (1990) followed up a sub-sample of the total series of 114 patients over six months, and they found that there were mild, residual impairments on verbal anterograde and retrograde memory tests in comparison with the performance of an age- and IQ-matched comparison group. However, Kritchevsky and colleagues (Kritchevsky, Squire and Zouzounis, 1988; Kritchevsky and Squire, 1989) found that complete recovery in performance on neuropsychological tests had occurred within one month of the acute episode, consistent with clinical 'lore'.

As mentioned above, epilepsy is the underlying cause of a TGA syndrome in a small minority of cases. Kapur (1990) has termed this phenomenon 'transient epileptic amnesia' (TEA). The main predictive factors for an epileptic basis to such attacks (where epilepsy has not previously been diagnosed) are the occurrence of multiple episodes and their relatively brief duration. In the Hodges and Warlow (1990) series, all four subjects who had had multiple attacks, lasting one hour or less, were subsequently found to have underlying epilepsy. Other authors have corroborated this finding (Miller *et al.*, 1987*a,b*; Kapur, 1990). Standard EEGs and CT scans may be normal, and the epileptic basis to the disorder may be revealed only on a sleep EEG (Kopelman, Panayiotopoulos and Lewis, 1994*a*). A PET study of such cases found no abnormality six months after commencement of treatment with an anticonvulsant (Kopelman *et al.*, 1994*a*).

Head injury

Head injury gives rise to the familiar pattern of memory loss, consisting of a brief period of retrograde amnesia (RA), which may last only a few seconds or minutes, a longer period of post-traumatic amnesia (PTA), and islets of preserved memory within the amnesic gap (Russell and Nathan, 1946; Lishman, 1987). Occasionally, PTA may occur without any RA, although this is more common in cases of penetrating lesions (Lishman, 1968; Newcombe, 1969). Sometimes, there is a particularly vivid memory for images or sounds occurring immediately before the injury, on regaining consciousness, or during a 'lucid' interval between the injury and the onset of PTA (Russell and Nathan, 1946; Lishman, 1987). As is well known, the duration of PTA is assumed to reflect the degree of underlying diffuse brain pathology; and rotational forces, such as can occur in a motor accident, are particularly likely to produce axonal tearing and generalised cognitive impairment. The length of PTA is predictive of eventual cognitive outcome (Brooks, 1984), psychiatric outcome (Lishman, 1968), and social outcome (Russell and Smith, 1961; Brooks, 1984). However, these relationships are weaker than is frequently assumed, and a problem is that the duration of PTA is often not documented adequately in the medical records. There appears to be a relationship with age such that older subjects tend to have a longer PTA and more serious deficits at a given PTA (Russell and Smith, 1961), whereas in subjects under 30, PTA is sometimes found to be less effective as a predictor of subsequent memory impairment (Brooks, 1972). In addition, contusion to the frontal and anterior temporal lobes is a common consequence of head injury and, recently, two sets of authors have attributed a disproportionate degree of retrograde memory loss, associated with only a mild degree of anterograde memory impairment, to damage in these structures (Kapur *et al.*, 1992; Markowitsch *et al.*, 1993).

ECT

Squire and his colleagues (Squire, 1977; Squire, Cohen and Nadel, 1984) have found that subjects tested within a few hours of ECT show a retrograde impairment for information from the preceding 1 to 3 years, and a pronounced anterograde deficit on both recall and recognition memory tests. Other authors have corroborated these findings (Weeks, Freeman and Kendall, 1980; Frith *et al.*, 1983), and there is general agreement that, 6 to 9 months after completion of a course of ECT, memory performance on objective tests returns to normal, apart from a persistent loss of material acquired within a few hours of the convulsions (Squire, 1977; Squire *et al.*, 1984; Weeks *et al.*, 1980; Frith *et al.*, 1983; Squire and Slater, 1983). However, *complaints* of memory impairment may persist, and can still be evident three years or more after the course of ECT (Squire and Slater, 1983). Squire and Slater found that these complaints focused upon the period for which there had been an initial retrograde and anterograde amnesia, as determined by neuropsychological tests, even though that memory loss was no longer evident on formal assessment. Freeman, Weeks and Kendell (1980) reported that those subjects who complain most about their memories do, in fact, perform poorer on objective tests than do those who complain less, but Squire and Slater (1983), using similar tests, did not find this. On the contrary, both Squire and Slater (1983) and Frith *et al.* (1983) found that the 'complainers' were the patients who, on other criteria, had recovered least well from their depression.

Neuropsychological studies have found that verbal memory appears to be particularly sensitive to disruption, and unilateral ECT to the non-dominant hemisphere produces considerably less memory impairment than bilateral ECT (Squire, 1977), making it important to identify the non-dominant hemisphere by a valid procedure (Kopelman, 1982). Various recent studies have attempted to minimise memory disruption by either changes in premedication or concomitant administration of other substances: the agents employed here included glycopyrrolate, physostigmine, thyroxine, nimodipine, vasopressin, naloxone, dexamethasone, ACTH, and caffeine infusion (d'Elia and Frederiksen, 1980; Horne *et al.*, 1984; Nasrallah *et al.*, 1986; Levin, Elizur and Korczyn, 1987; Sommer *et al.*, 1989; Coffey *et al.*, 1990; Mattes *et al.*, 1990; Stern *et al.*, 1991; Cohen and Swartz, 1991). In general, these agents have produced little or no benefit, and the most effective methods of avoiding memory deficit consist of electrode placement *either* over the frontal rather than the temporal lobes *or* over the non-dominant temporal lobe (Squire, 1977; Sackheim *et al.*, 1993).

Psychogenic amnesia

Psychogenic amnesia can involve situation-specific memory loss, as occurs for amnesia for offences, occasionally in post-traumatic stress disorder, and in amnesia for childhood sexual abuse. Secondly, the memory loss can involve a more global memory deficit, often accompanied by a loss of the sense of personal identity, such as occurs in a psychogenic 'fugue' state. Thirdly, there can be a more persistent psychologically based memory disorder, as occurs in a depressive pseudo-dementia, for example.The latter is the subject of a large literature in its own right, and will not be considered further here (see Watts, 1995 and Burt, Zember and Niederehe, 1995 for review).

Various forms of terminology are currently employed. The present writer favours the term 'psychogenic amnesia', because it does not make any assumptions about the degree to which memory loss results from unconscious processes ('hysterical amnesia'), rather than motivated/deliberate/conscious processes ('simulated' or 'factitious' amnesia). The term 'functional amnesia' is somewhat misleading in that there are, of course, deficits in function (or 'process') in organic amnesia, and the salient feature of psychogenic amnesia is that, in some sense, it is always 'dysfunctional'.

Psychogenic amnesia has been discussed in more detail in Kopelman (1995*b*).

Psychogenic fugue

A 'fugue state' refers, in essence, to a syndrome consisting of a sudden loss of all autobiographical memories and the sense of self or personal identity, usually associated with a period of wandering, for which there is a subsequent amnesic gap upon recovery (Kopelman, 1987*a*, 1995*b*). Fugue states usually last a few hours or days only. A review of the literature suggests that fugue states are always preceded by a severe, precipitating stress such as marital or emotional discord (Kanzer, 1939), bereavement (Schacter *et al.*, 1982), financial problems (Kanzer, 1939), a charge of offending (Wilson, Rupp and Wilson, 1950), or stress during wartime (Sergant and Slater, 1941; Parfit and Gall, 1944). Secondly, depressed mood is an extremely common antecedent for a psychogenic fugue state. In fact, many patients in a 'fugue' have been contemplating suicide just before the episode or do so following recovery from it (Abeles and Schilder, 1935; Stengel, 1941). The third factor that commonly precedes a fugue state is a history of a transient, organic amnesia: Stengel (1941) reported that 10% of his sample had a history of epilepsy, and Berrington, Liddell and Foulds (1956) reported that 16 of their 37 cases had previously experienced a severe head injury, and a further three cases had suffered a head injury of unknown severity. In brief, it appears that patients who have experienced a previous, transient organic amnesia, and who have become depressed and/or suicidal, are particularly likely to go into a 'fugue' in the face of a severe, precipitating stress.

The clinical and neuropsychological phenomena of psychogenic amnesia often bear interesting resemblances to organic amnesia. For example, there may be islets or fragments of preserved memory within the amnesic gap. A woman, who was due to meet her husband to discuss divorce, recalled that she was 'supposed to meet someone' (Kanzer, 1939). A young man, who slipped into a fugue following his grandfather's funeral, recalled a cluster of details from the year which he described (after recovery) as having been the happiest of his life (Schacter *et al.*, 1982). The subject may adopt a detached attitude to these memory fragments, describing them as 'strange and unfamiliar' (Coriat, 1907). In many cases, semantic knowledge remains intact, e.g. foreign languages, and the names of streets, towns, and famous people (Kanzer, 1939; Schacter *et al.*, 1982), whereas in others it is also implicated (Coriat, 1907; Abeles and Schilder, 1935; Kanzer, 1939). Similarly, performance at verbal learning tests has been reported as unaffected (Abeles and Schilder, 1935; Kopelman *et al.*, 1994*b*), mildly impaired (Schacter *et al.*, 1982), or more severely impaired (Gudjonsson and Taylor, 1985). Memory for skills is often preserved (e.g. Coriat, 1907), but in the Padola hearing in 1959 (Bradford and Smith, 1979), retention of a rudimentary knowledge of aerodynamics and of other skills (e.g. solving jigsaw puzzles) was taken as evidence against an organic amnesia – a frankly erroneous interpretation in the light of contemporary findings demonstrating preserved procedural memory in organic amnesia. Sometimes, memory retrieval may be facilitated by chance cues in the environment (e.g. Abeles and Schilder, 1935; Schacter *et al.*, 1982), but deliberate cuing is often unsuccessful (Coriat, 1907; Kanzer, 1939) and the results of Amytal abreaction are often disappointing (Lennox, 1943; Adatto, 1949; Kopelman *et al.*, 1994*b,c*).

Situation-specific amnesia

A common example is amnesia for an offence.This has been reported most commonly in cases of homicide, where rates of amnesia have been reported in between 25% and 45% of cases (Kopelman, 1987*b*, 1995*b*). However, claims of amnesia also arise following other types of crime, particularly violent crime, but also in shoplifting, fraud, and criminal damage. The factors that predispose to amnesia for crime resemble those that have been identified as producing impaired recall in eyewitness testimony – namely, violent crime, extreme emotional arousal (such as in a 'crime of passion'), severe alcohol abuse and intoxication, depressed mood, and occasionally acute psychosis (see Taylor and Kopelman, 1984). Aside from drug and alcohol abuse, organic factors are a rare cause of amnesia for crime but should always be excluded, e.g. epilepsy, hypoglycaemia, head injury, and sleep walking (Fenwick, 1990, 1993; Kopelman, 1995*b*).

The issue of whether the offender is deliberately simulating his amnesia always arises, but a number of factors suggest that many subjects claiming amnesia are not making it up, including the fact that many such offenders give themselves up as soon as they realise what they have done (Gudjonsson and MacKeith, 1983; Kopelman, 1995*b*).

The nature of psychogenic amnesia

Leaving aside deliberate simulation, various mechanisms have been proposed to account for psychogenic amnesia. These include repression, dissociative states, a failure of initial encoding, an encoding–retrieval interaction, and state- or context-dependent retrieval deficits. These various theories can be grouped into those that place emphasis on the failure of memory at the time of initial encoding, which may be particularly true of amnesic offenders where severe alcoholic or drug intoxication is implicated, and those that place emphasis on a failure of memory retrieval. The latter is possibly more true of those unpremeditated homicide cases, which take place in a state of extreme emotional arousal, although in these cases the possibility of an interaction between encoding and retrieval factors cannot be excluded.

On detailed assessment, subjects often show some degree of 'knowledge' or 'recognition' of certain memories without explicit recollection (Kopelman *et al.*, 1994*b*), in a manner analogous to that seen in studies of amnesic patients or healthy subjects who have failed to remember something (Gardiner and Parkin, 1990). For example, O'Connell (1960) pointed to the qualitative similarities between what he called the 'passive disregard' of those who deliberately put an unpleasant or traumatic memory to the back of their minds, and those subjects who, although claiming amnesia, describe the memory as being on the verge of 'forming a picture'. This suggests that there may be a continuum of levels of awareness in memory, and that patients with psychogenic amnesia do not necessarily fall at the extremes of either fully deliberate simulation or completely 'unconscious' amnesia. A number of recent case studies have illustrated these points in more detail (Kopelman *et al.*, 1994*b,c*).

The memory deficits in amnesic disorders

To some extent, these have been discussed in the preceding sections, and also in more detail in Chapter 5. However, a few general points may be useful. 'Storage' deficits can refer *either* to problems putting memories into the store *or* to accelerated forgetting from the store *or* to both (in which problems in initial storage result in a vulnerability to faster forgetting). Problems in putting information into storage are known, more generally, as 'acquisition' deficits, and these can broadly be of two types – (i) problems in 'psychological' processes of encoding, or (ii) dysfunction in an actual or hypothesised physiological process such as 'consolidation'. Problems in 'psychological' encoding could particularly involve either meaningful/semantic or contextual information; and both types of deficit have been postulated in the past (e.g. Cutting, 1978; Butters and Cermak, 1980; Mayes *et al.*, 1985). 'Physiological' deficits would include depletions in the cholinergic or serotoninergic neurotransmitter systems (e.g. Kopelman and Corn, 1988; Martin *et al.*, 1989). As discussed by Kopelman (1995*a*) and by Mayes (Chapter 5, this volume), there is little evidence that a deficit in encoding semantic information could account for amnesic disorders. Moreover, the low correlations between performance on tests of 'target' and 'context' memory respectively suggests that a deficit in encoding contextual information is also unlikely to be the fundamental basis to the disorder. However, as discussed by Mayes, retrieval processes are so closely entwined with encoding strategies that it also seems very unlikely that a 'pure' retrieval deficit causes the disorder.

As far as maintenance in the 'store' is concerned, there are numerous studies indicating that forgetting by amnesic patients is normal, after learning has been 'titrated' to match that of healthy subjects as closely as possible at a 10 minute delay (Huppert and Piercy, 1978*b*; Squire, 1981; Kopelman, 1985; Martone *et al.*, 1986; Freed, Corkin and Cohen, 1987; Freed *et al.*, 1989; McKee and Squire, 1992). These findings, which are unlikely to be the result of any artefact (Kopelman, 1995), were all obtained in patients with focal or generalised structural pathology giving rise to their amnesia, and the only exceptions are those patients with gross metabolic disruption following ECT or head injury (the latter 'within PTA') who show accelerated forgetting on similar tests (Squire, 1981; Levin, High and Eisenberg, 1988; Lewis and Kopelman, 1997).

By a process of exclusion, studies of patients with structural lesions have, therefore, generally been taken to imply a deficit in 'acquisition' or 'putting into store', presumably resulting from some unidentified dysfunction in an underlying process of physiological consolidation. However, the study by Kopelman and Stanhope, cited above, and those by Mayes and colleagues (Chapter 5) are highly consistent with one another in suggesting that there may be faster forgetting in amnesic patients, when tested on *free recall* measures at intervals *shorter* than 10 minutes (although *not* on recognition or cued recall measures over the same intervals). This suggests that *either* the acquisition deficit results in a relatively subtle secondary impairment in holding information within the store, detectable only on the most difficult tasks, *or* that there are two independent deficits involved – a major deficit in acquisition and a lesser problem in retention.

The retrograde deficit in memory in organic amnesia requires an additional explanation because there appear to be very low correlations between the severity of anterograde and retrograde amnesia (Shimamura and Squire, 1986; Kopelman, 1989, 1991; Parkin, 1991), and because it is well established that quite severe anterograde amnesia can exist in the absence of any retrograde loss (although the evidence that retrograde amnesia can occur without anterograde memory loss is much more tendentious). There is evidence that frontal pathology can give rise to retrograde memory loss (Baddeley and Wilson, 1986; Kopelman, 1991*a*; Della Sala *et al.*, 1993), and that temporal lobe lesions in various sites can also do so (De Renzi, Liotti and Nichelli, 1987; O'Connor *et al.*, 1992; Kapur, 1993). The likeliest possibility is that 'old' memories are stored in widely distributed neural networks across the frontal and temporal and (possibly) the parietal cortex. What is certainly agreed is that the limbic–diencephalic structures involved in laying down new memories are *not* the structures that 'store' them in the long-run.

There is debate as to whether or not the relative preservation of 'implicit' memory in amnesia implies independent 'memory systems', and the extent to which implicit memory is, in fact, spared. Although these issues are not completely resolved, knowledge of the expected patterns of breakdown in organic amnesia may sometimes help in the differentiation of psychologically based amnesia from that resulting from brain disorder.

Conclusions

Clinical and neuropsychological studies are identifying varying patterns of impairment within different clinical syndromes. Several examples of these have been discussed above in the context of the amnesic syndrome, degenerative dementia, transient and psychogenic amnesia. In addition, there has been recent research interest in the putative memory disorders of schizophrenia and depression, as well as increasing acknowledgement that autobiographical memory is central to notions such as 'self', personal identity, and development. It is no longer entirely flippant to suggest that, central to the study of psychiatric phenomena, is an understanding of memory and its disorders.

Acknowledgement

Dr Kopelman is grateful to Miss C. Hook for patiently typing the manuscript. He is supported by the West Lambeth Community Care Trust.

References

Abeles, M. and Schilder, P. (1935). Psychogenic loss of personal identity. *Archives of Neurology and Psychiatry*, **34**, 587–604.

Adatto, C.P. (1949). Observations on criminal patients during narcoanalysis. *Archives of Neurology and Psychiatry*, **62**, 82–92.

Albert, M.S., Butters, N. and Levin, J. (1979). Temporal gradients in the retrograde amnesia of patients with alcoholic Korsakoff's disease. *Archives of Neurology, Chicago*, **36**, 211–165.

Alexander, L. (1940). Wernicke's disease; identity of lesions produced experimentally by B1 avitaminosis in pigeons with haemorrhagic polioencephalitis occurring in chronic alcoholism in man. *American Journal of Pathology*, **16**, 61–70.

Alexander, L., Pijoan, M. and Myerson, A. (1938). Beri-beri and scurvy. *Transactions of the American Neurological Association*, **64**, 135–9.

Baddeley, A.D. and Wilson, B. (1986). Amnesia, autobiographical memory, and confabulation. In *Autobiographical Memory* (ed. D.C. Rubin), pp. 225–52. Cambridge: Cambridge University Press.

Baddeley, A.D., Logie, R., Bressi, S. *et al.* (1986). Dementia and working memory. *Quarterly Journal of Experimental Psychology*, **38A**, 603–18.

Baddeley, A.D., Bressi, S., Della Sala, S. *et al.* (1991). The decline of working memory in Alzheimer's Disease: a longitudinal study. *Brain*, **114**, 2521–42.

Beatty, W.W., Salmon, D.P., Butters, N. *et al.* (1988). Retrograde amnesia in patients with Alzheimer's disease or Huntington's disease. *Neurobiology of Aging*, **9**, 186–8.

Becker, J.T. (1988). Working memory and secondary memory deficits in Alzheimer's disease. *Journal of Clinical and Experimental Neuropsychology*, **10**, 739–53.

Becker, J.T., Bajulaiye, O. and Smith, C. (1992). Longitudinal analysis of a two-component model of the memory deficit in Alzheimer's disease. *Psychological Medicine*, **22**, 437–46.

Berrington, W.P., Liddell, D.W. and Foulds, G.A. (1956). A reevaluation of the fugue. *Journal of Mental Science*, **102**, 281–6.

Blass, J.P. and Gibson, G.E. (1977). Abnormality of a thiamine-requiring enzyme in patients with Wernicke-Korsakoff syndrome. *New England Journal of Medicine*, **297**, 1367–70.

Bradford, J. and Smith, S.M. (1979). Amnesia and homicide: the Podola case and a study of thirty cases. *Bulletin of the American Academy of Psychiatry and the Law*, **7**, 219–31.

Brooks, N. (1972). Memory and closed head injury. *Journal of Nervous and Mental Disease*, **155**, 350–5.

Brooks, N. (1984). Cognitive deficits after head injury. In *Closed Head Injury: Psychological, Social and Family Consequences* (ed. N. Brooks). Oxford: Oxford University Press.

Brooks, D.N. and Baddeley, A.D. (1976). What can amnesic patients learn? *Neuropsychologia*, **14**, 111–22.

Burt, D.B., Zember, M.J. and Niederehe, G. (1995). Depression and memory impairment: a meta-analysis of the association, its pattern, and specificity. *Psychological Bulletin*, **117**, 285–305.

Butters, N. and Cermak, L.S. (1980). *Alcoholic Korsakoff's Syndrome: An Information-processing Approach to Amnesia*. New York and London: Academic Press.

Butters, N., Salmon, D.P., Munro Cullum C. *et al.* (1988). Differentiation of amnesic and demented patients with the Wechsler Memory Scale – Revised. *The Clinical Neuropsychologist*, **2**, 133–48.

Cermak, L.S. (1984). The episodic-semantic distinction in amnesia. In *The Neuropsychology of Memory*, 1st edition (ed. L.R. Squire and N. Butters), New York and London: Guilford Press.

Chertkow, H., Bub., D., Bergman, H. *et al.* (1994). Increased semantic priming in patients with dementia of the Alzheimer's type. *Journal of Clinical and Experimental Neuropsychology*, **16**, 608–22.

Christensen, H. and Birrell, P. (1991). Explicit and implicit memory in dementia and normal ageing. *Psychological Research*, **53**, 149–61.

Christensen, H., Maltby, N., Jorm, A.F. *et al.* (1992). Cholinergic blockade as a model of the cognitive deficits in Alzheimer's disease. *Brain*, **115**, 1681–99.

Christensen, H., Kopelman, M.D., Stanhope, N. *et al.* (1997). Rates of forgetting in Alzheimer dementia. *Neuropsychologia*, in press.

Claparede, E. (1911). Recognition and 'me-ness'. (Recognition et moiite). *Archives Psychologique, Geneve*, **11**, 79–80.

Coffey, C.E., Figiel, G.S., Werner, R.D. and Saunders, W.B. (1990). Caffeine augmentation of ECT. *American Journal of Psychiatry*, **147**, 579–85.

Cohen, N.J. and Squire, L.R. (1981). Retrograde amnesia and remote memory impairment. *Neuropsychologia*, **19**, 337–56.

Cohen, M.R. and Swartz, C.M. (1991). Absence of nimodipine premedication effect on memory after electroconvulsive therapy. *Neuropsychobiology*, **24**, 165–8.

Coriat, I.H. (1907). The Lowell case of amnesia. *Journal of Abnormal Psychology*, **2**, 93–111.

Corkin, S. (1982). Some relationships between global amnesias and the memory impairments in Alzheimer's disease. In *Alzheimer's Disease: a Report of Research in Progress* (ed. S. Corkin, K.L. Davis, J.H. Growdon, E. Usdin, and R.J. Wurtman), pp. 149–63. New York: Raven Press.

Cutting, J. (1978). A cognitive approach to Korsakoff's syndrome. *Cortex*, **14**, 485–95.

Dannenbaum, S.E., Parkinson, S.R. and Inman, V.W. (1988). Short-term forgetting: comparisons between patients with dementia of the Alzheimer-type, depressed, and normal elderly. *Cognitive Neuropsychology*, **5**, 213–33.

d'Elia, G. and Frederiksen, S.O. (1980). ACTH4–10 and memory in ECT-treated and untreated patients. I. Effect on consolidation. *Acta Psychiatrica Scandinavica*, **62**, 418–28.

Della Sala, S., Laiacona, M., Spinnler, H. and Trivelli, C. (1993). Impaired autobiographical recollection in some frontal patients. *Neuropsychologia*, **31**, 823–40.

De Renzi, E., Liotti, M. and Nichelli, P. (1987). Semantic amnesia with preserveration of autobiographical memory. *Cortex*, **23**, 575–97.

De Wardener, H.E. and Lennox, B. (1947). Cerebral beriberi (Wernicke's encephalopathy): review of 52 cases in a Singapore PoW hospital. *Lancet*, **1**, 11–17.

Fenwick, P. (1990). Automatism, medicine and the law. *Psychological Medicine Monograph*, Supplement 17, Cambridge University Press.

Fenwick, P. (1993). Brain, mind and behaviour: some medico-legal aspects. *British Journal of Psychiatry*, **163**, 565–73.

Fisher, C.M. (1982). Transient global amnesia. *Archives of Neurology*, **39**, 605–8.

Freed, D.M., Corkin, S. and Cohen, N.J. (1987). Forgetting in H.M.: a second look. *Neuropsychologia*, **25**, 461–72.

Freed, D.M., Corkin, S., Growdon, J.H. and Nissen, M.J. (1989). Selective attention in Alzheimer's disease: characterizing cognitive subgroups of patients. *Neuropsychologia*, **27**, 325–39.
Freeman, C.P.L., Weeks, D. and Kendell, R.E. (1980). Electroconvulsive therapy. *British Journal of Psychiatry*, **137**, 8–37.
Frith, C.D., Stevens, M., Johnstone, E.C. *et al.* (1983). Effects of ECT and depression on various aspects of memory. *British Journal of Psychiatry*, **142**, 610–17.
Frith, C.D., Cahill, C., Ridley, R.M. and Baker, H.F. (1992). Memory for what it is and memory for what it means: a single case of Korsakoff's amnesia. *Cortex*, **28**, 53–67.
Gardiner, J.M. and Parkin, A.J. (1990). Attention and recollective experience. *Memory and Cognition*, **18**, 579–83.
Graf, P. and Schacter, D.L. (1985). Implicit and explicit memory for new associations in normal amnesic subjects. *Journal of Experimental Psychology: Learning, Memory and Cognition*, **11**, 501–18.
Graf, P., Squire, L.R. and Mandler, G. (1984). The information that amnesic patients do not forget. *Journal of Experimental Psychology: Learning, Memory and Cognition*, **10**, 164–78.
Graff-Radford, N.R., Damasio, H., Yamada, T. *et al.* (1985). Non-haemorrhagic thalamic infarction: clinical, neurological, and electrophysiological findings in four anatomical groups defined by computerised tomography. *Brain*, **108**, 485–516.
Graff-Radford, N.R., Tranel, D., Van Hoesen, G.W. and Brandt, J.P. (1990). Diencephalic amnesia. *Brain*, **113**, 1–26.
Guberman, A. and Stuss, D. (1983). The syndrome of bilateral paramedian thalamic infarction. *Neurology*, **33**, 540–6.
Gudjonsson, G.H. and MacKeith, J. (1983). A specific recognition deficit in a case of homicide. *Medicine, Science and the Law*, **23**, 37–40.
Gudjonsson, G.H. and Taylor, P.J. (1985). Cognitive deficit in a case of retrograde amnesia. *British Journal of Psychiatry*, **147**, 715–18.
Heathfield, K.W.G., Croft, P.B. and Swash, M. (1973). The syndrome of transient global amnesia. *Brain*, **96**, 729–36.
Hirst, W. (1982). The amnesic syndrome: descriptions and explanations. *Psychological Bulletin*, **91**, 435–60.
Hodges, J. and Oxbury, S.M. (1990). Persistent memory impairment following transient global amnesia. *Journal of Clinical and Experimental Neurology*, **12**, 904–20.
Hodges, J.R. and Ward, C.D. (1989). Observations during transient global amnesia: a behavioural and neuropsychological study of five cases. *Brain*, **112**, 595–620.
Hodges, J. and Warlow, C.P. (1990). The aetiology of transient global amnesia. *Brain*, **113**, 639–57.
Hodges, J.R., Patterson, K., Oxbury, S. and Funnell, E. (1992). Semantic dementia. Progressive fluent aphasia with temporal lobe atrophy. *Brain*, **115**, 1783–806.
Hodges, J.R., Salmon, D.P. and Butters, N. (1993). Recognition and naming of famous faces in Alzheimer's disease: a cognitive analysis. *Neuropsychologia*, **31**, 775–88.
Horne, R.L., Pettinati, H.M., Menken, M. *et al.* (1984). Dexamethasone in electroconvulsive therapy: efficacy for depression and post-ECT amnesia. *Biological Psychiatry*, **19**, 13–27.

Huff, F.J., Corkin, S. and Growdon, J.H. (1986). Semantic impairment and anomia in Alzheimer's disease. *Brain and Language*, **28**, 235–49.

Huppert, F.A. and Piercy, M. (1976). Recognition memory in amnesic patients: effect of temporal context and familiarity of material. *Cortex*, **12**, 3–20.

Huppert, F.A. and Piercy, M. (1978*a*). The role of trace strength in recency and frequency judgements by amnesic and control subjects. *Quarterly Journal of Experimental Psychology*, **30**, 347–54.

Huppert, F.A. and Piercy, M. (1978*b*). Dissociation between learning and remembering in organic amnesia. *Nature*, **275**, 317–18.

Huppert, F.A. and Piercy, M. (1979). Normal and abnormal forgetting in organic amnesia: effect of locus of lesion. *Cortex*, **15**, 385–90.

Jacobson, R.R. and Lishman, W. (1987). Selective memory loss and global intellectual deficits in alcoholic Korakoff's syndrome. *Psychological Medicine*, **17**, 649–55.

Jacobson, R.R., Acker, C.F. and Lishman, W.A. (1990). Patterns of neuropsychological deficit in alcoholic Korsakoff's syndrome. *Psychological Medicine*, **20**, 321–34.

Janowsky, J.S., Shimamura, A.P., Kritchevsky, M. and Squire, L.R. (1989). Cognitive impairment following frontal lobe damage and its relevance to human amnesia. *Behavioral Neuroscience*, **103**, 548–60.

Johnson, M.K., Kim, J.K. and Risse, G. (1985). Do alcoholic Korsakoff's Syndrome patients acquire affective reactions? *Journal of Experimental Psychology: Learning, Memory, and Cognition*, **11**, 22–36.

Jolliffe, N., Wortis, H. and Fein, H.D. (1941). The Wernicke syndrome. *Archives of Neurology and Psychiatry*, **46**, 569–97.

Joyce, E.M. and Robbins, T.W. (1991). Frontal lobe function in Korsakoff and non-Korsakoff alcoholics: planning and spatial working memory. *Neuropsychologia*, **29**, 709–23.

Kanzer, M. (1939). Amnesia: a statistical study. *American Journal of Psychiatry*, **96**, 711–16.

Kapur, N. (1990). Transient epiletic amnesia: a clinically distinct form of neurological memory disorder. In *Transient Global Amnesia and Related Disorders* (ed. H.J. Markowitsch). Lewiston, NY: Hogrefe and Huber.

Kapur, N. (1993). Focal retrograde amnesia in neurological disease. *Cortex*, **29**, 217–34.

Kapur, N., Ellison, D., Smith, M. *et al.* (1992). Focal retrograde amnesia following bilateral temporal lobe pathology: a neuropsychological and magnetic resonance study. *Brain*, **116**, 73–86.

Katz, D.I., Alexander, M.P. and Mandell, A.M. (1987). Dementia following strokes in the mesencephalon and diencephalon. *Archives of Neurology*, **44**, 1127–33.

Kopelman, M.D. (1982). Speech dominance, handedness and electro-convulsions. *Psychological Medicine*, **12**, 667–70.

Kopelman, M.D. (1985). Rates of forgetting in Alzheimer-type dementia and Korsakoff's syndrome. *Neuropsychologia*, **23**, 623–38.

Kopelman, M.D. (1986). The cholinergic neurotransmitter system in human memory and dementia: a review. *Quarterly Journal of Experimental Psychology*, **38A**, 535–573.

Kopelman, M.D. (1987*a*). Amnesia: organic and psychogenic. *British Journal of Psychiatry*, **150**, 428–42.

Kopelman, M.D. (1987*b*). Crime and amnesia: a review. *Behavioural Sciences and the Law*, **5**, 323–42.

Kopelman, M.D. (1989). Remote and autobiographical memory, temporal context memory, and frontal atrophy in Korsakoff and Alzheimer patients. *Neuropsychologia*, **27**, 437–60.

Kopelman, M.D. (1991*a*). Frontal lobe dysfunction and memory deficits in the alcoholic Korsakoff syndrome and Alzheimer-type dementia. *Brain*, **114**, 117–37.

Kopelman, M.D. (1991*b*). Non-verbal, short-term forgetting in the alcoholic Korsakoff syndrome and Alzheimer-type dementia. *Neuropsychologia*, **29**, 737–47.

Kopelman,M.D. (1994). Working memory in the amnesic syndrome and degenerative dementia. *Neuropsychology*, **8**, 555–62.

Kopelman, M.D. (1995*a*). The Korsakoff syndrome. *British Journal of Psychiatry*, **166**, 154–73.

Kopelman, M.D. (1995*b*). The assessment of psychogenic amnesia. In *Handbook of Memory Disorders* (ed. A. Baddeley, B. Wilson and F. Watts), pp. 427–48. London: John Wiley and Sons.

Kopelman, M.D. (1996). Transient disorders of memory and consciousness. In *Neuropsychiatry: A Comprehensive Textbook* (ed. B.S. Fogel, R.B. Schiffer and S.M. Rao), pp. 615–24. Baltimore: Williams and Wilkins.

Kopelman, M.D. (1997). Comments on Mayes and Downes: What do theories of the functional deficit(s) underlying amnesia have to explain? *Memory*, **5**, 105–14.

Kopelman, M.D. and Corn, T.H. (1988). Cholinergic 'blockade' as a model for cholinergic depletion: a comparison of the memory deficits with those of Alzheimer-type dementia and the alcoholic Korsakoff syndrome. *Brain*, **111**, 1079–110.

Kopelman, M.D. and Stanhope, N. (1997). Rates of forgetting in organic amnesia following temporal lobe, diencephalic, or frontal lobe lesions. *Neuropsychology*, **11**, 343–56.

Kopelman, M.D. Panayiotopoulos, C.P. and Lewis, P. (1994*a*). Transient epileptic amnesia differentiated from psychogenic 'fugue': neuropsychological, EEG and PET findings. *Journal of Neurology, Neurosurgery and Psychiatry*, **57**, 1002–4.

Kopelman, M.D., Christensen, H., Puffett, A. and Stanhope, N. (1994*b*). The Great Escape: a neuropsychological study of psychogenic amnesia. *Neuropsychologia*, **32**, 675–91.

Kopelman, M.D., Green, R.E.A., Guinan, E.M. *et al.* (1994*c*). The case of the amnesic intelligence officer. *Psychological Medicine*, **24**, 1037–45.

Korsakoff, S.S. (1887). Disturbance of psychic function in alcoholic paralysis and its relation to the disturbance of the psychic sphere in multiple neuritis of non-alcoholic origin. Quoted by Victor, M., Adams, R.D. and Collins, G.H. (1971). In *The Wernicke–Korsakoff Syndrome*. Oxford: Blackwell.

Korsakoff, S.S. (1889*a*). Psychic disorder in conjunction with peripheral neuritis. Translated and republished by M. Victor and P.I. Yakovlev (1955). *Neurology*, **5**, 394–406.

Korsakoff, S.S. (1889*b*). Etude médico-psychologique sur une forme des maladies de la mémoire. *Revue Philosophie*, **20**, 501–30.

Kritchevsky, M. and Squire, L.R. (1989). Transient global amnesia: evidence for extensive, temporally graded retrograde amnesia. *Neurology*, **39**, 213–18.

Kritchevsky, M., Squire, L.R. and Zouzounis, J.A. (1988). Transient global amnesia: characterization of anterograde and retrograde amnesia. *Neurology*, **38**, 213–19.

Leng, N.R.C. and Parkin, A.J. (1988). Double dissociation of frontal dysfunction in organic amnesia. *British Journal of Clinical Psychology*, **27**, 359–62.

Leng, N.R.C. and Parkin, A.J. (1989). Aetiological variation in the amnesic syndrome: comparisons using the Brown-Peterson task. *Cortex*, **25**, 251–9.

Lennox, W.G. (1943). Amnesia, real and feigned. *American Journal of Psychiatry*, **99**, 732–43.

Levin, Y., Elizur, A. and Korczyn, A.D. (1987). Physostigmine improves ECT-induced memory disturbances. *Neurology*, **37**, 871–5.

Levin, H., High, W.M. and Eisenberg, H.M. (1988). Learning and forgetting during post-traumatic amnesia in head-injured patients. *Journal of Neurology, Neurosurgery and Psychiatry*, **51**, 14–20.

Lewis, P. and Kopelman, M.D. (1997). Forgetting rates in psychiatric disorders. Submitted for Publication.

Lishman, W.A. (1968). Brain damage in relation to psychiatric disability after head injury. *British Journal of Psychiatry*, **114**, 373–410.

Lishman, W.A. (1987). *Organic Psychiatry: The Psychological Consequences of Cerebral Disorder*, 2nd edition. Oxford: Blackwell Scientific Publications Ltd.

Mair, W.G.P., Warrington, E.K. and Weiskrantz, L. (1979). Memory disorder in Korsakoff's psychosis; a neuropathological and neuropsychological investigation of two cases. *Brain*, **102**, 749–83.

Markowitsch, H.J., Calabrese, P., Haupts, M. *et al.* (1993). Searching for the anatomical basis of retrograde amnesia. *Journal of Clinical and Experimental Neuropsychology*, **15**, 947–67.

Martin, A. (1990). Neuropsychology of Alzheimer's disease: the case for subgroups. In *Modular Deficits in Alzheimer-Type Dementia* (ed. M.F. Schwartz), pp. 143–75. Cambridge, Massachusetts: MIT Press.

Martin,A. (1992*a*). Degraded knowledge representations in patients with Alzheimer's disease: implications for models of semantic and repetition priming. In *Neuropsychology of Memory*, 2nd edition (ed. L.R. Squire and N. Butters), pp. 220–32. New York: Guilford Press.

Martin, A. (1992*b*). Semantic knowledge in patients with Alzheimer's disease: evidence for degraded representations. In *Memory Functioning in Dementia* (ed. L. Backman), pp. 119–34. Amsterdam: North Holland Press.

Martin, A. and Fedio, P. (1983). Word production and comprehension in Alzheimer's disease: a breakdown of semantic knowledge. *Brain and Language*, **19**, 323–41.

Martin, A., Brouwers, P., Lalonde, F. *et al.* (1986). Towards a behavioral typology of Alzheimer's patients. *Journal of Clinical and Experimental Neuropsychology*, **8**, 594–610.

Martin, P.R., Adinoff, B., Eckardt, M.J. *et al.* (1989). Effective pharmacotherapy of alcoholic amnestic disorder with fluvoxamine. *Archives of General Psychiatry*, **46**, 617–21.

Martone, M., Butters, N., Payne, M. *et al.* (1984). Dissociations between skill learning and verbal recognition in amnesia and dementia. *Archives of Neurology*, **41**, 965–70.

Martone, E., Butters, N. and Trauner, D. (1986). Some analyses of forgetting of pictorial material in amnesic and demented patients. *Journal of Clinical and Experimental Neuropsychology*, **8**, 161–78.

Mattes, J.A., Pettinati, H.M., Stephens, S. *et al.* (1990). A placebo-controlled evaluation of vasopressin for ECT-induced memory impairment. *Biological Psychiatry*, **27**, 289–303.

Mayes, A.R. (1992). Automatic memory processes in amnesia: how are they mediated? In *The Neuropsychology of Consciousness*, (ed. A.D. Milner and M.D. Rugg), pp. 235–62. London: Academic Press.

Mayes, A.R., Meudell, P.R. and Pickering, A. (1985). Is organic amnesia caused by a selective deficit in remembering contextual information? *Cortex*, **21**, 167–202.

Mayes, A.R., Meudell, P.R., Mann, D. and Pickering, A. (1988). Location of lesions in Korsakoff's syndrome: neuropsychological and neuropathological data on two patients. *Cortex*, **24**, 367–88.

McCool, B.A., Plonk, S.G., Martin, P.R. and Singleton, C.K. (1993). Cloning of human transketolase cDNAs and comparison of the nucleotide sequence of the coding region in Wernicke–Korsakoff and non-Wernicke–Korsakoff individuals. *Journal of Biological Chemistry*, **268**, 1397–404.

McEntee, W.J., Biber,M.P., Perl, D.P. and Benson, D.F. (1976). Diencephalic amnesia: a reappraisal. *Journal of Neurology, Neurosurgery and Psychiatry*, **39**, 436–41.

McKee, R.D. and Squire, L.R. (1992). Equivalent forgetting rates in long-term memory for diencephalic and medial temporal lobe amnesia. *Journal of Neuroscience*, **12**, 3765–72.

Meudell, P. and Mayes, A. (1982). Normal and abnormal forgetting: some comments on the human amnesic syndrome. In *Normality and Pathology in Cognitive Functions* (ed. A.W. Ellis), pp. 203–38. London: Academic Press.

Miller, J.W., Petersen, R.C., Metter, E.J. *et al.* (1987*a*). Transient global amnesia: clinical characteristics and prognosis. *Neurology*, **37**, 733–7.

Miller, J.W., Yanagihara, T., Petersen, R.C. and Klass, D. (1987*b*). Transient global amnesia and epilepsy. Electroencephalographic distinction. *Archives of Neurology*, **44**, 629–33.

Morris, R.G. (1986). Short-term forgetting in senile dementia of the Alzheimer's type. *Cognitive Neuropsychology*, **3**, 77–97.

Morris, R.G. (1994). Working memory in Alzheimer-type dementia. *Neuropsychology*, **8**, 544–54.

Moscovitch, M. (1982). Multiple dissociation of function in amnesia. In *Human Memory and Amnesia* (ed. L.S. Cermak), pp. 337–760. Hillsdale, New Jersey: Lawrence Erlbaum.

Nasrallah, H.A., Varney, N., Coffman, J.A. *et al.* (1986). Opiate antagonism fails to reverse post-ECT cognitive deficits. *Journal of Clinical Psychiatry*, **47**, 555–6.

Nebes, R.D. (1992). Cognitive dysfunction in Alzheimer's disease. In *The Handbook of Ageing and Cognition* (ed. F.I.M. Craik and T.A. Salthouse), pp. 373–446. Hillsdale, NJ: Erlbaum.

Nebes, R.D. and Brady, C.B. (1989). The effect of semantic and syntactic structure on verbal memory in Alzheimer's disease. *Brain and Language*, **36**, 301–13.

Nebes, R., Martin, D. and Horn, L. (1984). Sparing of semantic memory in Alzheimer's disease. *Journal of Abnormal Psychology*, **93**, 321–30.

Newcombe, F. (1969). *Missile Wounds of the Brain*. Oxford: Oxford University Press.

Ober, B.A. and Shenaut, G.K. (1994). Semantic priming in Alzheimer's disease: meta-analysis and theoretical evaluation. In *Age Differences in Word and Language Processing* (ed. P.A. Allen and T.R. Bashore). Amsterdam: North-Holland.

O'Connell, B.A. (1960). Amnesia and homicide. *British Journal of Delinquency*, **10**, 262–76.
O'Connor, M., Butters, N., Miliotis, P. *et al.* (1992). The dissociation of anterograde and retrograde amnesia in a patient with herpes encephalitis. *Journal of Clinical and Experimental Neuropsychology*, **14**, 159–78.
Ostergaard, A.L. (1994). Dissociations between word priming effects in normal subjects and patients with memory disorders: multiple memory systems or retrieval? *Quarterly Journal of Experimental Psychology: Section A: Human Experimental Psychology*, **47**, 331–64.
Parfitt, D.N. and Gall, C.M.C. (1944). Psychogenic amnesia: the refusal to remember. *Journal of Mental Science*, **90**, 511–27.
Parkin, A.J. (1991). Recent advances in the neuropsychology of memory. In *Memory: Neurochemical and Abnormal Perspectives* (ed. J. Weinman and J. Hunter), pp. 141–62. London: Harwood Academic Publishers.
Parkin, A.J. (1992). Functional significance of aetiological factors in human amnesia. In *The Neuropsychology of Memory*, 2nd edition (ed. L.R. Squire and N. Butters), pp. 122–9. New York: Guilford Press.
Parkin, A.J. and Leng, N.R.C. (1988). Comparative studies of human amnesia: syndrome or syndromes? In *Information Processing by the Brain* (ed. H. Markowitsch), pp. 107–23. Toronto: Hans Huber.
Parkin, A.J., Montaldi, D., Leng, N.R.C. and Hunkin, N.M. (1990). Contextual cueing effects in the remote memory of alcoholic Korsakoff patients and normal subjects. *The Quarterly Journal of Experimental Psychology*, **42A**, 585–96.
Parkin, A.J., Rees, J.E., Hunkin, N.M. and Rose, P.E. (1994). Impairment of memory following discrete thalamic infarction. *Neuropsychologia*, **32**, 39–52.
Partridge, F.M., Knight, R.G. and Feehan, M.J. (1990). Direct and indirect memory performance in patients with senile dementia. *Psychological Medicine*, **20**, 111–18.
Perani, D., Bressi, S., Cappa, S.F. *et al.* (1993). Evidence of multiple memory systems in the human brain. A [^{18}F]FDG PET metabolic study. *Brain*, **116**, 903–20.
Russell, W.R. and Nathan, P.W. (1946). Traumatic amnesia. *Brain*, **69**, 280–300.
Russell, W.R. and Smith, A. (1961). Post-traumatic amnesia in closed head injury. *Archives of Neurology*, **5**, 4–29.
Sackheim, H.A., Prudic, J., Devanand, D.P. *et al.* (1993). Effects of stimulus intensity and electrode placement on the efficacy and cognitive effects of ECT. *New England Journal of Medicine*, **328**, 839–46.
Sagar, H.J., Sullivan, E.V., Gabrielli, J.D.E. *et al.* (1988). Temporal ordering and short-term memory deficits in Parkinson's disease. *Brain*, **111**, 525–39.
Sargant, W. and Slater, E. (1941). Amnesic syndromes in war. *Proceedings of the Royal Society of Medicine*, **34**, 757–64.
Schacter, D.L. (1994). Paper presented at the *3rd International Conference on Practical Aspects of Memory*, Maryland, USA.
Schacter, D.L. and Graf, P. (1986). Preserved learning in amnesic patients: perspectives from research on direct priming. *Journal of Clinical and Experimental Neuropsychology*, **8**, 727–43.
Schacter, D.L., Wang, P.L., Tulving, E. and Freeman, M. (1982). Functional retrograde amnesia: a quantitative case study. *Neuropsychologia*, **20**, 523–32.
Schacter, D.L., Harbluk, J.L. and McLachan, D.R. (1984). Retrieval without recollection: an experimental analysis of source amnesia. *Journal of Verbal Learning and Verbal Behavior*, **23**, 593–611.

Shimamura, A.P. and Squire, L.R. (1984), Paired-associate learning and priming effects in amnesia: a neuropsychological study. *Journal of Experimental Pychology: General*, **133**, 556–70.

Shimamura, A.P. and Squire, L.R. (1986). Korsakoff's syndrome: a study of the relation between anterograde amnesia and remote memory impairment. *Behavioral Neuroscience*, **100**, 165–70.

Shimamura, A.P., Salmon, D.P., Squire, L.R. and Butters, N. (1987). Memory dysfunction and word priming in dementia and amnesia. *Behavioral Neuroscience*, **101**, 347–51.

Shimamura, A.P., Jernigan, T.L. and Squire, L.R. (1988). Korsakoff's syndrome: radiological (CT) findings and neruopsychological correlates. *Journal of Neuroscience*, **8**, 4400–10.

Shimamura, A.P., Janowsky, J.S. and Squire, L.R. (1990). Memory for the temporal order of events in patients with frontal lobe lesions and amnesic patients. *Neuropsychologia*, **28**, 803–13.

Shoqeirat, M.A., Mayes, A., MacDonald, C. *et al.* (1990). Performance on tests sensitive to frontal lobe lesions by patients with organic amnesia: Leng and Parkin revisited. *British Journal of Clinical Psychology*, **29**, 401–8.

Sommer, B.R., Satlin, A., Friedman, L. and Cole, J.O. (1989). Glycopyrrolate versus atropine in post-ECT amnesia in the elderly. *Journal of Geriatric Psychiatry and Neurology*, **2**, 18–21.

Speedie, L.J. and Heilman, K.M. (1982). Amnesic disturbance following infarction of the left dorsomedial nucleus of the thalamus. *Neuropsychologia*, **20**, 597–604.

Squire, L.R. (1977). ECT and memory loss. *American Journal of Psychiatry*, **134**, 997–1001.

Squire, L.R. (1981). Two forms of human amnesia: an analysis of forgetting. *Journal of Neuroscience*, **1**, 635–40.

Squire, L.R. (1982). Comparisons between forms of amnesia: some deficits are unique to Korsakoff's syndrome. *Journal of Experimental Psychology, Learning, Memory, Cognition*. **8**, 560–72.

Squire, L.R. and Slater, P.C. (1983). ECT and complaints of memory dysfunction: a prospective three-year follow-up study. *British Journal of Psychiatry*, **142**, 1–8.

Squire, L.R., Cohen, N.J. and Nadel, L. (1984). The medial temporal region and memory consolidation: a new hypothesis. In *Memory Consolidation* (ed. H. Weingartner and E. Parker). Hillsdale, NJ: Erlbaum Associates.

Squire, L.R., Haist, F. and Shimamura, A.P. (1989). The neurology of memory: quantitative assessment of retrograde amnesia in two types of amnesic patients. *Journal of Neuroscience*, **9**, 828–39.

Stengel, E. (1941). On the aetiology of the fugue states. *Journal of Mental Science*, **87**, 572–99.

Stern, R.A., Nevels, C.T., Shelhorse, M.E. *et al.* (1991). Antidepressant and memory effects of combined thyroid hormone treatment and electroconvulsive therapy: preliminary findings. *Biological Psychiatry*, **30**, 623–7.

Sullivan, E.V., Corkin, S. and Growdon, J.H. (1986). Verbal and non-verbal short-term memory in patients with Alzheimer's disease and in healthy elderly subjects. *Developmental Neuropsychology*, **2**, 387–400.

Taylor, P.J. and Kopelman, M.D. (1984). Amnesia for criminal offences. *Psychological Medicine*, **14**, 581–8.

Tulving, E. and Schacter, D.L. (1990). Priming and human memory systems. *Science*, **247**, 301–6.

Victor, M., Adams, R.D. and Collins, G.H. (1971). *The Wernicke-Korsakoff Syndrome*, 1st edition. Philadelphia: F.A. Davis Co.

Von Cramon, D.Y., Hebel, N. and Schuri, U. (1985). A contribution to the anatomical basis of thalamic amnesia. *Brain*, **108**, 997–1008.

Warrington, E.K. and Weiskrantz, L. (1970). Amnesic syndrome: consolidation or retrieval? *Nature*, **228**, 628–30.

Warrington, E.K. and Weiskrantz, L. (1982). Amnesia – a disconnection syndrome? *Neuropsychologia*, **20**, 233–48.

Watts, F.N. (1995). Depression and anxiety. In *Handbook of Memory Disorders* (ed. A. Baddeley, B. Wilson and F. Watts), pp. 293–317. John Wiley and Sons.

Weeks, D., Freeman, C.P.L. and Kendall, R.E. (1980). ECT, 3: enduring cognitive deficits. *British Journal of Psychiatry*, **137**, 26–37.

Weingartner, H., Rudorfer, M.V., Buchsbaum, M.S. and Linnoila, M. (1983). Effects of serotonin on memory impairments produced by ethanol. *Science*, **221**, 472–3.

Weiskrantz,L. (1985). On issues and theories of the human amnesic syndrome. In *Memory Systems of the Brain*. (ed. N.M. Weinberger, J.L. McGaugh and G. Lynch), pp. 380–415. New York and London: Guilford Press.

Weiskrantz, L. and Warrington, E.K. (1979). Conditioning in amnesia patients. *Neuropsychologia*, **17**, 187–94.

Whitty, C., Stores, G. and Lishman, W.A. (1977). Amnesia in cerebral disease. In *Amnesia*, 2nd edition (ed. C.W.M. Whitty and O.L. Zangwill), London and Boston: Butterworths.

Wilson, G., Rupp, C. and Wilson, W.W. (1950). Amnesia. *American Journal of Psychiatry*, **106**, 481–5.

Winocur, G., Oxbury, S., Roberts, R. *et al.* (1984). Amnesia in a patient with bilateral lesions to the thalamus. *Neuropsychologia*, **22**, 123–43.

Witt, E.D. (1985). Neuroanatomical consequences of thiamine deficiency: a comparative analysis. *Alcohol and Alcoholism*, **20**, 201–21.

Section IV

Brain disease and mental illness

7

Psychiatric manifestations of demonstrable brain disease

MARIA A. RON

The brain and the mind: a complex relationship

We are able to visualise the brain at rest, image it when active, map and quantify neurotransmitter receptors and study its *in vivo* chemistry using a variety of methods that have recently become available. Despite these breathtaking advances, the pathophysiological basis of mental illness remains largely unresolved and the same applies to our understanding of how psychiatric symptoms arise in the context of established brain pathology.

The application of new imaging techniques to the study of neurological and psychiatric conditions has highlighted the complexity of these interactions. Severe psychotic symptoms can be present in patients with structurally normal brains and the imaging abnormalities described in patients with schizophrenia or affective psychosis tend to be subtle and static. On the other hand, gross brain pathology may occur without psychiatric counterparts, suggesting that the brain abnormalities we are currently able to visualise are neither sufficient nor necessary to cause psychosis and that other biological or environmental factors may play a crucial role. As the lack of specificity and limited repertoire of psychiatric responses to brain disease has become evident so has the complexity of the brain circuits subserving behaviour. To make sense of this wealth of information and to understand its clinical significance has become a major challenge for those working in the field of mental illness.

This chapter will discuss the psychiatric manifestations of established brain disease, trying to compare symptoms and pathophysiological mechanisms with those of primary psychiatric illness. It is hoped that a better understanding of brain and mind interactions in this setting will clarify the mechanisms operating in primary psychiatric illness. Affective disorder, schizophrenia-like psychoses and obsessive-compulsive disorder will be the main foci of the chapter.

Affective symptoms in neurological disease

Affective symptoms, especially those of depression and anxiety, are very common in patients with neurological disease. Recent studies using standardised psychiatric interviews have reported a prevalence of around 40% for Parkinson's disease (Cummings, 1992) and MS (Ron and Logsdail, 1989), far in excess of those expected in patients with a similar degree of physical disability but without brain disease. In stroke the frequency of affective disorders is somewhat lower and two recent community based studies (House *et al.*, 1990; Burvill *et al.*, 1995) have reported an incidence of symptoms of depression and anxiety of around 25% in the first six months after stroke. The presence of affective symptoms appears higher in patients with widespread as opposed to focal pathology and in those with progressive rather than static disability.

Using the DSM-IV criteria these affective symptoms come under the generic diagnosis of 'mood disorder due to a medical condition'. In most patients, however, this causal link is difficult to prove and the diagnosis often hinges on the observed high prevalence of mood disorder in certain neurological illness. The full range of symptoms observed in primary affective illness has been reported in patients with neurological disease, but there is good agreement from studies of patients with MS (Ron and Logsdail, 1989), Parkinson's disease (Cummings, 1992), and stroke (House *et al.*, 1990, Burvill *et al.*, 1995) that the symptoms that form the 'melancholia' core (i.e., diurnal variation, self-blame, etc.) are less common in these patients who generally express feelings of irritability, sadness without self-blame, poor concentration and subjective anxiety. The severity of symptoms tends to be mild to moderate and only half of the patients reported in these studies fulfilled the criteria for major depression, the diagnosis of dysthymia, a milder, more chronic mood disturbance, being more appropriate for the rest.

The natural history of affective symptoms in neurological patients is difficult to ascertain from the largely cross-sectional studies, although clinical observation suggests that a chronic course or one with recurrent episodes is common in progressive neurological conditions such as MS or Parkinson's disease. An exception to this lack of information is the outcome of depression and anxiety in stroke patients, carefully charted by recent community based studies. The Oxford (House *et al.*, 1990) and Perth (Burvill *et al.*, 1995) community stroke studies have suggested that the peak incidence for depression and anxiety occurs during the first six months and that their incidence decreases markedly after that. In the Perth study, a year after stroke, the prevalence of dysthymia was similar to that of the general population and half of those who initially fulfilled the criteria for major depression had recovered.

The neuroanatomy of primary affective disorders

The interest in structural brain abnormalities in affective illness has lagged behind that lavished on schizophrenia. Early studies using CT remarked on the presence of ventricular and sulcal enlargement in populations of depressed patients compared to controls (Dolan, Calloway and Mann, 1985; Dolan, *et al.*, 1986). Important differences have nevertheless been reported between the structural brain abnormalities present in schizophrenic and affective psychoses using volumetric techniques. Thus Harvey *et al.* (1994), using volumetric MRI measurements, failed to detect in bipolar patients the reduction in cortical volume present in schizophrenics, suggesting important differences between the two groups. The presence of MRI hyperintensities in the periventricular white matter is another intriguing finding in patients with affective disease (Dupont *et al.*, 1990). The cause of these lesions, which may be commoner in those with treatment-resistant depression, is unclear, but a vascular aetiology remains a strong possibility.

Functional imaging studies have been far more important in highlighting the role that fronto-subcortical circuits play in affective illness. Bench *et al.* (1992) using PET reported significant decrements in blood flow in the left anterior cingulate and left dorsolateral prefrontal cortex (DLPFC) in depressed patients compared to healthy controls. In addition, in those with cognitive impairment, decrements were also observed in the medial temporal gyrus. SPET studies have reported similar findings and have suggested that the reversible reduction of blood flow in the basal ganglia may represent a state-related abnormality, whilst the persistent 'hypofrontality' is more likely to be a trait marker (Goodwin *et al.*, 1993).

The neuroanatomy of affective disorders in neurological disease

The role of fronto-subcortical circuits in neuropsychiatric disorders has recently been reviewed by Mega and Cummings (1994) and is dealt with elsewhere in the book (Chapter 1). These circuits involve frontal areas, striatum, globus pallidus, substantia nigra and thalamus. The spatial closeness of these circuits, especially at subcortical levels, and their dependence on the same neurotransmitter systems, result in lesions often involving more than one system and in similar clinical manifestations resulting from lesions interrupting these circuits at different sites.

Affective symptoms are particularly likely to occur with cortical or subcortical lesions involving the basotemporal limbic or basal ganglia–thalamo–cortical pathways. In Parkinson's disease depression is likely to result from the primary degeneration of mesocorticolimbic dopaminergic neurones, which in turn leads to dysfunction of the orbito-frontal cortex and serotonergic neurones in the dorsal raphe. Whilst in Huntington's disease involvement of the dorsomedial caudate is likely to be central in the causation of affective symptoms.

Some support for this hypothesis comes from the studies of Mayberg *et al.* (1990, 1992, 1994), who compared changes in brain glucose metabolism in depressed and euthymic patients with basal ganglia disease. Reduced glucose metabolism was observed in frontal and temporal areas in depressed patients with Parkinson's disease or Huntington's disease compared with controls. This pattern was similar to that found in primary depression and the degree of metabolism reduction was correlated with the severity of depression. This suggests a common final path involving selective disruption of cortico-striatal and baso-temporal limbic pathways and leading to depression in conditions with different pathological sites.

In stroke, the link between site of lesion and the presence of depression has been more elusive. Methodological flaws in the design of some uncontrolled studies are partly to blame. In addition the distant effects of a given lesion cannot be visualised with structural imaging. Starkstein *et al.* (1987) reported a close association between depression and left anterior lesions, especially when the caudate was involved. In such patients the incidence of depression was considered to be around 90% and serotonergic mechanisms were postulated. However these studies are open to criticism because of the narrow inclusion criteria, often excluding aphasic patients, the small sample size and the inaccuracies of lesion localisation. More recently community-based studies (Sharpe *et al.*, 1990), with more representative populations, have failed to find a correlation between depressive symptomatology and lesion localization, suggesting that lesions differently placed can cause similar affective symptoms. It remains to be determined whether similar distant effects of stroke can be detected using functional imaging in those patients with post-stroke depression.

Clinico-pathological correlations become more tenuous in patients with widespread brain disease such as MS. In our MS study (Ron and Logsdail, 1989), although the prevalence of depression was much higher than in disabled controls without brain disease, the correlations with lesion load as detected by MRI were low. This points to the difficulties in estimating the functional role of a given brain lesion and highlights the importance of genetic and environmental factors in the genesis of depression even in those with demonstrable brain disease. Thus in MS patients bipolar disorder may be commoner in those with a family history of the disease, whilst post-stroke depression in the Perth study (Burvill *et al.*, 1995) was commoner and more severe in those who had previously been depressed.

The recognition of affective symptoms in neurological patients is of considerable practical importance not only because hospital stay is likely to be longer and costs higher, but because long-term survival may also be impaired. In the Perth study (Burvill *et al.*, 1995) mortality rates a year after stroke were twice as high in those initially depressed and three times as high in those with anxiety symptoms compared to those free from psychiatric symptoms.

Other affective accompaniments of neurological disease

Two rarer affective accompaniments of brain disease are worth mentioning here: secondary mania and pathological crying and laughter.

Secondary mania

This is defined as the occurrence of manic symptoms in the absence of previous history of affective disorder and in the presence of primary brain disease or systemic disease affecting the brain. The clinical features of secondary mania are poorly characterised, partly due to the fact that the syndrome is rare and that it merges imperceptibly with 'fixed' personality changes that occur in various types of brain disease.

Cummings and Mendez (1984) have reviewed the reported cases of mania following a variety of brain insults adding some cases of their own. Different pathologies including trauma, tumours, neurodegenerative and vascular disease were represented in the series and diencephalic and basal forebrain lesions, particularly right-sided, were commoner. The evolution of clinical symptoms was variable and whilst in some cases symptoms remitted spontaneously or after removal of tumours, in others a chronic or a cyclic manic-depressive course ensued. Cognitive impairment, unilateral neglect or denial of illness and amnesia for the episode were often reported. A more recent study (Starkstein *et al.*, 1991), comparing patients with mania and bipolar disorder following brain injury, found no differences in demographic features and interval between insult and symptoms in the two groups, but whilst those with bipolar episodes tended to have subcortical lesions involving the caudate and right thalamus, those with mania had larger cortical lesions in orbito-frontal and baso-temporal regions disrupting fronto-limbic connections. A third of those with secondary mania had previous depressive episodes suggesting that factors other than brain pathology may be relevant in producing these symptoms. Cognitive impairment was also common and more marked in those with manic depressive symptoms, despite the fact that lesions were larger in the manic group. Elation, pressure of speech, hyperactivity, grandiose delusions and insomnia were the commonest symptoms and a family history of psychiatric disorder was present in a quarter of all cases. In our own small series of MS patients with clear episodes of mania (Feinstein, du Boulay and Ron, 1992) psychotic symptoms occurred many years after the onset of MS. A predominance of lesions around the temporal horns and trigone was seen in these patients compared to non-psychotic MS patients matched for disability and total MRI lesion load. However, the distribution of MRI lesions in manic patients was indistinguishable from that found in those who developed schizophrenia-like psychoses, suggesting that other factors may be relevant in determining the type of psychosis.

Secondary mania is difficult to separate from the personality change that occurs in close head injury or diseases such as MS. Disinhibition, euphoria, lack of social judgement, irritability and aggression, tactlessness and jocularity are symptoms common to both and in the presence of cognitive impairment, the course of the symptoms, waxing and waning in mania and fixed in personality disorder, are diagnostically useful. Both syndromes also overlap with the manifestations of frontal pathology, although in severe head injury, as in MS, diffuse axonal pathology can be seen throughout the neuraxis and it would be inaccurate to ascribe symptoms to frontal pathology alone. It seems more likely that a frontal disconnection syndrome could occur as a consequence of diffuse white matter disease or, as has been postulated by Stuss and Gow (1992), widespread white matter disease could manifest as a failure of the more vulnerable cognitive skills of reasoning, planning and cognitive flexibility (i.e., frontal lobe impairment) whilst overlearned activities may be better preserved. Support for this hypothesis accrues from our studies in MS patients (Ron and Logsdail, 1989), which found a clear correlation between the presence of ‘euphoria’, a fixed mood abnormality without the psychomotor changes observed in mania, and the overall MRI lesion load.

Pathological crying and laughing or emotionalism

Many aspects of the physiology of emotional control remain to be determined, but a distributed network comprising the brain stem, limbic and paralimbic structures and neocortex is involved (Black, 1982, Derryberry and Tucker, 1992). Descending pathways facilitate the patterned responses of endocrine, autonomic and motor systems regulated by the brain stem, whilst ascending pathways produce a preparatory modulation of the cortex to facilitate perceptual and cognitive processing. Noradrenergic, dopaminergic and serotonergic fibres are involved in the process.

Pathological crying or laughing was clearly described in the writings of Kinnear Wilson (1924) as '. . . a sequal to and consequence of a recognisable cerebral lesion or lesions in which attacks of involuntary, irresistible laughing or crying, or both, have come into the foreground of the clinical picture'. He distinguished these symptoms from the depression that often accompanies neurological disease. Many terms have been used to describe the symptoms (i.e., emotional lability or incontinence, emotionalism, forced crying, pseudo-bulbar affect, etc.). This complex terminology has been used to describe the same core phenomena, although the extent, location and multiplicity of lesions can modify the clinical expression. Thus mood incongruent emotionalism may be commoner with bulbar or bilateral upper motor neurone lesions, whilst unilateral or bilateral lesions affecting the basal forebrain and medial temporal lobe are more likely to produce mood congruent symptoms. Some support for this hypothesis comes from the study of Arroyo *et al.* (1993) in patients with gelastic epilepsy, a type of epilepsy where laughter is part of the seizures. Lesions in medial temporal structures were common in those in whom mirth accompanied laughter during the seizures, whilst mirthless laughter occurred in one patient with an anterior cingulate focus. Mood congruent emotionalism was also the rule in the first-ever stroke patients studied by House *et al.* (1989), in whom these episodes were usually triggered by sad or sentimental events and were under some degree of voluntary control.

Emotionalism may follow single, but more often multiple, lesions of variable localization. In the series reported by Poeck (1969) single lesions were present in a third of patients who came to post-mortem. The lesions extended to subcortical regions in all cases and the anterior limb of the internal capsule, caudate, putamen and thalamus were often involved. The largest series of patients in whom lesion localisation was attempted clinically, with imaging or at autopsy, was reported by Sackheim *et al.* (1982) who described a significant association between the presence of right-sided lesions and isolated laughter. Crying, which occurred much more often, was twice as likely to be associated with left-sided lesions, whilst mixed episodes of crying and laughter were always associated with bilateral pathology. In this series single lesions were also present in a third of the patients.

Pathological crying and laughing has been observed in many neurological conditions (i.e., brain tumours, Parkinson's disease, Wilson's disease, head injury), but has been best characterised in stroke, MS and motor neurone disease. House *et al.* (1989) reported a prevalence of around 20% during the first six months following the first-ever stroke, decreasing to 11% a year later. Emotionalism was commoner with left fronto-temporal lesions (57%), than with lesions in other localisations (19%) and it was closely associated with the presence of depression. In MS, early studies (Cottrell and Wilson, 1926) described emotionalism as an almost universal feature, but a 10% prevalence suggested by recent reports (Minden and Schiffer, 1990), is more likely to be accurate. Emotionalism is rare during the early stages of MS and commoner during relapses. In motor neurone disease a prevalence of around 50% has been reported (Gallagher, 1989), especially in those with bulbar involvement, in whom it can be an early feature of the illness.

In gelastic epilepsy the laughter observed during seizures is unprovoked, stereotyped and inappropriate, usually lasting for seconds, but may last longer if associated with complex partial seizures. Loss of memory for the attacks, automatisms and other motor symptoms are a frequent accompaniment. Dacrystic (crying) seizures are even rarer, but may occur in the same patients. In the cases reviewed by Sackheim *et al.* (1982) uncontrollable laughter resulted from desinhibition or excitation of the left hemisphere or from right-sided destructive lesions. In patients with dacrystic seizures right hemisphere lesions were always present.

Schizophrenia-like psychoses in neurological disease

Psychotic symptoms similar to those observed in schizophrenia also occur in patients with brain disease. The association between schizophrenia and epilepsy was highlighted a long time ago by Slater, Beard and Glithero (1963) and Davison and Bagley (1969) collected the previously reported cases in association with a variety of neurological conditions. Schizophrenic symptoms are less common than mood disorders in neurological patients and their prevalence and clinico-pathological correlates less well documented. However, awareness of this association, in particular with temporal lobe epilepsy, has been important in directing the search for structural abnormalities in primary schizophrenia and is likely to remain an area of research interest.

Using current diagnostic classifications (DSM-IV) 'psychotic disorder due to a general medical condition' is the diagnosis applied to schizophrenia-like illness in neurological patients. As in the case of mood disorders, the diagnosis is only made when a causal connection with the medical disorder can be made. This link is once again very difficult to establish and the clinician has to rely on indirect evidence. Pointers to an association are the fact that schizophrenic symptoms are commoner in certain neurological conditions (e.g., temporal lobe epilepsy), the late onset of psychosis in these patients and the absence of other alternative explanations for the symptoms. The difficulty in separating these psychoses from primary schizophrenia has been highlighted in recent years by the detection in the latter of structural and functional brain abnormalities, often accompanied by cognitive impairment.

There is considerable overlap of symptomatology between primary and secondary schizophrenia. Although early studies (Cutting, 1987), had highlighted clinical differences and their diagnostic value, carefully controlled studies have, by contrast, emphasised the similarities. Johnstone *et al.* (1988) examined a large sample of schizophrenic patients who met standard diagnostic criteria, looking for the presence of underlying systemic or brain disease. Comparison between those with organic illness and the rest disclosed a more advanced age of onset in the organic group, but nuclear symptoms of schizophrenia were present in both groups. No significant differences in the frequency of individual symptoms was detected between the two groups, although visual hallucinations tended to be commoner in those with organic illness. These findings are similar to those described in our sample of patients with demonstrable brain disease (Feinstein and Ron, 1990). In our sample lack of insight and delusions of persecution were the commonest symptoms and their frequency did not differ from that reported by the International Pilot Study of Schizophrenia. An interesting feature of our sample was the presence of affective symptomatology in over a third of the patients and the relative instability of the diagnosis over time. Thus eight out of 53 patients deserved a diagnosis of affective psychosis when seen four years later. Although these changes may have been in part due to the retrospective evaluation of the initial mental state, our observation agrees with that of Toone, Garralda and Ron (1982) who also found similar diagnostic inconsistencies in epileptics with schizophrenia-like psychosis over time. The variability of psychotic symptomatology may be one of the hallmarks of the psychoses arising in the context of established brain pathology.

The neuroanatomy of primary schizophrenia

The structural abnormalities that can be detected in the brains of schizophrenics with modern imaging methods are dealt with elsewhere in this book (Chapters 2 and 8). Suffice it to say here that since the early descriptions of enlarged ventricles and cortical sulci appeared in the literature (Johnstone *et al.*, 1976), many other studies have confirmed these findings, even if the proportion of patients in whom these abnormalities are present is still uncertain. Many studies have focused on the structural abnormalities present in medial temporal structures (e.g., Suddath *et al.*, 1990), but more recent studies have suggested that structural abnormalities are widespread. Thus Harvey *et al.* (1993) have reported a diffuse loss of cortical volume that appears to be specific to schizophrenia. At post-mortem, cytoarchitectural disruption and loss of neuronal density, without accompanying gliosis, have been described in hippocampal and adjacent areas (Altschuler, 1987; Conrad *et al.*, 1993) and similar abnormalities have also been described in the dorsolateral, prefrontal and cingulate cortices (Benes *et al.*, 1991). Recently, the application of proton magnetic resonance spectroscopy (MRS) has provided the means to explore *in vivo* some of these abnormalities (see Chapter 13). The study of the neuronal marker *N*-acetylaspartate (NAA) is of particular interest, as it provides an *in vivo* measure of neuronal integrity. In our study (Maier *et al.*, 1995), a significant left-sided hippocampal depletion of NAA was found in schizophrenics compared to controls. The loss of NAA was not related to age or disease duration and this suggests that at least some of these neuropathological abnormalities are static. It remains to be determined whether similar abnormalities are present in other brain areas and whether they are pathognomonic to schizophrenia.

In addition to these subtle abnormalities, other brain lesions have unexpectedly been found in schizophrenics who meet standard diagnostic criteria. The prevalence of these abnormalities is under 10% (Johnston, McMillan and Crow, 1987; Lewis, 1990), being perhaps commoner in older, institutionalised patients. In the published series, lesions were of variable pathology, but equally distributed between the right and left hemispheres. The significance of these abnormalities is uncertain and whilst some (i.e., small infarct) occurred in all probability when schizophrenic symptoms were well established, others (i.e., cavum of the septum pellucidum) are likely to be neurodevelopmental abnormalities.

As in affective illness, white matter hyperintensities have also been reported in schizophrenia. Although their number may not be increased when compared to a healthy population, there is some evidence that their area may be more extensive than in controls (Persaud *et al.*, 1997).

Functional imaging (PET) studies have emphasised the role of prefrontal limbic circuits in schizophrenia (Weinberger, Berman and Zec, 1986) and hypofrontality in response to activation has often been reported. Different patterns of resting cerebral blood flow have also been found in patients with different constellations of symptoms. Liddle *et al.* (1992) reported reductions in prefrontal blood flow in patients with the syndrome of 'psychomotor poverty' (poverty of speech, flatness of affect, decreased spontaneous movement) and in those with the 'disorganisation' syndrome (i.e., thought disorder and inappropriate affect), whilst reduced blood flow in mid temporal regions was found in those with delusions and hallucinations. More recent PET activation studies (Frith *et al.*, 1995), have suggested that a loss of functional connectivity between prefrontal and temporal cortices may be a key feature in schizophrenia. Abnormalities in the activation of this fronto-temporal circuit may, in turn, result in secondary dopaminergic failure.

It has so far proved difficult to incorporate in a unitary theory of schizophrenia the findings of structural and functional imaging studies, but a correlation between hypofrontality, ventricular enlargement and reduced hippocampal volume has now been reported (Weinberger *et al.*, 1994).

Schizophrenia-like psychosis or secondary schizophrenia in neurological disease

The occurrence of symptoms of schizophrenia in patients with demonstrable, often longstanding, brain disease has been recognised for a long time. Davison and Bagley (1969) gathered reported cases who exhibited psychotic symptoms such as thought disorder, shallow or incongruous affect, delusions or hallucinations in the context of established brain disease. The symptoms exhibited by these patients were indistinguishable from those of schizophrenia, although the authors pointed out that flattened and incongruous affect was commoner in those who exhibited these symptoms at an early age. The design of this classic study, which gathered patients with different types of brain pathology, did not allow determination of whether the incidence of schizophrenia in these patients was greater than chance. Lesion localisation was tentative in many cases, but pathology in the left temporal and diencephalic regions seemed to be overrepresented.

Many of the findings of this early study were confirmed in the National Hospital series (Feinstein and Ron, 1990) of 53 patients with schizophrenia-like psychosis secondary to demonstrable brain pathology and in whom lesion localisation was made using CT and EEG. Patients with focal epilepsy, with or without demonstrable structural pathology, were overrepresented in this sample, pointing to an association between psychosis and epilepsy discussed elsewhere in the book (Chapter 10). Right and left-sided lesions were equally common and schizophrenic symptomatology was observed in a wide range of neurological conditions (i.e., MS, Parkinson's disease, brain tumours, head injury, stroke, etc.). The onset of psychosis in these patients occurred at a more advanced age than in primary schizophrenia when the neurological disease was well established. Symptoms were often persistent and three-quarters of patients were still psychotic when re-examined or had been so during the four-year follow-up period, but on the whole the duration of these psychotic episodes seem to be shorter than in primary schizophrenia and patients rarely received depot medication. Younger patients with non-psychotic premorbid symptoms and those with psychiatrically ill first-degree relatives were more likely to remain psychotic at follow-up. This constellation of predictors, similar to that operating in primary schizophrenia, suggests that factors other than brain disease are relevant in the aetiology of secondary schizophrenia. So far, no studies have been performed comparing patients with affective or schizophrenic symptoms in the setting of brain disease and it remains to be determined why affective or schizophrenic symptoms develop following the same neurological diseases or with lesions that, at first sight, appear indistinguishable in type and localisation.

Obsessive-compulsive symptoms in neurological disease

Obsessive-compulsive disorder (OCD) is characterised by the presence of obsessions which are intrusive thoughts or impulses which the subject attempts to resist, and by compulsions which are repetitive, stereotyped, purposeful actions performed in response to obsessions or to avert a dreaded event or situation. Data from a large epidemiological study from the USA (Karno *et al.*, 1988) suggest that obsessions and compulsions do not always occur together. In this study, the frequency of OCD, when prevalence rates were adjusted for the presence of other psychiatric conditions, has been estimated to be around 2%. Despite preservation of insight, the disorder often causes significant disability.

Obsessions and compulsions have been described in association with a variety of neurological conditions affecting the basal ganglia and the orbito-frontal cortex. These conditions include, amongst others, head injury, anoxia, carbon monoxide or manganese poisoning, epilepsy, encephalitis lethargica, neuroacanthocytosis, Parkinson's disease, Huntington's disease (see Cummings and Cunningham, 1992 for a review). Similar symptoms have also been described in other conditions such as

Tourette's syndrome (Pauls *et al.*, 1986), Alzheimer's disease (Burns, Jacoby and Levy, 1990), Pick's disease (Tonkonogy, Smith and Barreira, 1994) and in focal cortical degenerations (Lawrence *et al.*, 1994), particularly when the frontal and temporal lobes were involved.

There has been considerable debate as to whether the obsessional symptoms experienced by patients with neurological disease are similar to those in primary OCD. As in other psychiatric syndromes arising in the context of brain disease, the similarities in symptomatology with the primary disorder are greater than the differences. However, in patients with cognitive impairment obsessions are reported less often than compulsions, either because they are rarer or because it is more difficult to access the mental state in these patients. Repetitive actions are, on the other hand, very common, but unlike in primary OCD, patients with neurological disease may not always recognise their absurdity or excessiveness and anxiety may only be experienced when others try to prevent these actions. In less cognitively impaired patients, compulsions may have more ritualistic, even pleasurable connotations (i.e., in some patients with Tourette's syndrome).

The neuroanatomy of primary and secondary OCD

A variety of soft neurological signs and minor brain imaging abnormalities have been described over the years in OCD patients, although there are no post-mortem studies to indicate that neuropathological abnormalities are present in OCD. Hollander *et al.* (1990) highlighted the difficulties in coordination and visuospatial tasks and the presence of subtle movement disorders. The greater frequency of these abnormalities in the left side of the body, together with mild impairment of visual memory, pointed to right hemisphere abnormalities. More severe 'obsessional slowness' has also been described in these patients, often accompanied by other subtle motor disturbances and complex tics (Hymas *et al.*, 1991). In addition, some neuropsychological studies (Flor-Henry *et al.*, 1979; Behar *et al.*, 1984), have suggested poor performance in executive tasks.

Structural imaging studies using CT and MRI have reported conflicting results. The earlier findings of ventricular enlargement (Behar *et al.*, 1984) have not been replicated by other studies (Luxenberg *et al.*, 1988) and the same applies to reduction of caudate volume (Luxenberg *et al.*, 1988; Robinson *et al.*, 1995) not found by others (Kellner *et al.*, 1991).

Important, albeit indirect, information about the brain structures subserving OCD accrues from the neurosurgical treatments that have proved successful over the years. Although data derive principally from uncontrolled follow-up studies, there is evidence that subcaudate tractotomy and limbic leucotomy, which involve subcortical prefrontal and cingulate lesions (Chiocca and Martuza, 1990; Poynton, Bridges and Bartlett, 1988), are effective treatments for OCD. The role of fronto-striatal circuits has been further emphasized in functional imaging studies. Baxter *et al.* (1987), using PET, described increased metabolism in the left orbital gyrus and caudate nuclei. The metabolism in the latter, increased further in those patients who responded to behavioural or pharmacological treatment (Baxter *et al.*, 1992). A similar increase in metabolism in the orbito-frontal cortex, but not in the striatum has been found in OCD patients with obsessional slowness (Sawle *et al.*, 1991). The heightened orbito-frontal metabolism has been interpreted as reflecting dysfunction of attentional mechanisms, which could in turn result in a failure of the sensory gating mechanism subserved by the caudate, despite the concurrent metabolic increases in this area. Through mechanisms that remain to be elucidated, treatment appears to restore the appropriate interaction between the various components of the orbito-frontal striatum circuit. Timing of post-treatment studies and choice of therapy may explain the differences in the patterns of activation reported in recovered patients. Thus Insel (1992) has suggested that decreased metabolic activity in the caudate may occur first and be followed by decreased activity in orbito-frontal and cingulate cortices. Longitudinal studies are likely to answer this important question.

More recently PET activation studies have examined changes in cerebral blood flow when patients were exposed to feared stimuli and during neutral conditions. McGuire *et al.* (1994) and Rauch *et al.* (1994) found an increase in blood flow in the inferior prefrontal and striatum, but it remains to be determined whether these changes relate specifically to OCD or to the anxiety that invariably accompanies exposure to feared stimuli.

In patients with OCD in the context of neurological disease, altered functioning of the orbito-frontal, anterior cingulate cortex and striatum is also likely, but few studies have set out to confirm this. Similarly, the differences in symptomatology with primary OCD may be explained by the presence of pathology in other brain areas. However, a SPET study of patients with Tourette's syndrome with and without obsessional symptoms has so far failed to find any significant differences in the pattern of brain metabolism attributable to the presence of these symptoms (George *et al.*, 1992).

Conclusions

A wide range of psychiatric symptoms similar to those observed in primary psychiatric illness is also present in patients with brain disease. The similarities are greater than the differences in the symptomatology exhibited by these patients and it seems likely that dysfunction of the same cortico-subcortical circuits is central in the causation of symptoms in both groups. The link between the psychiatric symptoms and the neurological disease is often difficult to establish and environmental and genetic factors predisposing to psychiatric disease may, in some cases, be as important as brain disease in causing abnormalities of mood and behaviour. The presence of psychiatric symptoms in patients with neurological disease plays an important role in the survival, overall disability, and outcome of rehabilitation and their detection and treatment, although often neglected, is of considerable importance. The study of patients with neurological disease has provided significant insights into the pathophysiology of primary psychiatric disease and will continue to do so.

References

Altshuler, L.L. (1987). Hippocampal pyramidal cell orientation in schizophrenia. *Archives of General Psychiatry*, **44**, 1094–8.

Arroyo, S., Lesser, R.P., Gordon, B. *et al.* (1993). Mirth, laughter and gelastic seizures. *Brain*, **116**, 757–80.

Baxter, L.R., Phelps, M.E., Mazziotta, J.C. *et al.* (1987). Local cerebral glucose metabolite rates in obsessive-compulsive disorder. *Archives of General Psychiatry*, **44**, 211–18.

Baxter, L.R., Schwartz, J.M., Bergman, K.S. *et al.* (1992). Caudate glucose metabolic rate changes with both drug and behaviour therapy for obsessive compulsive disorder. *Archives of General Psychiatry*, **49**, 681–9.

Behar, D., Rapoport, J.L., Berg, C.J. *et al.* (1984). Computerised tomography and neuropsychological test measures in adolescents with obsessive-compulsive disorder. *American Journal of Psychiatry*, **141**, 363–9.

Bench, C.J., Friston, K.J., Brown, R.G. *et al.* (1992). The anatomy of melancholia – focal abnormalities of cerebral blood flow in major depression. *Psychological Medicine*, **22**, 607–15.

Benes, F.M., McSparren, J., Bird, E.D. *et al.* (1991). Deficits in small interneurones in prefrontal and cingulate cortices of schizophrenic and non-schizophrenic patients. *Archives of General Psychiatry*, **48**, 996–1001.

Black, D.W. (1982). Pathological laughter: a review of the literature. *Journal of Nervous and Mental Disease*, **170**, 67–71.

Burns, A., Jacoby, R. and Levy, R. (1990). Psychiatric phenomenology in Alzheimer's disease IV: Disorders of behaviour. *British Journal of Psychiatry*, **157**, 86–94.

Burvill, P.W., Johnson, G.A., Jamrozik, K.D. *et al.* (1995). Prevalence of depression after stroke: The Perth community stroke study. *British Journal of Psychiatry*, **166**: 320–7.

Chiocca, E.A. and Martuza, R.L. (1990). Neurosurgical therapy of the obsessional-compulsive disorder. In *Obsessive-compulsive Disorders: Theory and Management* (ed. M.A. Jenike, L. Baer, W.E. Minichello *et al.*) St. Louis: Mosby Year Book.

Conrad, A.J., Abebe, T., Austin, R. *et al.* (1993). Hippocampal pyramidal cell disarray in schizophrenia as a bilateral phenomenon. *Archives of General Psychiatry*, **48**, 413–17.

Cottrell, S.S. and Wilson, S.A.K. (1926). The affective symptomatology of disseminated sclerosis. *Journal of Neurology and Psychopathology*, **7**, 1–30.

Cummings, J.L. (1992). Depression and Parkinson's disease: A review. *American Journal of Psychiatry*, **149**, 443–54.

Cummings, J.L. and Cunningham, K. (1992). Obsessive compulsive disorder in Huntington's disease. *Biological Psychiatry*, **31**, 263–70.

Cummings, J.L. and Mendez, M.F. (1984). Secondary mania with focal cerebrovascular lesions. *American Journal of Psychiatry*, **141**, 1084–7.

Cutting, J. (1987). The phenomenology of acute organic psychosis. Comparisons with acute schizophrenia. *British Journal of Psychiatry*, **151**, 324–32.

Davison, K. and Bagley, C.R. (1969). Schizophrenia-like psychoses associated with organic disorders of the central nervous system: a review of the literature. In *Current Problems in Neuropsychiatry* (ed. R.N. Herrington). British Journal of Psychiatry Special publication No 4. Ashford, Kent: Hedley Brothers.

Derryberry, D. and Tucker, D.M. (1992). Neural mechanisms of emotion. *Journal of Consulting and Clinical Psychology*, **60**, 329–38.

Dolan, R.J., Calloway, S.P. and Mann, A.H. (1985). Cerebral ventricular size in depressed subjects. *Psychological Medicine*, **15**, 873–8.

Dolan, R.J., Calloway, S.P., Thacker, P. and Mann, A.H. (1986). The cerebral cortical appearance in depressed subjects. *Psychological Medicine*, **16**, 775–9.

Dupont, R.M., Jernigan, T.L., Butters, N. *et al.* (1990). Subcortical abnormalities detected in bipolar affective disorder using magnetic resonance imaging. *Archives of General Psychiatry*, **47**, 55–9.

Feinstein, A. and Ron, M.A. (1990). Psychosis associated with demonstrable brain disease. *Psychological Medicine*, **20**, 793–803.

Feinstein, A., du Boulay, G. and Ron, M.A. (1992). Psychotic illness in multiple sclerosis. A clinical and magnetic resonance imaging study. *Psychological Medicine*, **161**, 680–5.

Flor-Henry, P., Yeudall, L.T., Koles, Z.J. and Howarth, B.G. (1979). Neuropsychological and power-spectral EEG investigations of the obsessive-compulsive syndrome. *Biological Psychiatry*, **14**, 119–30.

Frith, C.D., Friston, K.J., Herold, S. *et al.* (1995). Regional brain activity in chronic schizophrenic patients during the performance of a verbal fluency task. *British Journal of Psychiatry*, **167**, 343–9.

Gallagher, J.P. (1989). Pathological laughter and crying in ALS: a search for their origin. *Acta Neurologica Scandinavica*, **80**, 114–17.

George, M.S., Trimble, M.R., Costa, D.C. *et al.* (1992). Elevated frontal cerebral blood flow in Gilles de la Tourette syndrome: a 99-Tc-HMPAO SPECT study. *Psychiatric Research*, **45**, 143–51.

Goodwin, G.M., Austin, M.P., Dougall, N. *et al.* (1993). State changes in brain activity shown by the uptake of 99-Tc-exametazime with single photon emission tomography in major depression before and after treatment. *Journal of Affective Disorder*, **29**, 243–53.

Harvey, I., Ron, M.A., du Boulay, G. *et al.* (1993). Reduction of cortical volume in schizophrenia on magnetic resonance imaging. *Psychological Medicine*, **23**, 591–604.
Harvey, I., Persaud, R., Ron, M.A. *et al.* (1994). Volumetric MRI measurements in bipolars compared with schizophrenics and healthy controls. *Psychological Medicine*, **24**, 689–99.
Hollander, E., Schieffman, E., Cohen, B. *et al.* (1990). Signs of central nervous system dysfunction in obsessive-compulsive disorder. *Archives of General Psychiatry*, **47**, 27–32.
House, A., Dennis, M., Molyneux, A. *et al.* (1989). Emotionalism after stroke. *British Medical Journal*, **298**, 991–4.
House, A., Dennis, M., Warlow, C. *et al.* (1990). Mood disorders after stroke and their relation to lesion localization. A CT scan study. *Brain*, **113**, 1113–29.
Hymas, N., Lees, A., Bolton, D. *et al.* (1991). The neurology of obsessional slowness. *Brain*, **114**, 2203–33.
Insel, T. (1992). Toward a neuroanatomy of obsessive-compulsive disorder. *Archives of General Psychiatry*, **49**, 739–44.
Johnstone, E.C., Crow, T.J., Frith, C.D. *et al.* (1976). Cerebral ventricular size and cognitive impairment in chronic schizophrenia. *Lancet*, **ii**, 924–6.
Johnstone, E.C., McMillan, J.F. and Crow, T.J. (1987). The occurrence of organic disease of possible or probable aetiological significance in a population of 268 cases of first episode schizophrenia. *Psychological Medicine*, **17**, 371–9.
Johnstone, E.C., Cooling, N.J., Frith, C.D. *et al.* (1988). Phenomenology of organic and functional psychoses and the overlap between them. *British Journal of Psychiatry*, **153**, 770–6.
Karno, M., Golding, J.M., Sorenson, S.B. and Burnam, M.A. (1988). The epidemiology of obsessive-compulsive disorder in five US communities. *Archives of General Psychiatry*, **45**, 1094–9.
Kellner, C.H., Jolley, R.R., Holgate, R. *et al.* (1991). Brain MRI in obsessive-compulsive disorder. *Psychiatry Research*, **36**, 45–9.
Lawrence, R., Ron, M.A., Tyrrell, P. and Rossor, M.N. (1994). Psychiatric symptoms in patients with focal cortical degeneration. *Behavioural Neurology*, **7**, 153–8.
Lewis, S.W. (1990). Computerized tomography in schizophrenia 15 years on. *British Journal of Psychiatry*, Suppl. 9, 16–24.
Liddle, P.F., Friston, K.J., Frith, C.D. *et al.* (1992). Patterns of cerebral blood flow in schizophrenia. *British Journal of Psychiatry*, **160**: 179–86.
Luxenberg, J.S., Swedo, S.E., Flament, M.F. *et al.* (1988). Neuroanatomical abnormalities in obsessive-compulsive disorder detected with quantitative x-ray computed tomography. *American Journal of Psychiatry*, **145**, 1089–93.
Maier, M., Ron, M.A., Barker, G.J. and Tofts, P.S. (1995). Proton magnetic resonance spectroscopy: an in vivo method of estimating hippocampal neuronal depletion in schizophrenia. *Psychological Medicine*, **25**, 1201–9.
Mayberg, H.S., Starkstein, S.E., Sadzot, B. *et al.* (1990). Selective hypometabolism in the inferior frontal lobe in depressed patients with Parkinson's disease. *Annals of Neurology*, **28**, 57–64.
Mayberg, H.S., Starkstein, S.E., Peyser, C.E. *et al.* (1992). Paralimbic frontal lobe hypometabolism in depression associated with Huntington's disease. *Neurology*, **42**, 1791–7.
Mayberg, H.S. (1994). Frontal lobe dysfunction in secondary depression. *Journal of Neuropsychiatry and Clinical Neurosciences*, **6**, 428–42.

McGuire, P.K., Bench, C.J., Frith, C.D. *et al.* (1994). Functional anatomy of obsessive compulsive phenomena. *British Journal of Psychiatry*, **164**, 159–68.

Mega, M.S. and Cummings, J.L. (1994). Frontal-subcortical circuits and neuropsychiatric disorders. *Journal of Neuropsychiatry and Clinical Neurosciences*, **6**, 358–70.

Minden, S.L. and Schiffer, R.B. (1990). Affective disorders in multiple sclerosis: a review and recommendations for clinical research. *Archives of Neurology*, **47**, 98–104.

Pauls, D.L., Towbin, K.E., Leckman, J.F. *et al.* (1986). Gilles de la Tourette's syndrome and obsessive-compulsive disorder: evidence supporting a genetic relationship. *Archives of General Psychiatry*, **43**, 1180–2.

Persaud, R., Russouw, H., Harvey, I. *et al.* (1997). Focal signal hyperintensity in schizophrenia (in press).

Poeck, K. (1969). Pathophysiology of emotional disorders associated with brain damage. In *Handbook of Clinical Neurology*, Vol 3 (ed. P.J. Vinken and G.W. Bruyn), pp. 343–67. Amsterdam: North-Holland Publishing Co.

Poynton, A., Bridges, P.K. and Bartlett, J.R. (1988). Psychosurgery in Britain now. *British Journal of Neurosurgery*, **2**, 297–306.

Rauch, S.L., Jenike, M.A., Alpert, N.M. *et al.* (1994). Regional cerebral blood flow measured during sympton provocation in obsessive compulsive disorder using oxygen 15-labeled carbon dioxide and positron emission tomography. *Archives of General Psychiatry*, **51**, 62–70.

Robinson, D., Wu, H., Ashari, M. *et al.* (1995). Reduced caudate nucleus volume in obsessive compulsive disorder. *Archives of General Psychiatry*, **52**, 393–8.

Ron, M.A. and Logsdail, S.J. (1989). Psychiatric morbidity in multiple sclerosis: an MRI study. *Psychological Medicine*, **19**, 887–95.

Sackeim, H.A., Greenberg, M.S., Weiman, A.L. *et al.* (1982). Hemispheric asymmetry in the expression of positive and negative emotions: neurological evidence. *Archives of Neurology*, **39**, 210–18.

Sawle, G., Hymas, N., Lees, A. and Frackowiack, R. (1991). Obsessional slowness: functional studies with positron emission tomography. *Brain*, **114**, 2191–202.

Sharpe, M., Howton, K., House, A. *et al.* (1990). Mood disorders in long-term survivors of stroke: association with brain lesion localization and volume. *Psychological Medicine*, **20**, 815–28.

Slater, E., Beard, A.W. and Glithero, E. (1963). The schizophrenia-like psychoses of epilepsy. *British Journal of Psychiatry*, **109**, 95–150.

Starkstein, S.E., Robinson, R.G. and Price, T.R. (1987). Comparison of cortical and subcortical lesions in the production of post-stroke mood disorders. *Brain*, **110**, 1045–59.

Starkstein, S.E., Fedoroff, P., Berthier, M.L. and Robinson, R.G. (1991). Manic-depressive and pure manic states after brain lesions. *Biological Psychiatry*, **29**, 149–58.

Stuss, D.T. and Gow, C.A. (1992). 'Frontal dysfunction' after traumatic brain injury. *Neuropsychiatry, Neuropsychology and Behavioural Neurology*, **5**, 272–82.

Suddath, R.L., Christison, G.W., Fuller Torrey, E. *et al.* (1990). Anatomical abnormalities in the brains of monozygotic twins discordant for schizophrenia. *The New England Journal of Medicine*, **322**, 789–94.

Tonkonogy, J.M., Smith, T.W. and Barreira, P.J. (1994). Obsessive-compulsive disorder in Pick's disease. *Journal of Neuropsychiatry and Clinical Neurosciences*, **6**, 176–80.

Toone, B.K., Garralda, E.M. and Ron, M.A. (1982). The psychoses of epilepsy and the functional psychoses. A clinical and phenomenological evaluation. *British Journal of Psychiatry*, **141**, 256–61.

Weinberger, D.R., Berman, K.F. and Zec, R.F. (1986). Physiologic dysfunction of the dorsolateral prefrontal cortex in schizophrenia. I. Regional cerebral blood flow evidence. *Archives of General Psychiatry*, **43**, 114–24.

Weinberger, D.R., Aloia, M.S., Goldberg, T.E. and Berman, K.F. (1994). The frontal lobes and schizophrenia. *The Journal of Neuropsychiatry and Clinical Neurosciences*, **6**, 419–27.

Wilson, S.A.K. (1924). Some problems in neurology. II. Pathological laughing and crying. *Journal of Neurology and Psychopathology*, **16**, 99–333.

8

Structural brain imaging in the psychoses

SHÔN LEWIS

Introduction

For much of the 20th century, Western psychiatry has viewed schizophrenia and manic depressive disorder as the two main examples of 'functional psychosis'. In contrast to the organic psychoses, such as delirium and dementia, the functional psychoses were seen essentially as disorders of mind rather than brain. If there were at some level assumed to be brain abnormalities, these were a considerable way 'downstream', comprising as it were disturbances of software, rather than hardware. Although this was not the view held by Emil Kraepelin when he first delineated schizophrenia, it arose on the one hand out of the ascendency, particularly in North America, of psychobiological and psychoanalytic formulations in psychiatry and, on the other hand, from the lack of suitable tools to test the null hypothesis: that there was no underlying structural disorder of the brain. Post-mortem investigations in schizophrenia were reported in the first half of the 20th century, but the lack of a clear hypothetical focus to direct investigations and the absence of proper control groups led to the abandonment of this approach in the 1950s. Visual imaging of brain structure during life was, at about the same time, becoming a possibility largely through the technique of pneumoencephalography (PEG). PEG essentially used the low electron density of air to act as an X-ray contrast medium, by introducing small volumes of air into the ventricles of the brain via a spinal tap. Plain X-rays of the skull with the patient tipped into a variety of positions would then enable the internal contours of much of the ventricular system to be delineated. The procedure was lengthy, painful and hazardous. Nonetheless, during the 1950s and early 1960s a handful of European studies used PEG to measure ventricular size in schizophrenia. Although these studies suggested that, in chronic schizophrenia, some degree of lateral ventricular enlargement was present, they attracted little attention.

It was not until the second half of the 1970s that *in vivo* structural brain imaging using non-invasive, painless, relatively safe techniques became available. X-ray computed tomography (CT) owed its development in the main to the advent of fast computers, rather than any specifically radiological advances. CT was central in schizophrenia research in confirming a biological focus for investigations into cause and mechanisms. As well as the importance of structural imaging in redrawing the proper focus for investigation, the research findings have also been critical in generating hypotheses about the nature of brain abnormalities in schizophrenia. The development and deployment of these lines of evidence arising out of structural imaging research using CT and magnetic resonance imaging, particularly in schizophrenia, will be examined further here.

Early pitfalls

At its simplest level, the usual CT study of schizophrenia involved scanning a sample of schizophrenic patients, scanning a sample of non-schizophrenic controls, and measuring various parameters of the images obtained. However, early on it became clear that any differences seen between patient and control groups were in the main quantitative rather than qualitative. Moreover, these changes were usually minor in degree, with considerable overlap between groups. Studies were soon seen to vary widely in the reported prevalence of abnormal findings and the most reasonable explanation of this lay in variation in the selection of patients, the choice of controls, and the methods of measurement.

Most studies used operational diagnostic criteria to define the patient group, but still differed widely in patients' demographic and treatment characteristics. There is now much evidence that these factors do influence the prevalence of abnormalities found (Owen and Lewis, 1986). Epidemiological samples such as first-episode patients (Turner, Toone and Brett-Jones, 1986) or consecutive admissions from a defined catchment area (Iacono *et al.*, 1988), are to be preferred.

The use of exclusion criteria also varied in the earlier studies. Those more commonly applied were histories of neurological disease, mental retardation, an upper age limit, and concurrent physical illness. Evidence of heavy alcohol consumption is also a common exclusion criterion, although definitions varied from 'abuse' to 'alcoholism'; some studies only excluded alcohol abuse if of 'aetiological significance to the psychiatric disorder' despite evidence that it is a potent confounding variable however defined (Ron, 1983). Elsewhere, exclusion criteria comprised female gender, abnormal findings on electro-encephalography (EEG), left-handedness and others whose theoretical justification was often unclear.

The rigorous selection of controls in a structural imaging study is at least as important as characterising the patient group. Although the use of normalised neurological controls was defended (Raz, Raz and Bigler, 1988), Smith & Iacono (1986) reviewed the literature and showed that reported ventricular size was significantly smaller in neurological control groups than in healthy volunteer control groups. The use of neurological controls was probably a major source of type 1 error. This view was supported by these authors' own prospective study. This used both types of controls and showed that comparisons with the neurological control group led to an overestimate of the prevalence of abnormalities in the schizophrenic patients (Smith *et al.*, 1988). The ideal control group would seem to be healthy volunteers matched at least for age and sex, prospectively scanned on the same machine during the same period. Psychiatric screening and determination of alcohol consumption is needed. Any exclusion criteria used in the patient group should also be used in the controls.

The third source of variation between studies was in the techniques of measurement used. The structures most commonly measured were the lateral cerebral ventricles. The most popular index of lateral ventricular size has been the ventricle:brain ratio (VBR) first proposed by Synek and Reuben (1976). The VBR expresses the area of the lateral ventricles as measured on the same slice. Its rationale was that, since people with large heads will normally have large ventricles, this ratio would control for differences in head size. It assumed firstly that there is a linear relationship between ventricle size and head size in the general population, and secondly that head size in schizophrenic patients is no different from that in controls. In fact, neither assumption is watertight (Harvey *et al.*, 1990) although VBR does seem to be a valid indicator of the total volume of the lateral ventricles.

Actual measurement of areas has been performed in two ways. Mechanical planimetry used an articulated device to trace manually around the edge of the structure on the photographic film. However, this relied on visual inspection and, particularly where ventricles are small, the grey areas at the interface between fluid and brain can give rise to real problems in deciding where the edges of the ventricle actually lie: the so-called partial-volume effect. This method was superseded by various automated or semi-automated techniques. These have theoretical and practical advantages in that they use the original digital CT data and, although the partial-volume problem is not wholly overcome, have very high inter-rater reliability.

By the early 1990s there were over 50 controlled studies in the world literature that examined some aspect of brain structure in schizophrenic patients using CT. A critical review needs to consider only those studies in which controls were prospectively ascertained healthy volunteers, scanned concurrently with the patient group. The 21 studies meeting these criteria have been reviewed (Lewis, 1990). Most of these were the more recent studies. In comparison with less well-controlled studies, a relatively high proportion of these studies failed to show significant CT abnormalities in schizophrenic patients. Of these 21 studies, nine could not demonstrate lateral ventricular enlargement in the patient group and a further three showed this at only marginal degrees of statistical significance.

Besides lateral ventricular size, studies increasingly looked for a difference in other cerebral fluid spaces, in particular enlargement of the third ventricle and cerebral cortical sulci. Several studies reported an enlarged third ventricle or enlarged cortical sulci in the absence of significant lateral ventricular changes. Other claims, such as enlarged cerebellar sulci, widened Sylvian and interhemispheric fissures, and asymmetry of occipital pole size, have not been well replicated.

The disparity even between well-controlled studies again points to the likelihood of methodological confounding factors. Although the studies reviewed had as their minimum requirement a control group of prospectively scanned healthy volunteers, the decision about which variables should be matched between patients and controls is still at issue. Certainly, age and sex should be matched. In addition, there is evidence that other demographic factors can influence measures of brain structure: social class height, ethnicity (Nimgaonkar, Wessley and Murray, 1988) and educational level (DeMayer *et al.*, 1988), for example.

Another issue left in need of further clarification by CT was the specificity of reported abnormalities to schizophrenia. Most of the changes in schizophrenia have also been reported in other severe 'functional' psychiatric disorders, including affective disorders, obsessive-compulsive disorder and anorexia nervosa.

Focal lesions

As well as the minor degrees of enlargement of ventricles and sulci found in the majority of studies there are a handful of reports in the literature of gross focal brain lesions in schizophrenia: aqueduct stenosis (Reveley and Reveley, 1983), arachnoid and septal cysts (Kuhnley *et al.*, 1981; Lewis and Mezey, 1985), and agenesis of the corpus callosum (Lewis *et al.*, 1988).

Four studies enable an estimate to be made of the prevalence of such focal lesions on brain imaging in schizophrenia. Owens *et al.* (1980), in their series of 136 schizophrenic patients, found 'unsuspected intracranial pathology' as a focal finding on CT in 12 cases (9%), excluding lesions due to leucotomy. Five of these 12 were aged over 65. Lewis (1987) examined a series of 228 Maudsley Hospital patients who met Research Diagnostic Criteria for schizophrenia and who had been consecutively scanned for clinical reasons. Patients with a history of epilepsy or intracranial surgery, or who were aged over 65 at the time of scan, were excluded. The original scan reports were examined and the films of those not unequivocally normal were reappraised by a neuroradiologist blind to the original report. In 41 patients the scan showed a definite intracranial abnormality. This was in the nature of enlarged fluid spaces in 28 cases, but in 13 patients (6%) there was a discrete focal lesion. These 13 lesions varied widely in location and probable pathology, although left temporal and right parietal regions were most commonly implicated. The third study (Lewis and Reveley, in preparation) was an attempt to examine a geographically defined sample of schizophrenic patients, ascertained as part of a large, multidisciplinary survey (Brugha *et al.*, 1988). All catchment area residents who, on a particular census day, were aged 18–65 and were in regular contact with any psychiatric day service were approached. Of 120 eligible people, 83 consented to CT and psychiatric interview. Fifty of these met RDC for schizophrenia or schizoaffective disorder. In four of these 50 patients were found clinically unsuspected focal lesions: low density in the right caudate head; a left occipitotemporal porencephalic cyst; low-density regions in the right parietal lobe; agenesis of the corpus callosum (described further by Lewis *et al.*, 1988). None of 50 matched healthy volunteers showed focal pathology on CT. Using MRI, O'Callaghan and colleagues (1990) found definite focal neurodevelopmental lesions in 4 of 47 prospectively scanned cases of schizophrenia: one had partial agenesis of the corpus callosum.

Given the differences in the nature of the patient samples, these three studies are in rough agreement about the prevalence of unexpected focal (usually neurodevelopmental) abnormalities on CT: between 6% and 9%.

Clinical correlates of CT abnormalities

Given that a proportion of schizophrenic patients do have modest enlargement of lateral and third ventricles and cortical sulci, on CT, can this subgroup be identified in terms of a particular clinical picture? Studies that have compared patients with abnormal versus normal CT, in terms of lateral ventricular size, on a range of clinical variables, use a strategy that does not strictly require a normal control group, although the dividing line between normal and abnormal ventricular size is necessarily arbitrary, often being expressed in terms of greater than one or two standard deviations of a patient or control group mean. The distribution of VBR in most patient groups is positively skewed, although there is little evidence to suggest this is in reality a bimodal distribution.

For most clinical variables mooted at one time or another to be related to ventricular enlargement, there is little in the way of convincing replication. The appealing notion that negative symptoms and poor treatment response are characteristics of schizophrenia with ventricular enlargement does not have consistent support. The only associations that have more positive than negative replications are those of tardive dyskinesia and, most particularly, impaired performance on neuropsychological tests, although the specific areas of cognitive impairment tend to vary from study to study (reviewed by Lewis, 1990).

There is some evidence that abnormalities on CT scans are actually predicted by an atypical clinical picture. Harvey *et al.* (1990) found that their subgroup of unspecified functional psychoses had particular enlarged ventricles, and unusual symptoms such as delusional misidentification are often associated with CT abnormalities. In the CT study of 228 schizophrenic patients referred to earlier (Lewis, 1987) the subgroup with unequivocally abnormal scans had a significantly greater frequency of changing clinical diagnosis, suggesting an atypical presentation.

The natural history and aetiology of CT abnormalities

The lack of an association between length of illness and degree of lateral ventricular enlargement suggested that this enlargement is not progressive, neither in the sense of reflecting a neurodegenerative disorder, nor as being an artefact of continuing treatment or institutional care. This view received support from the demonstration of significant ventricular enlargement in young, first-episode patients. Direct evidence for the non-progressive nature of ventricular enlargement on CT is available from several follow-up studies that have re-scanned patients after periods of up to seven years. The implication from the apparently non-progressive nature of the CT scan changes, which is reinforced by the increasing number of reports of congenital focal lesions as noted above, is that they represent early neurodevelopmental abnormalities. Clues about this have been sought by trying to show an association between CT abnormalities and indicators either of a genetic diathesis or of early neurodevelopment damage; specifically, manifest family history of psychiatric disorder, or history of pregnancy and birth complications. The early hypothesis, that ventricular enlargement was largely confined to those patients with no evident family history (Murray, Lewis and Reveley, 1985; Lewis *et al.*, 1987), in the end received mixed experimental support and was probably too simplistic. However, almost all of the studies to look for an association with manifest family history lacked adequate statistical power. A metanalysis of these studies (Vita *et al.*, 1994) showed there to be an overall effect of family history, with sporadic patients showing larger ventricles. In a study designed to overcome the problem of limited power, Owen, Lewis and Murray (1989) compared ventricular size in 48 schizophrenic patients with no such history in first-degree relatives, 48 schizophrenic patients with no such history in first- or second-degree relatives, and the same number of healthy controls. The three groups were matched for age and sex. Significant ventricular enlargement was found in those without a family history, as predicted. However, those patients with a family history positive for schizophrenia also showed significant enlargement, against expectations, whereas a family history of affective disorder was associated with normal ventricular size. Studies with CT and MRI within multiply affected pedigrees may elucidate this issue, particularly with respect to the hypothesis that ventricular enlargement might be part of an 'endophenotype' demonstrable in obligate carriers as well as probands.

Several studies have demonstrated a raised rate of obstetric complications in the histories of schizophrenic patients compared with other psychiatric patients, well siblings, or unrelated controls (Lewis, 1989; Eagles *et al.*, 1990). This has led to the hypothesis that obstetric complications could be a risk factor for schizophrenia with abnormal CT findings, but results are conflicting (Lewis, 1990).

Thus, the story of X-ray CT in schizophrenia research is at the same time enlightening and salutary. As a technique, its inception coincided with the renaissance of biological psychiatry in the 1970s and a torrent of early studies were more or less agreed that ventricular enlargement characterised a large proportion of patients with schizophrenia. Subsequently, there were reported several large, properly controlled studies that signalled caution about the initial enthusiasm. It is still fair to conclude that relative enlargement of third and lateral ventricles, and cortical sulci, is found in some schizophrenic patients, but the extent of these changes is probably not as marked as first thought. The failure of several rigorous studies to demonstrate these changes has yet to be explained. Variations in sampling methods of patients seems increasingly to be an important factor when appropriate control groups are used. What factors determine the various structural brain parameters in the general population remains an under-researched area and it is becoming obvious that a range of interacting demographic factors such as age, sex, socio-economic status, race, educational level, and alcohol consumption are important. A further caveat is that lateral ventricular enlargement has also been reported in controlled studies of severe affective disorders and the specificity of these changes to schizophrenia, or to psychosis in general, remains to be shown conclusively. In the light of this, it is perhaps not surprising that the search for clinical correlates of CT changes in schizophrenia has been disappointing, although a relationship with tardive dyskinesia and neuropsychological impairments does seem to exist. One important consequence of this research has been the reappraisal of the natural history of CT abnormalities, where they exist, with the emergence of the view that these are long-standing, non-progressive changes, similar to those seen in other neurodevelopmental disorders (Weinberger, 1987).

Magnetic resonance imaging

The baton has now been passed to magnetic resonance imaging as the definitive *in vivo* structural brain-imaging technique. MRI has the advantage of not using ionising radiation, and its high resolution, good tissue contrast and multiplanar abilities make it the technique of choice in looking at medial brain structures.

Nuclear magnetic resonance was first used as a technique back in the 1940s. However, it is only since the 1980s that the application of this technique to biological tissue in general, and the human body in particular, has been widely available to the clinical research community. Atomic nuclei comprise positively charged protons and a neutral neutrons. Nuclei rotate and so, having both charge and spin, generate a magnetic field of finite strength and direction. When in an external magnetic field, interaction between the two fields induces a secondary 'wobbling' motion around the primary axis of spin: this is called 'precession'. Every isotope has its own frequency of precession within an external magnetic field of certain strength. Hydrogen, being very abundant in biological tissue, is the most important contributor to the magnetic resonance signal. Within a one Tesla magnetic field the hydrogen nucleus resonates at 42 Mhz. What this means is that, if an external radio frequency signal is transmitted at this frequency, the spinning protons will be brought into phase. After the radio frequency pulse stops, the magnetization vector returns to its original direction by a process of 'relaxation'. By convention, the time taken to relax back to the original state is determined by two time constants: T_1 and T_2. Energy emitted during various points of the relaxation process is picked up by detectors and used to create images 'weighted' to T_1 or T_2 parts of the relaxation curve.

The first studies that applied structural MRI to schizophrenia were essentially aiming to replicate the main finding generated by CT research: enlarged fluid spaces, particularly lateral and third ventricles. The higher resolution structural imaging with MRI enabled lateral ventricular volume measurements to be made more easily. In a way reminiscent of the CT studies, the earlier studies noted a larger effect size than did the later studies. In a careful first episode study, Degreef *et al.* (1992) found a 26% increase in lateral ventricular volume in 40 patients compared to controls. The left temporal horn particularly was found to be enlarged and the degree of enlargement correlated with both positive and negative symptoms in their sample.

It was soon realised that the sensitivity of MRI allowed more interesting hypotheses to be tested in schizophrenia. With CT research, the ventricular system had been the centre of scientific attention largely because it was one of the only things that could be measured objectively on CT. The ability of MRI to image in several planes and to differentiate between different compartments of brain tissue led on to measurement of discrete brain structure, rather than fluid spaces. The different dispositions of hydrogen atoms in grey and white matter, largely dictated by differences in water content, allowed volumetric measurements of the two compartments independently. This had not been possible with CT, partly because the electron density of the two tissues was similar, and partly because artefacts generated by nearby bone stopped realistic measurement of the cerebral cortex.

Some artefacts of area and volume measurements applicable to CT are still constraints with MRI. In particular, the partial volume artefact can still be a difficulty especially when measuring small structures or convoluted surfaces. The increasing use of very thin, contiguous slices down to 1–2 mm as well as rapid image acquisition techniques that collect a complete three-dimensional dataset, rather than a set of slices, allows for resegmentation and reconstruction in other planes.

After initial studies replicating fluid volume enlargement, a large number of studies appeared that concentrated on measuring medial temporal lobe structures. Suddath *et al.* (1990) reported a study of identical twins discordant for schizophrenia in which the affected twin consistently showed lateral and third ventricular enlargement compared to the unaffected co-twin, as well as reduced volume of temporal lobe grey matter including hippocampus. Reduced volume of the hippocampus–amygdala complex and parahippocampal gyrus is now a fairly well replicated finding in schizophrenia compared to healthy volunteer controls. Some studies have claimed that this reduction is more pronounced on the left than the right side in schizophrenia (Bogerts *et al.*, 1990; Suddath *et al.*, 1990) but the balance of evidence suggests that the decrease is bilateral. As with lateral ventricular enlargement, the findings have held up in samples of young first episode schizophrenic patients (Bogerts *et al.*, 1990).

Although decreased volumes in temporal lobe structures are probably bilateral in schizophrenia, correlates with clinical symptoms have been shown with decreased grey matter volume on the left. More or less intriguing associations between reduced superior temporal gyrus volume on the left with auditory hallucinations (Barta *et al.*, 1990) and reduced posterior superior temporal gyrus volume and thought disorder (Shenton *et al.*, 1992) have been reported.

With MRI, the list of anecdotal reports of neurodevelopmental lesions of a gross nature in association with schizophrenia has lengthened. Interestingly, developmental anomalies of mid-line structures are increasingly commonly reported. The original case series of cysts of the septum pelucidum found in schizophrenia with CT (Lewis and Mezey, 1985) has been replicated in at least one MRI study (Degreef *et al.*, 1992). Several further cases of partial or complete agenesis of the corpus collosum have been reported (Swayze *et al.*, 1990). Quantitative measures of corpus collosum area on saggital MRI images have been reported in an increasing number of studies, with little in the way of concensus. Increased area, decreased area and distorted shape have all been reported.

The question now remains whether the small but definite decreases in temporal lobe grey matter are truly limited to the temporal lobe in schizophrenia. Theoretical considerations have focused attention on this area, but recent MRI volumetric studies have suggested that more widespread volumetric decreases in grey matter are present. Harvey *et al.* (1993) controlled for a variety of anthropometric and demographic variables, including height, parental social class, age and gender, to show a small (6%) but significant reduction in diffuse cerebral cortical grey matter volume, but not white matter volume, in schizophrenic patients compared to controls. Zipursky and colleagues (1992) in a careful study reported the same finding, of a generalised reduction in grey matter volume in schizophrenia compared to healthy controls. Zipursky and colleagues had a second control group of age-matched alcohol dependent subjects. In this group, grey matter volume was also reduced but in the presence of a proportional reduction in white matter volume also. This finding suggests that a global neurodegenerative process is not at work. Importantly, the findings seem to be specific to schizophrenia rather than psychosis in general. Both Harvey *et al.* (1993) and Schlaepfer *et al.* (1994) found grey matter volume reduction in schizophrenic patients, but not in bipolar patients, compared to controls. In the Schlaepfer study, volumes of association cortex in dorsolateral prefrontal cortex, superior temporal gyrus and inferior parietal lobule, were particularly reduced, leading to the interpretation that heteromodal association cortex was principally affected.

Tomorrow's research

These most recent findings with structural MRI in schizophrenia support a hypothesis that it results from a disorder of development of cerebral cortex, perhaps particularly association cortex, arising largely out of genetic factors. The cells that make up the central nervous system descend from ectodermally derived neural tube cells. With a few exceptions, such as the cerebellum, cell proliferation occurs in a germinal, periventricular zone containing a growing area of post-mitotic cells. Neurogenesis is driven by gene products intrinsic to cells and by extrinsic factors such as growth factors. A cascade of gene–environment interactions controls cell migration to and within the cortex, thalamocortical axon development, apoptosis (cell death) and a series of further events. The cerebral cortical dysgenesis that seems to have been demonstrated by brain imaging in schizophrenia will be shown to have its origins in the genetic and epigenetic events controlling brain development.

References

Andreasen, N.C., Olsen, S.A., Dennert, J.W. *et al.* (1982). Ventricular enlargement in schizophrenia: relationship to positive and negative symptoms. *American Journal of Psychiatry*, **139**, 297–302.

Barta, P.E., Pearlson, G.D., Powers, R.E. *et al.* (1990). Auditory hallucinations and smaller superior temporal gyral volume in schizophrenia. *American Journal of Psychiatry*, **147**, 1457–62.

Bogerts, B., Ashtari, M., Degreef, G. *et al.* (1990). Reduced temporal limbic structure volumes on magnetic resonance images in first episode schizophrenia. *Psychiatry Research: Neuroimaging*, **35**, 1–13.

Bogerts, B., Lieberman, J., Ashtari, M. *et al.* (1993). Hippocampus–amygdala volumes and psychopathology in chronic schizophrenia. *Biological Psychiatry*, **33**, 236–46.

Brugha, T.S., Wing, J.K., Brewin, L.R. *et al.* (1988). The problems of people in long termpsychiatric care. An introduction to the Camberwell High Contact Survey. *Psychological Medicine*, **18**, 457–68.
Casanova, M.F., Prasad, C.N., Waldman, I. *et al.* (1990). No difference in basal ganglia mineralization between schizophrenic and non-schizophrenic patients: a quantitive CT study. *Biological Psychiatry*, **27**, 138–42.
Degreef, G., Ashtari, M., Bogerts, B. *et al.* (1992). Volumes of ventricular system subdivisions measured from magnetic resonance images in first-episode schizophrenic patients. *Archives of General Psychiatry*, **49**, 531–7.
DeMyer, M.K., Gilmor, R.L., Hendrie, H.C. *et al.* (1988). Magnetic resonance brain images in schizophrenic and normal subjects: influence of diagnosis and education. *Schizophrenia Bulletin*, **14**, 21–38.
Eagles, J.M., Gibson, I., Bremner, M.H. *et al.* (1990). Obstetric complications in DSM-3 schizophrenics and their siblings. *Lancet*, **335**, 1139–41.
Francis, A.F. (1979). Familial basal ganglia calcification and schizophreniform psychosis. *British Journal of Psychiatry*, **133**, 360–2.
Harvey, I., Williams, M., Toone, B.K. *et al.* (1990). The ventricle-brain ratio (VBR) in functional psychoses: the relationship of lateral ventricular and total ventricular area. *Psychological Medicine*, **20**, 55–62.
Harvey, I., Ron, M.A., Du Boulay, G. *et al.* (1993). Reduction of cortical volume in schizophrenia on magnetic resonance imaging. *Psychological Medicine*, **23**, 591–604.
Iacono, W.G., Smith, G.N., Morean, M. *et al.* (1988). Ventricular and sulcal size at the onset of psychosis. *American Journal of Psychiatry*, **145**, 820–4.
Kuhnley, E.J., White, D.H. and Granoff, A.L. (1981). Psychiatric presentation an arachnoid cyst. *Journal of Clinical Psychiatry*, **42**, 167–9.
Lewis, S.W. (1987). Schizophrenia with and without intracranial abnormalities on CT scan. Unpublished MPhil thesis, University of London.
Lewis, S.W. (1989). Congenital risk factors for schizophrenia. *Psychological Medicine*, **19**, 5–13.
Lewis, S.W. (1990). Computed tomography in schizophrenia 15 years on. *British Journal of Psychiatry*, **157** (Suppl 9), 16–24.
Lewis, S.W. and Mezey, G.C. (1985). Clinical correlates of septum pellucidium cavities: an unusual association with psychosis. *Psychological Medicine*, **15**, 43–54.
Lewis, S.W., Reveley, A.M., Reveley, M.A. *et al.* (1987). The familial-sporadic distinction as a strategy in schizophrenia research. *British Journal of Psychiatry*, **151**, 306–13.
Lewis, S.W., Reveley, M.A., David, A.S. *et al.* (1988). Agenesis of the corpus callosum and schizophrenia. *Psychological Medicine*, **18**, 341–7.
Luchins, D.J. (1982). Computed tomography in schizophrenia: disparities in the prevalence of abnormalities. *Archives of General Psychiatry*, **39**, 859–60.
Meltzer, H.Y., (1986). A comparison of CT findings in acute and chronic ward schizophrenics. *Psychiatry Research*, **17**, 7–14.
Murray, R.M., Lewis, S.W. and Reveley, A.M. (1985). Towards an aetiological classification of schizophrenia. *Lancet*, **i**, 1023–6.
Nimgaonkar, V.L., Wessley, S. and Murray, R.M. (1988). Prevalence of familiality, obstetric complications and structural brain damage in schizophrenic patients. *British Journal of Psychiatry*, **153**, 191–7.
O'Callaghan, E., Larkin, C. and Waddington, J.L. (1990). Obstetric complications in schizophrenia and the validity of maternal recall. *Psychological Medicine*, **20**, 89–94.

Owen, M.J. and Lewis, S.W. (1986). Lateral ventricular size in schizophrenia. *Lancet*, **ii**, 223–4.

Owen, M.J., Lewis, S.W. and Murray, R.M. (1989). Family history and cerebral ventricular enlargement in schizophrenia: a case control study. *British Journal of Psychiatry*, **154**, 629–34.

Owens, D.G.C., Johnstone, E.C., Bydder, G.M. *et al.* (1980). Unsuspected organic disease in chronic schizophrenia demonstrated by computed tomography. *Journal of Neurology, Neurosurgery and Psychiatry*, **43**, 1065–9.

Pearlson, G.D., Garbacz, D.J., Moberg, P.J. *et al.* (1985). Symptomatic, familial, perinatal and social correlates of computerised axial tomography (CAT) changes in schizophrenics and bipolars. *Journal of Nervous and Mental Disease*, **173**, 42–50.

Philpot, M. and Lewis, S.W. (1990). Psychopathology of basal ganglia calcification. *Behavioural Neurology*, **2**, 227–34.

Raz, S., Raz, N. and Bigler, E.D. (1988). Ventriculomegaly in schizophrenia: is the choice of controls important? *Psychiatry Research*, **24**, 71–7.

Reveley, A.M. and Reveley, M.A. (1983). Aqueduct stenosis and schizophrenia. *Journal of Neurology, Neurosurgery and Psychiatry*, **46**, 18–22.

Ron, M.A. (1983). *The Alcoholic Brain: CT Scan and Psychological Findings.* Psychological Medicine in Monograph Supplement 3. Cambridge: Cambridge University Press.

Schlaepfer, T.E., Harris, G.J., Tien, A.Y. *et al.* (1994). Decreased regional cortical gray matter volume in schizophrenia. *American Journal of Psychiatry*, **151**, 842–8.

Shenton, M.E., Kikinis, R. Jolesz, F.A. *et al.* (1992) Left-lateralized temporal lobe abnormalities in schizophrenia and their relationship to thought disorder: a computerized, quantitative MRI study. *New England Journal of Medicine*, **327**, 604–12.

Smith, G.N. and Iacono, W.G. (1986). Lateral ventricular size in schizophrenia and choice of control group. *Lancet*, **i**, 1450.

Smith, G.N., Iacono, W.G., Moreau, M. *et al.* (1988). Choice of comparison group and computerised tomography findings in schizophrenia. *British Journal of Psychiatry*, **153**, 667–74.

Suddath, R.L., Christison, G.W., Torrey, E.F. *et al*, (1990). Anatomical abnormalities in the brains of monozygotic twins discordant for schizophrenia. *New England Journal of Medicine*, **322**, 789–94.

Swayze, W., Andreasen, N.C., Erhardt, J.C. *et al.* (1990). Development abnormalities of the corpus callosum in schizophrenia: an MRI study. *Archives of Neurology*, **47**, 805–8.

Synek, V. and Reuben, J.R. (1976). The ventricular–brain ratio using planimetric measure of EMI scans. *British Journal of Psychiatry*, **49**, 233–7.

Turned, S.W., Toone, B.K. and Brett-Jones, J.R. (1986). Computerised tomographic scan changes in early schizophrenia preliminary findings. *Psychological Medicine*, **16**, 219–25.

Vita, A., Dieci, M., Giobbio, G.M. *et al.* (1994). A reconsideration of the relationship between cerebral structural abnormalities and family history of schizophrenia. *Psychiatry Research*, **53**, 41–55.

Weinberger, D.R. (1987). Implications of normal brain development for pathogenesis of schizophrenia. *Archives of General Psychiatry*, **44**, 660–9.

Zipursky, R.B., Lim, K.O. and Sullivan, E.V. (1992). Widespread cerebral grey matter volume in schizophrenia. *Archives of General Psychiatry*, **49**, 195–205.

Zipurski, R.B., Marsh, L., Lim, K.O. *et al.* (1994). Volumetric assessment of temporal lobe structures in schizophrenia. *Biological Psychiatry*, **35**, 501–16.

Section V

Epilepsy: biology and behaviour

9

Behaviour in chronic experimental epilepsies

JOHN G.R. JEFFERYS & JANE MELLANBY

Introduction

Epilepsies can cause significant behavioural problems. Trimble (Chapter 10) outlines the major issues presented by this problem in humans. Complex partial seizures, perhaps more commonly known as temporal lobe epilepsy, present most of the psychological consequences of epilepsy. Several factors could be responsible in clinical cases: the electrophysiological abnormality of the focus itself, side-effects of drug treatments, and the behavioural effects of structural lesions that may either have caused, or been the consequence of, repeated seizures. Clinical cases do not lend themselves to fundamental analysis because of their variability in aetiology, history, drug treatment, and so on. Animal models provide much better controlled and repeatable conditions, and can replicate many of the features of clinical epilepsies. Several animal models are available of temporal lobe epilepsy. Chronic models provide the most scope to explore behavioural consequences, so we will consider four of those that are available.

Experimental models

1. Perhaps the best known model of temporal lobe epilepsy is *kindling*. Here a stimulus is repeated regularly every few hours to every few days. The stimulus typically is a brief train of electrical pulses delivered to amygdala or hippocampus, but alternatively can be a systemic injection of a convulsant drug. In conventional use, the first stimulus causes a minimal behavioural response, and usually a brief local afterdischarge. Responses progressively increase until they become epileptic, progressing through the five stages of Racine (1972). Once established, kindling is remarkably persistent. On the other hand it is difficult to kindle to spontaneous seizures. In general there is minimal loss of neurones,

although there may be more subtle structural changes. Hippocampal and amygdalar kindling can cause long-lasting impairments of learning and memory (Leung *et al.*, 1990; Stone and Gold 1988; Leung and Shen 1991; Lopes da Silva, Gorter and Wadman, 1986), although other studies of kindling show only a transient effect (Cain *et al.*, 1993; McNamara *et al.*, 1993; Robinson, McNeill and Reed, 1993).

2. More intense, or more rapidly repeated stimuli can cause prolonged epileptic discharges or *status epilepticus*. These often cause selective losses of neurones, for instance in the hippocampal hilus, CA3 or CA1 regions. A seizure-free period follows recovery from status epilepticus, but a relapse into spontaneous seizures occurs a month or two later, and this persists indefinitely (Sloviter, 1991; Bekenstein and Lothman, 1993). The model therefore is of epilepsy and not just of seizures. While this is a promising model for studying basic mechanisms of epilepsies, little behavioural work has been performed. However, lesions in the hippocampus would have behavioural consequences of the kind documented in the basic psychological literature on these regions (O'Keefe and Nadel, 1978; Nadel, 1991; Rawlins *et al.*, 1993; Rawlins, 1985).
3. *Kainic acid* is a glutamatergic agonist that causes seizures acutely, and may also produce lesions in the hippocampal CA3 region and elsewhere. These lesions can in turn lead to chronic epileptic foci in adjacent regions (Cavalheiro, Riche and Le Gal La Salle, 1982). Here there is evidence of behavioural disturbances after intrahippocampal injection of kainic acid in cat. During seizures animals show a 'defensive rage' reaction while interictally they are emotionally labile, or hyperreactive (Griffith, Endel and Bandler, 1987). These behavioural changes wear off following several seizure-free days, showing that they are related to the electrophysiology of the active focus rather than to the lesion, and also providing some encouragement that behavioural problems can be reversed by good seizure control.
4. The intracerebral *tetanus toxin model* of focal epilepsy usually does not cause lesions. Seizures and other epileptic discharges occur spontaneously and intermittently over long periods. The model provides an opportunity to study the progression of recurrent seizure activity at the levels of the EEG, behaviour, cellular physiology, histology and molecular biology. During the remission phase it also provides a chance to measure the long-term behavioural and other functional consequences of recurrent seizures. It has been particularly extensively exploited in the analysis of the behavioural consequences of epileptic foci. It also is the model that interests us most and we will describe it in some detail.

Tetanus toxin model

Injecting a single small dose of tetanus toxin into the brains of rats or cats leads to chronically recurring epileptic discharges. Rats develop spontaneous focal and secondarily generalised seizures 3–7 days after they receive 5–20 mouse LD_{50} of toxin into the hippocampus. Typically seizures last <2 minutes, and recur intermittently (at a frequency of up to 30/day) for the following 3–4 weeks. Continuous video recordings over this period show that the frequency of fits waxes and wanes usually showing several peaks and troughs in 3 weeks. The incidence of motor fits shows a diurnal rhythm, with more fits occurring during the hours of light (when the rats sleep most). This parallels the observation in humans where more fits occur at night (when humans sleep most). Figure 9.1 illustrates the rhythm related to the light–dark cycle in 23 male rats and nine female rats and the absence of a diurnal rhythm in five females exposed to continuous lighting. Simultaneous video filming and recordings from implanted electrodes reveal electrographic seizures apparently identical with some of those which are associated with motor fits and interictal spikes in the absence of clear motor signs, and these can be seen over a longer period than the motor fits (Hawkins and Mellanby 1987; Mellanby *et al.*, 1977). Frequently, motor fits are the culmination of a period of electrographic seizures and there then follows a cessation of motor fits for 1 or 2 days. Motor fits are associated with electrographic discharges of longer duration. Over the weeks of the syndrome the length of discharges waxes and wanes but in the later stages the discharges become shorter and eventually cease (Figure 9.2). Motor fits stop by 3–4 weeks after injection. Epileptiform spikes occur throughout the active phase and continue for a period after the seizure activity stops. The EEG returns to normal by 6–8 weeks. In the longer term a minority of animals will relapse (Mellanby, 1993).

Spontaneous and electrically evoked epileptic activity also occurs reliably in hippocampal slices prepared from these rats and maintained *in vitro* (Jefferys, 1989; Empson and Jefferys, 1993; Whittington and Jefferys, 1994). However the 'seizures' are only of short duration compared with those seen *in vivo* (Finnerty and Jefferys, 1993). Work on such slices confirmed that the initial action of the toxin is to block synaptic inhibition mediated by $GABA_A$ receptors, but also showed that this is followed by recovery of GABA release, with epileptic activity sustained by the apparent failure of inhibitory neurones to respond adequately to synaptic excitation (Whittington and Jefferys, 1994). This 'dormant interneurone' mechanism has now been implicated in three chronic epilepsies, and should be considered as a likely contender for a role in clinical epilepsies (Sloviter, 1991;

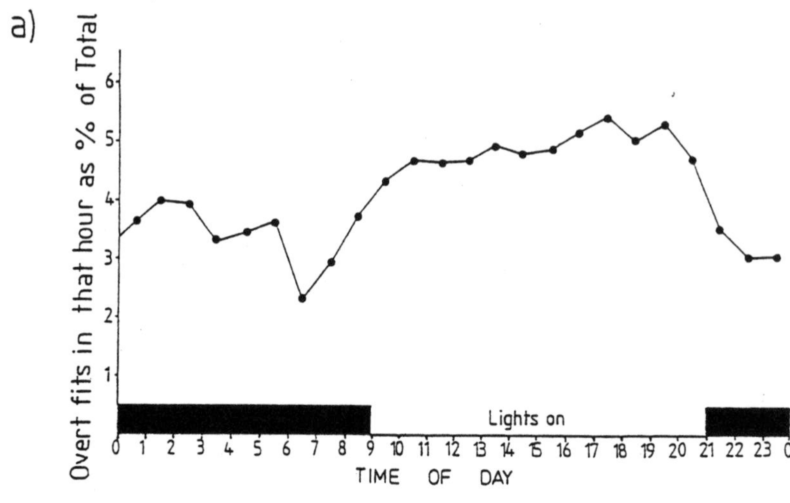
a)
Overt fits in that hour as % of Total
Lights on
TIME OF DAY

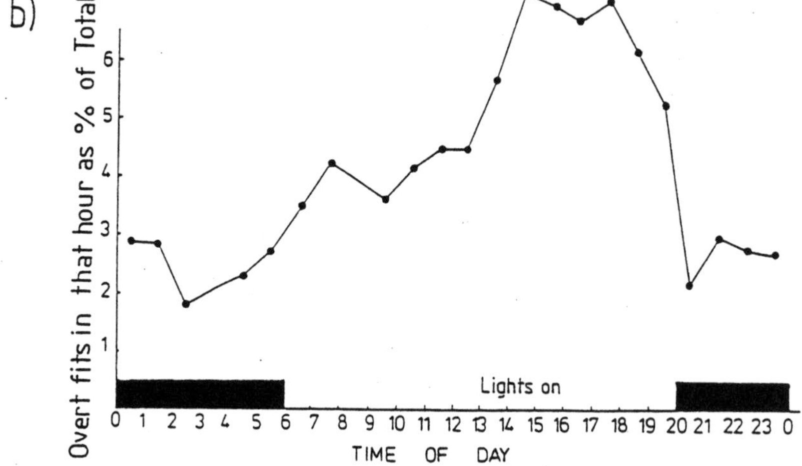
b)
Overt fits in that hour as % of Total
Lights on
TIME OF DAY

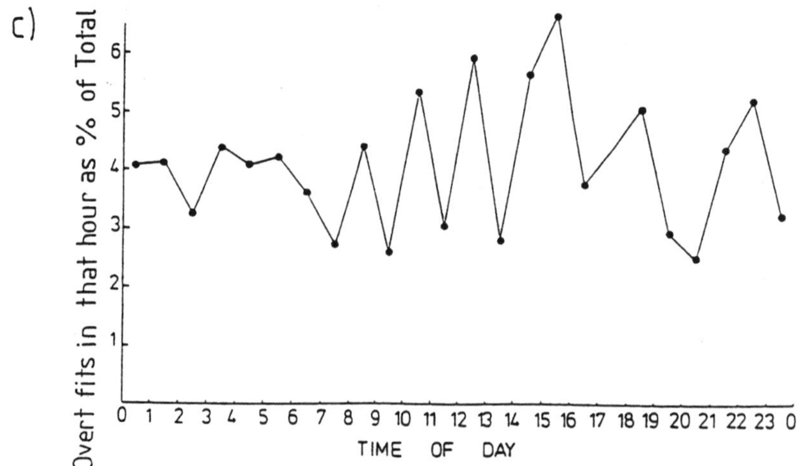
c)
Overt fits in that hour as % of Total
TIME OF DAY

Empson and Jefferys, 1993; Bekenstein and Lothman, 1993; Whittington and Jefferys, 1994). A second mechanism is conspicuous by its recurrence in chronic models, namely the sprouting of new excitatory axons (Mathern *et al.*, 1993; Sundstrom, Mitchell and Wheal, 1993; Ben-Ari and Represa 1990; Sutula *et al.*, 1988; Trauck and Nadler 1985). We suspect that it may occur in the tetanus toxin model, and are testing this now.

Rats that receive comparable doses of intracortical tetanus toxin behave differently. Motor signs are not obvious, although they have been studied in much less detail so far (Mellanby *et al.*, 1977; George and Mellanby, 1975). Interictal spikes certainly appear on the EEG, and epileptic activity is prominent in brain slices (Brener *et al.*, 1991). These epileptic foci are essentially permanent, being found at least 9 months after the initial injection. Toxin injection into the amygdala produces fits similar to those after intrahippocampal injection (limbic fits) but the same dose of toxin produces fewer fits in the amygdala (J. Mellanby and B. Nicholls, unpublished). The behavioural changes have not been investigated in detail in the amygdala-injected rats but there are some differences from those after hippocampal injection.

In cats tetanus toxin induces foci that can be permanent both in the neocortex and in the hippocampus (Louis, Williamson and Darcey, 1990; Darcey and Williamson, 1992). The management of the model in the cat is more difficult than with rats. It frequently requires some anticonvulsant therapy, at least in the early stages. In some cases repeated injections of toxin were needed to produce a chronic epileptic focus. This manoeuvre has not been reported in the rat, and may increase the yield of limbic foci persisting >3 months after injection.

Behaviours associated with chronic experimental epilepsies

Description of ictal behaviours

In humans temporal lobe fits usually are preceded by 'auras' that are reported to involve a strong emotional component, most often fear

Figure 9.1. Diurnal rhythm in motor fit frequency. The rats had received bilateral tetanus toxin into the ventral hippocampus on day 0. They were filmed continuously with time-lapse video for 23 days and the numbers of motor fits counted from the video records. For each rat, the percentage of its total fits that occurred in each hour of the 24 hours was calculated. Mean values for the group were then plotted. (a) Mean values for 28 male rats kept in 12 hours light/12 hours dark. (b) Mean for nine female rats kept in 14 hours light/10 hours dark. (c) Mean values for five female rats kept in continuous light (from Hawkins, 1985).

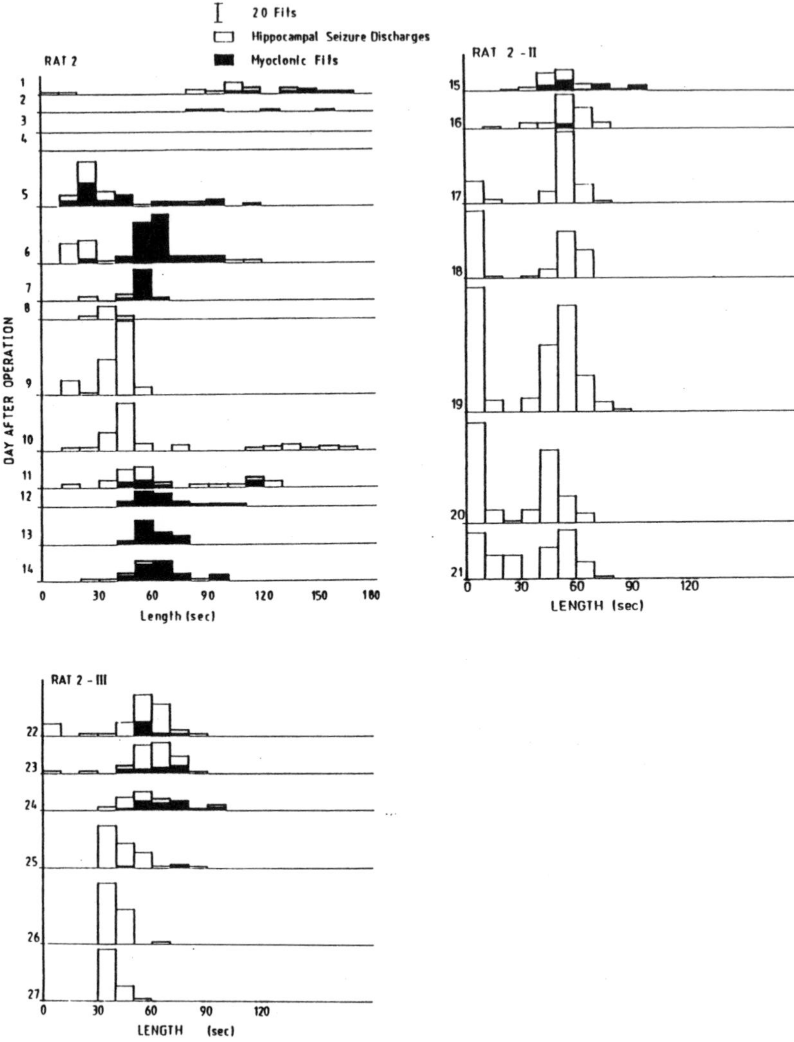

Figure 9.2. The distribution of the duration of seizures for each day of the syndrome. The rat had received an injection of tetanus toxin into the left ventral hippocampus on day 0 and at the same operation recording electrodes were implanted 1 mm above the injection site. The duration of each seizure was measured and they were arranged in 10 s 'bins'. The overall columns indicate the number of seizures whether or not accompanied by a motor fit; the filled areas denote those where obvious motor signs occurred (from Hawkins, 1985).

accompanied by unpleasant alimentary sensations and/or feelings of *déjà vu*, but also occasionally ecstasy (Dostoevsky, 1913). This stage is associated with fast spiking on the EEG. In tetanus toxin-induced epilepsy there may be a parallel since just before a fit the rats usually take up a stance that bears all the appearance of the 'freezing' response to a fear-promoting stimulus, with the ears laid back and the body hunched. This stage is associated also with fast activity on the EEG. Seizures due to intrahippocampal tetanus toxin have much in common with seizures kindled from the hippocampus or amygdala. After the initial behavioural arrest, seizures progress to vibrissal and facial twitching, forelimb myoclonus, and eventually to rearing and falling fits (a clonic-tonic sequence, characteristic of stage 5 of kindling).

In clinical limbic epilepsy the fits are often followed by a period of disorientation and confusion involving an altered state of consciousness or fugue state which may last for hours (Impey and Mellanby, 1994). Limbic seizures induced in rats, or in other laboratory animals, by kindling or intrahippocampal tetanus toxin also cause postictal behaviours. Rats often remain immobile for some minutes after a fit but then they may become hyper-reactive and act aggressively if disturbed.

Seizures have long-lasting effects on brain function. In humans these postictal deficits include cortical dysfunctions such as Todd's paralysis. These can last for minutes to days. Rats have similar behavioural deficits. Neocortical seizures can cause behavioural arrest and decreased locomotion. These effects may be side-effects of endogenous seizure suppression mechanisms. Opioid systems are implicated in postictal suppression of kindled seizures, and in at least some of the behaviours during this period. However, opioids have paradoxical effects on the hippocampus where they are convulsant due to their selective actions on interneurones (see also 'Learning and memory' below).

Activity and social interaction

During the active epilepsy, rats characteristically are hyper-reactive to handling and other external stimuli such as loud noises: they will leap vertically and dash about energetically. This response has been roughly quantified and has been shown to stop at around the same time that the rat ceases to have seizure activity in the hippocampus (Hawkins and Mellanby, 1987). A more quantitative assessment of hyper-reactivity, using the open field test (Walsh and Cummins, 1976), in which the locomotion and other activities of rats is measured on a raised platform in the presence of loud noise and flashing lights, confirmed the increased reactivity during but not after recovery from epilepsy (Mellanby *et al.*, 1981). In contrast, neither during (2–3 weeks) nor after (3 months) the epileptic phase was there evidence of increased spontaneous locomotor activity measured in the home cage (Mellanby *et al.*, 1981). The reactiveness to handling was associated with sporadic attacks on the handler or inanimate objects introduced into the cage. Such behaviour, although appearing to be aggressive, may represent a response more related to extreme fearfulness (Blanchard *et al.*, 1979). This interpretation has been supported by observation of the social interactions between epileptic rats and their non-epileptic peers in the home intruder test (File *et al.*, 1979). In this test, a normal but unfamiliar rat is introduced into the epileptic rat's own cage and the interactions between the animals observed and scored as aggressive (nip, box, wrestle, kick, leap on, push, follow, climb on) passive (lying on back, run away, climb under, freeze) or non-interactive (groom, explore, eat, drink) over a 10 minute period. With two normal rats, it is usually the 'home rat' that shows more aggressive and less passive responses. However, with actively epileptic home rats (3 weeks after operation) and normal intruders, the epileptic rats were more passive and less aggressive than the intruders (Mellanby *et al.*, 1985). This finding could be interpreted as suggesting that the behaviour of the epileptic rat in some way elicited aggressive behaviour from the intruder rat. This suggestion is further supported by observations in experiments in which cages of epileptic and control rats have been continuously filmed throughout the period of active epilepsy. In one such experiment, there were three cages of rats, each containing two epileptic and one control rat. Over a period of 28 days from the injection of toxin, 442 aggressive interactions were observed of which 324 (73%) were by the control rat on one of the toxin-injected rats ($P<0.01$; Anne-Katherine Brink; unpublished). Figure 9.3 illustrates the pattern of aggression and submission exhibited by a typical control and a typical epileptic rat in the above experiment. This social response of the epileptic rats and their peers is reminiscent of the finding of Delgado (1963) that in colonies of monkeys (*Macaca mulatta*), a dominant male will fall to the bottom of the social hierarchy if it is made epileptic, and may have a parallel in social treatment of some people with epilepsy. Attempts to see whether a comparable effect to that in monkeys can be induced by the tetanus toxin injection in rats have been unsuccessful since we have found that rats do not appear to form stable hierarchies when caged in groups of four. However, the passive response to an intruder rat still persisted at 6 months after toxin injection (J. Mellanby and L. Impey, unpublished).

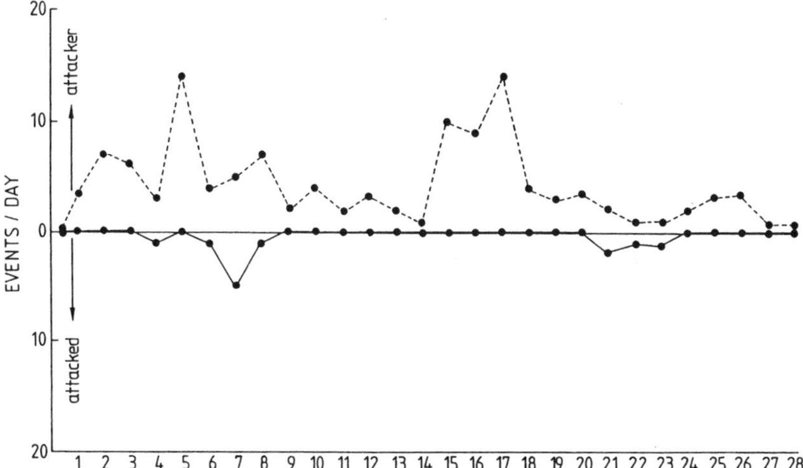

Figure 9.3. Aggressive interaction between control and toxin-injected rats. The (female) rat had received a unilateral injection of tetanus toxin (or vehicle) into the ventral hippocampus on day 0. The rats were caged in threes: two toxin-injected and one control. They were filmed continuously for 28 days and the numbers of times that one rat attacked another counted. The graphs show the data from two typical rats, one toxin-injected (solid lines) and one control (dashed lines), and illustrate that the control was more often the aggressor and the toxin-injected rat the attacked (from Ann-Katherine Brink, unpublished).

Sexual behaviour and reproduction

The very long-term study of 100 children with epilepsy carried out by Ounsted's group (Lindsay, Ounsted and Richards, 1979), showed that men who had fits during puberty were likely to be sexually indifferent in adult life and did not usually reproduce. The possibility that this could be modelled in the tetanus toxin-induced epilepsy was tested by inducing epilepsy in 15 male rats at 21 days of age leading to their having limbic fits during the immediately prepubertal and pubertal period (and injecting 15 control rat similarly with neutralised toxin). Five months later, each rat was housed with two female rats for 4 days (to allow one complete oestrous cycle in the female) and the pregnancy and production of young followed. No deficiency in male potency was found, the females housed with control or ex-epileptic rats all producing successful litters. In contrast to the lack of effect of the epilepsy on the behaviour of the males, it did disturb the reproductive physiology and behaviour of females. Firstly, during the period of overt motor fits (but not after recovery), the oestrous cycle was disrupted (Mellanby *et al.*, 1993) in all the epileptic females (and only very transiently just after the operation in the

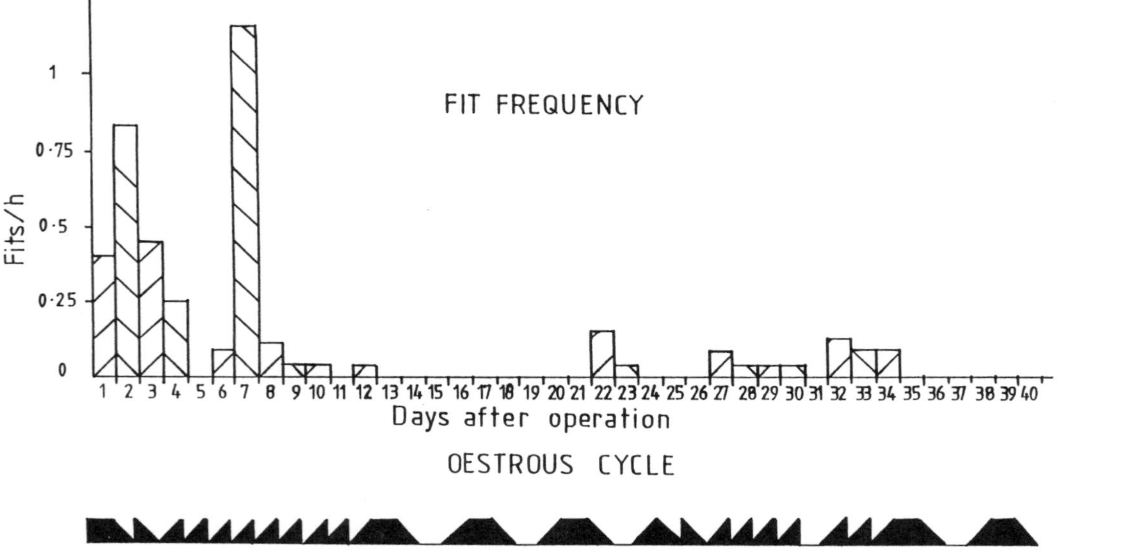

Figure 9.4. The relationship between fit frequency and the disruption of the oestrus cycle. The female rat has received a unilateral injection of tetanus toxin into the ventral hippocampus on the morning of pro-oestrus (day 0). It was filmed continuously to enable counting of motor fits. Vaginal smears were taken daily and examined microscopically to assess the stage of the oestrus cycle (from J. Dwyer, unpublished).

controls). Figure 9.4 shows one example of the rather close relationship between disturbance of the cycle and the occurrence of fits in a toxin-injected female rat. We have previously shown that as the epilepsy wanes the seizure activity fails to spread outside the hippocampus (Hawkins and Mellanby, 1987). The finding that the effect on the oestrous cycle did not long outlast the occurrence of overt fits suggests that it results when the seizure activity spreads, presumably to the hypothalamus and related areas. Of further interest was the finding that during a period after overt fits had stopped, when the oestrous cycle had returned, the female rats were apparently less sexually attractive to males. Thus, when housed with a male on the evening of pro-oestrus (their sexually attractive time) there were fewer mounts, intromissions and ejaculations despite there not being any increase (actually a decrease) in acts of resistance on the part of the females. The matings were also less likely to result in the production of young. The numbers in the litters of the ex-epileptic rats that did produce young were not smaller than with control animals but the mothers did not care adequately for them so that fewer survived and those that did were small and scruffy. This effect on the females did not however last into a second pregnancy (8 weeks after the first) and was also found to depend on the level of apparent stress in the breeding rooms – it was only found where the animals were kept in a noisy environment with much coming and going of staff.

Ingestive behaviour and body weight

During the early part of the epileptic syndrome produced by hippocampal toxin injection, the rats always lose more weight than their controls (Mellanby *et al.*, 1981). The weight is however rapidly regained by around 2 weeks after the operation. Over the next 3–4 months, it is very reproducibly found that the toxin-injected rats gain weight at a slightly faster rate than do their controls and so by 6 weeks later they may be 10% heavier. Apparently such a tendency to increased weight gain after remission of fits is quite often seen clinically (G. Glaser, personal communication) and might presumably be related to long-term changes produced in the hypothalamic feeding initiation and/or termination mechanisms by the spread of seizure activity into the area (Hawkins and Mellanby, 1987).

With toxin injection into the amygdala, changes in eating behaviour are seen. H. Brace (unpublished) found that some of these rats showed bouts of 'paroxysmal eating' during the first few days after toxin injection. This behaviour was reminiscent of the apparent activation of a motivational system seen in stimulus-bound or stimulus-rebound eating elicited by electrical stimulation of parts of the limbic system in monkeys (MacLean and Delgado, 1953) and in rats (Valenstein, Cox and Kakolewski, 1969; Milgram, 1969). Because of this curious observation, various aspects of feeding behaviour were studied in amygdala-injected rats and compared with that of hippocampally injected rats. Neither group ate more overall than their controls but the amygdala rats showed a block of neophobia for unfamiliar palatable food such as chocolate buttons and harvest crunch breakfast cereal, while still finding bitter food (e.g. orange peel) aversive (J. Mellanby, M. Oliva and A. Peniket, unpublished).

Learning and memory

The majority of the behavioural characterisation of the epileptic syndrome has involved the investigation of the rats' ability to learn and remember. The hippocampus is considered to have an important, if not yet fully understood role in learning and memory (O'Keefe and Nadel, 1978; Olton, Becker and Handelman, 1979; Rawlins, 1985; Sutherland and Rudy, 1989; Nadel, 1991; Rawlins *et al.*, 1993). Seizure activity within the limbic system therefore might be expected to impair learning and memory. During the active phase of the epilepsy (1, 2 and 4 weeks after induction), rats were impaired in their ability to perform a light discrimination task in a Y-maze (involving running to the lit arm to escape a weak electric shock) which they had learned before the toxin injection (George and Mellanby, 1982). This was shown to be a memory deficit rather than just a performance deficit since rats that had received extra training sessions throughout the epileptic period before final re-test at 4 weeks were not impaired while those re-tested for the first time at 4 weeks were (Mellanby and George, 1979). The memory deficit outlasts the active epilepsy and therefore cannot be ascribed only to current interference with the functioning of the hippocampus. We have reported a weak correlation between the deficit in the memory for the light-discrimination task and the numbers of overt fits which the rats had previously experienced – and this correlates with the total number of hippocampal seizure discharges that they had experienced (Mellanby, Hawkins and Wilks, 1984). Carbamazepine (20–60 mg/kg p.o., t.d.s.) is a fairly effective antiepileptic drug in this model (Hawkins, Mellanby and Brown, 1985). It appears to block the spread of seizure activity to motor areas rather than reduce the number of seizure discharges within the hippocampus (Hawkins and Mellanby, 1987). In experiments where the number of fits was reduced by carbamazepine, the memory deficit seen after recovery was reduced (Hawkins *et al.*, 1985).

In many ways the post-epileptic rats behave as if they have partial hippocampal lesions – they are impaired on reversal learning (both of the light-discrimination task and of place learning in the Y-maze), they are impaired in learning a delayed alternation task in a T-maze (where they have to learn to alternate their choices between trials to obtain food pellets, (Mellanby *et al.*, 1982), and they are impaired in learning two spatial tasks, the radial arm maze (Brace, Jefferys and Mellanby, 1985) and the circular platform task (Jefferys and Williams, 1987). In the radial arm maze they have to learn to visit each of a number (8–16) of positions just once within a trial in order to obtain food pellets, while in the circular platform task they need to learn the location of the hole leading to a comfortable dark tunnel. Thus these tasks involve both working memory (where they have been on this particular trial on the radial arm maze) and reference memory (where reward may be found on both tasks). This pattern of deficits fits with the proposed functions of the hippocampus in working and spatial memory. If the epilepsy is causing a general reduction in efficacy of hippocampal function then it would also be expected to interfere with learning other hippocampal tasks such as delayed responses with long latency (DRL). It has been found that the rats have difficulty in withholding responses in this test, in which they have to wait 20 seconds after each response before pressing the lever again if they are to succeed in getting the food pellets (Nicholls, 1994, and J. Tanner, unpublished) and in those experiments where control rats learn the task effectively, the rats with toxin in the hippocampus are slower to learn it.

It would thus seem that the rats are impaired in learning hippocampal tasks but are also impaired in a simultaneous discrimination (the light-discrimination task in the Y-maze), which is a task on which hippocampally damaged animals are not usually thought of as being impaired. It could indeed be argued that the recovered rats simply show mild impairment in most behavioural tasks – they are just not as effective as normal animals. They are not however globally impaired since their short-term memories appear to be intact. This conclusion is drawn from the observation that when learning the light-discrimination task they tend to use more perseverative strategies (e.g. most commonly, go to the position that was right last time) than do their controls (George and Mellanby, 1982). This, which is similar to the finding of Kimble (1975) with hippocampally lesioned rats, shows that they can use strategies that require them to hold information for a few seconds – i.e. short-term memory comparable to human digit span, which is intact in humans with bilateral hippocampal lesions (Baddeley and Warrington, 1970). Furthermore, they are not impaired in initial learning of a simple position task in the Y-maze – indeed they are actually significantly better at it than their controls, learning it in less than half the number of trials (Mellanby *et al.*, 1982).

Mechanisms of behavioural changes

We have described how a range of animal models of epilepsy show cognitive and other behavioural impairments. These studies show that the behaviours associated with epilepsies, especially those in temporal lobe epilepsies, can result from epileptic activity, and cannot be entirely attributed to the side-effects of anti-epileptic drugs or to other factors that affect people with chronic diseases. These animal studies also allow us to start to identify the mechanisms of behavioural disturbances in epilepsies.

Perhaps the most obvious cause for behavioural change is the loss of neurones in the lesions often found in human epileptic foci. Clearly a large lesion in the hippocampus or amygdala will cause similar behavioural impairments however it is caused. On the other hand structural lesions are not necessary for impairments of learning and memory. In neither kindling nor in the tetanus toxin model is there much evidence of histopathology to explain the long-lasting cognitive dysfunction. The hippocampal tetanus toxin model, as used by us, causes sporadic histopathology. Following dorsal injections ~10% of rats have focal losses of CA1 pyramidal neurones (Jefferys *et al.*, 1992), while ventral injections result in 30% of rats with extensive loss of pyramidal neurones in the CA1 region of the hippocampus, generally at sites in the dorsal hippocampus, remote from the injection (Shaw, Perry and Mellanby, 1994; Mellanby, 1993). Rather more common is the activation of microglia, which occurs in 63% of rats and which could signal more limited neuronal damage, such as deafferentiation and/or withering of the dendrites. One strain of rat also was susceptible to acidophylic damage to its neurones following injection of tetanus toxin into the dorsal hippocampus (Jefferys *et al.*, 1992), which suggests genetic or environmental risk factors in pathology. However, gross structural damage does not account for the impairment in learning and memory since no correlation was found between cell loss in dorsal CA1 and such deficits (J. Mellanby and L.E. Sundstrom, unpublished). The modest neuropathology in the face of frequent seizures is remarkable, and may be due to their limited duration of <2 minutes (Hawkins and Mellanby 1987). On the other hand, the extent of the neopathological changes is affected by the dose of toxin; much higher doses (>200 times) reliably cause lesions close to the injection site, and also result in a high mortality rate (Bagetta *et al.*, 1990).

The phenomenon of long-term synaptic potentiation (LTP) in the hippocampus and other parts of the brain is a model and possibly also a mechanism of learning and memory. One hypothesis to explain the memory deficits (that is deficits seen in subsequently performing tasks learned before the induction of epilepsy) in the tetanus toxin model is that seizure activity disrupts established LTP and hence disrupts memory (George and Mellanby, 1982). A comparable long-term disruption of the memory for the radial arm maze task has been demonstrated for <1 month after hippocampal kindling (Lopes da Silva *et al.*, 1986; Leung *et al.*, 1990; Leung and Shen, 1991). It has furthermore been reported that new learning may be impaired if LTP is first saturated by repetitive stimulation (McNaughton *et al.*, 1986). Both the spontaneous seizure activity seen in the tetanus toxin model and the kind of stimuli used in kindling would be expected to be able to induce LTP and hence in principle such saturation. However, there is conflicting evidence about the effect of kindling on subsequent learning (Bliss and Richter Levin, 1993). Several studies suggest that deficits in learning spatial tasks (water maze and radial arm maze) may only occur for short periods after the application of the kindling stimulation (Cain *et al.*, 1993; McNamara *et al.*, 1993; Robinson *et al.*, 1993). By 24 hours after the stimulation there is no longer impairment and it appears therefore that in these experiments it was the recent seizure activity that impaired the learning and that the kindled state itself is not detrimental to learning. Thus it would appear that while the disruption of established memories in the tetanus toxin model may be comparable to the effect of kindled seizures, the disruption of new learning, at times long after the seizure activity has remitted, highlights a marked difference between the two models. This may be related to the fact that in the toxin model there has been active damping of seizures associated with a decrease in hippocampal evoked responses, with selective reductions in the population spikes recorded in CA3 and CA1 and DG *in vivo*, and a reduction in inhibition (Brace *et al.*, 1985; Jefferys and Williams, 1987; Mellanby and Sundstrom, 1987). In the tetanus toxin model we have shown that the ability to produce and maintain LTP remain intact, at least for periods of <4 hours in anaesthetised rats (Brace *et al.*, 1985; Jefferys and Williams, 1987). Evoked responses recorded *in vitro* also revealed prolonged, bilateral abnormalities in toxin-injected rats: population spike depression in CA3, enhancement in dentate, and no change in CA1 (Whittington and Jefferys, 1994). The cellular mechanisms of these changes remain to be resolved, but they must be enduring because both the physiological and behavioural post-epileptic deficits last for many months, essentially for the remainder of the rats' expected lifespan.

In the long-term, a significant minority of rats with intrahippocampal tetanus toxin (~10%) may relapse into seizures, whose cellular mechanisms have not yet been resolved, but a predisposition may be associated with an early loss of CA1 pyramidal cells in the dorsal hippocampus (Mellanby, 1993). In contrast, chronic foci in the cat do not appear to be associated with any gross neuronal loss (Louis *et al.*, 1990; Darcey and Williamson 1992)).

Conclusion

The existence of behavioural consequences of experimental chronic epilepsies in laboratory animals shows that they are not necessarily due to anticonvulsants, nor to social stigma, but that they have a biological basis. The effects of tetanus toxin-induced epilepsy on behaviour can be divided into those associated with seizure activity spreading outside the focal area, producing motor fits, those associated with more focal epileptic activity and those persisting after remission from epileptiform electrographic signs. During the period where motor fits occur, the rats are hyper-reactive, and this is similar to the effect of kindling stimulation, they are impaired in both learning and memory, their social behaviour is passive and in females the oestrous cycle is disrupted. Most of these changes are still seen during the period of more focal seizure activity but the oestrous cycle is rapidly re-established. However, the females are less sexually attractive to males and when they do mate and produce young they fail to care for them properly. After seizure activity stops, the sexual and parenting behaviour returns to normal and the rats cease to be hyper-reactive to handling. However, the deficits in learning hippocampal tasks and the passive social behaviour remain after recovery and are presumably both related to the permanent changes in hippocampal physiology that have occurred in response to the epilepsy.

Acknowledgements

The authors' work is supported by the Wellcome Trust, Ciba Geigy, the British Epilepsy Research Foundation, the Marie Stopes Fund and St. Hilda's College.

References

Baddeley, A.D. and Warrington, E.K. (1970). Amnesia and the distinction between long and short-term memory. *Journal of Verbal Learning and Verbal Behaviour*, **9**, 176–89.

Bagetta, G., Knott, C., Nisticó, G. and Bowery, N.G. (1990). Tetanus toxin produces neuronal loss and a reduction in $GABA_A$ but not $GABA_B$ binding sites in rat hippocampus. *Neuroscience Letters*, **109**, 7–12.

Bekenstein, J.W. and Lothman, E.W. (1993). Dormancy of inhibitory interneurons in a model of temporal lobe epilepsy. *Science*, **259**, 97–100.

Ben-Ari, Y. and Represa, A. (1990). Brief seizure episodes induce long-term potentiation and mossy fibre sprouting in the hippocampus. *Trends in the Neurosciences*, **13**, 312–18.

Blanchard, D.C., Blanchard, R.J., Lee, E.M. and Nakamura, S. (1979). Defensive behaviors in rats following septal and septal–amygdala lesions. *Journal of Comparative Physiological Psychology*, **93**, 378–90.

Bliss, T.V.P. and Richter Levin, G. (1993). Spatial learning and the saturation of long-term potentiation. *Hippocampus*, **3**, 123–5.

Brace, H.M., Jefferys, J.G.R. and Mellanby, J. (1985), Long-term changes in hippocampal physiology and in learning ability of rats after intrahippocampal tetanus toxin. *Journal of Physiology*, **368**, 343–57.

Brener, K., Chagnac-Amitai, Y., Jefferys, J.G.R. and Gutnick, M.J. (1991). Chronic epileptic foci in neocortex: *in vivo* and *in vitro* effects of tetanus toxin. *European Journal of Neuroscience*, **3**, 47–54.

Cain, D.P., Hargreaves, E.L., Boon, F. and Dennison, Z. (1993). An examination of the relations between hippocampal long-term potentiation, kindling, afterdischarge, and place learning in the water maze. *Hippocampus*, **3**, 153–64.

Cavalheiro, E.A., Riche, D.A. and Le Gal La Salle, G. (1982). Long-term effects of intrahippocampal kainic acid injection in rats: a method for inducing spontaneous recurrent seizures. *Electroencephalography and Clinical Neurophysiology*, **53**, 581–9.

Darcey, T.M. and Williamson, P.D. (1992). Chronic/semichronic limbic epilepsy produced by microinjection of tetanus toxin in cat hippocampus. *Epilepsia*, **33**, 402–19.

Delgado, J.M.R. (1963). Effect of brain stimulation on task-free situations. *Electroencephalography and Clinical Neurophysiology Supplement*, **24**, 260–80.

Dostoevsky, F. (1913). *The Idiot*. London: Heinemann.

Empson, R.M. and Jefferys, J.G.R. (1993). Inhibitory synaptic function in primary and secondary chronic epileptic foci induced by intrahippocampal tetanus toxin in the rat. *Journal of Physiology*, **465**, 595–614.

File, S.E., Deakin, J.F.W., Longden, A. and Crow, T.J. (1979). An investigation of the role of the locus coeruleus in anxiety and agonistic behaviour. *Brain Research*, **169**, 411–20.

Finnerty, G.T. and Jefferys, J.G.R. (1993). Spontaneous epileptiform activity in freely moving rats with epileptic foci induced by tetanus toxin. *Journal of Physiology*, **467**, 319P.

George, G. and Mellanby, J. (1975). Cephalic tetanus in rats. *Proceedings of the IV International Conference on Tetanus*. Dhaka.

George, G. and Mellanby, J. (1982). Memory deficits in an experimental hippocampal epileptiform syndrome in rats. *Experimental Neurology*, **75**, 678–89.

Griffith, N., Endel, J. and Bandler, R. (1987). Ictal and enduring interictal disturbances in emotional behavior in an animal model of temporal-lobe epilepsy. *Brain Research*, **400**, 360–4.

Hawkins, C.A. (1985). Studies in an animal model of temporal lobe epilepsy. DPhil thesis, Oxford University.

Hawkins, C.A., Mellanby, J. and Brown, J. (1985). Antiepileptic and antiamnesic effect of carbamazepine in experimental limbic epilepsy. *Journal of Neurology, Neurosurgery and Psychiatry*, **48**, 459–68.

Hawkins, C.A. and Mellanby, J.H. (1987). Limbic epilepsy induced by tetanus toxin: a longitudinal electroencephalographic study. *Epilepsia*, **28**, 431–44.

Impey, M. and Mellanby, J. (1994). Epileptic phenomena as a source of creativity: the work of Alfred Kubin (1877–1959). *Journal of Moral and Social Studies*, **7**, 153–71.

Jefferys, J.G.R. (1989). Chronic epileptic foci *in vitro* in hippocampal slices from rats with the tetanus toxin epileptic syndrome. *Journal of Neurophysiology*, **62**, 458–68.

Jefferys, J.G.R. and Williams, S.F. (1987). Physiological and behavioural consequences of seizures induced in the rat by intrahippocampal tetanus toxin. *Brain*, **110**, 517–32.

Jefferys, J.G.R., Evans, B.J., Hughes, S.A. and Williams, S.F. (1992). Neuropathology of the chronic epileptic syndrome induced by intrahippocampal tetanus toxin in the rat: preservation of pyramidal cells and incidence of dark cells. *Neuropathology and Applied Neurobiology*, **18**, 53–70.

Kimble, D.P. (1975). Choice behavior in rats with hippocampal lesions. In *The Hippocampus* (ed. R.L. Isaacson and K.H. Pribram), pp. 309–26. New York: Plenum Press.

Leung, L.S. and Shen, B. (1991). Hippocampal CA1 evoked response and radial 8-arm maze performance after hippocampal kindling. *Brain Research*, **555**, 353–7.

Leung, L.S., Boon, K.A., Kaibara, T. and Innis, N.K. (1990). Radial maze performance following hippocampal kindling. *Behavioural Brain Research*, **40**, 119–29.

Lindsay, J., Ounsted, C. and Richards, P. (1979). Long-term outcome in children with temporal lobe seizures. II: Marriage, parenthood and sexual indifference. *Developmental Medicine and Child Neurology*, **21**, 433–40.

Lopes da Silva, F.H., Gorter, J.A. and Wadman, W.J. (1986). Kindling of the hippocampus induces spatial memory deficits in the rat. *Neuroscience Letters*, **63**, 115–20.

Louis, E.D., Williamson, P.D. and Darcey, T.M. (1990). Chronic focal epilepsy induced by microinjection of tetanus toxin into the cat motor cortex. *Electroencephalography and Clinical Neurophysiology*, **75**, 548–57.

MacLean, P.D. and Delgado, J.M.R. (1953). Electrical and chemical stimulation of frontotemporal portion of limbic system in the waking animal. *Electroencephalography and Clinical Neurophysiology*, **5**, 91–100.

Mathern, G.W., Cifuentes, F., Leite, J.P. *et al.* (1993). Hippocampal EEG excitability and chronic spontaneous seizures are associated with aberrant synaptic reorganization in the rat intrahippocampal kainate model. *Electroencephalography and Clinical Neurophysiology*, **87**, 326–39.

McNamara, R.K., Kirkby, R.D., DePape, G.E. *et al.* (1993). Differential effects of kindling and kindled seizures on place learning in the Morris water maze. *Hippocampus*, **3**, 149–52.

McNaughton, B.L., Barnes, C.A., Rao, G. *et al.* (1986). Long-term enhancement of hippocampal synaptic transmission and the acquisition of spatial information. *Journal of Neuroscience*, **6**, 563–71.

Mellanby, J. (1993). Tetanus toxin as a tool for investigating the consequences of excessive neuronal excitation. In *Botulinum and Tetanus Neurotoxins* (ed. B.R. DasGupta), pp. 291–7. Plenum Press: New York.

Mellanby, J. and George, G. (1979). Tetanus toxin and experimental epilepsy in rats. In *Advances in Cytopharmacology* (ed. B. Ceccarelli and F. Clementi), pp. 401–8. New York: Raven Press.

Mellanby, J.H. and Sundstrom, L. (1987). Long-term reduction in inhibition in rat dentate gyrus after intrahippocampal tetanus toxin. *Journal of Physiology*, **382**, 89P.

Mellanby, J., George, G., Robinson, A. and Thompson, P. (1977). Epileptiform syndrome in rats produced by injecting tetanus toxin into the hippocampus. *Journal of Neurology, Neurosurgery and Psychiatry*, **40**, 404–14.

Mellanby, J., Strawbridge, P., Collingridge, G.I. *et al.* (1981). Behavioural correlates of an experimental hippocampal epileptiform syndrome in rats. *Journal of Neurology, Neurosurgery and Psychiatry*, **44**, 1084–93.

Mellanby, J., Renshaw, M., Cracknell, H. *et al.* (1982). Long-term impairment of learning ability in rats after an experimental hippocampal epileptic syndrome. *Experimental Neurology*, **75**, 690–9.

Mellanby, J., Hawkins, C.A. and Wilks, L. (1984). The relationship between seizures and amnesia in experimental epilepsy. *Acta Neurologica Scandinavica*, **69**, 118–24.

Mellanby, J., Hawkins, C., Baillie-Hamilton, S. *et al.* (1985). Kindling, behaviour and anticonvulsant drugs. In *Psychopharmacology of Epilepsy* (ed. M.R. Trimble), pp. 17–31. London: John Wiley.

Mellanby, J., Dwyer, J., Hawkins, C.A. and Hitchen, C. (1993). Effect of experimental limbic epilepsy on the estrus cycle and reproductive success in rats. *Epilepsia*, **34**, 220–7.

Milgram, N.W. (1969). Effect of hippocampal stimulation on feeding in the rat. *Physiology and Behaviour*, **4**, 665–70.

Nadel, L. (1991). The hippocampus and space revisited. *Hippocampus*, **1**, 221–9.

Nicholls, B. (1994). An investigation of the long term effects of experimental limbic epilepsy on the exploratory behaviour of rats. Unpublished thesis. D.Phil, University of Oxford.

Nicholls, B., Springham, A. and Mellanby, J. (1992). The playground maze: a new method for measuring directed exploration in the rat. *Journal of Neuroscience Methods*, **43**, 171–80.

O'Keefe, J. and Nadel, L. (1978). *The Hippocampus as a Cognitive Map*. Oxford: Oxford University Press.

Olton, D.S., Becker, J.T. and Handelman, G.E. (1979). Hippocampus, space and memory. *Behavioral and Brain Sciences*, **2**, 315–65.

Racine, R.J. (1972). Modification of seizure activity by electrical stimulation. II. Motor seizure. *Electroencephalography and Clinical Neurophysiology*, **32**, 281–94.

Rawlins, J.N.P. (1985). Associations across time – the hippocampus as a temporary memory store. *Behavioral and Brain Sciences*, **8**, 479–97.

Rawlins, J.N., Lyford, G.L., Seferiades, A. *et al.* (1993). Critical determinants of nonspatial working memory deficits in rats with conventional lesions of the hippocampus or fornix. *Behavioural Neuroscience*, **107**, 420–33.

Robinson, G.B., McNeill, H.A. and Reed, G.D. (1993). Comparison of the short- and long-lasting effects of perforant path kindling on radial maze learning. *Behavioural Neuroscience*, **107**, 988–95.

Shaw, J.A.G., Perry, V.H. and Mellanby, J. (1994). MHC class II expression by microglia in tetanus toxin-induced experimental epilepsy in the rat. *Neuropathology and Applied Neurobiology*, **20**, 392–8.

Sloviter, R.S. (1991). Permanently altered hippocampal structure, excitability, and inhibition after experimental status epilepticus in the rat: the 'dormant basket cell' hypothesis and its possible relevance to temporal lobe epilepsy. *Hippocampus*, **1**, 41–66.

Stone, W.S. and Gold, P.E. (1988). Amygdala kindling effects on sleep and memory in rats. *Brain Research*, **449**, 135–40.

Sundstrom, L.E., Mitchell, J. and Wheal, H.V. (1993). Bilateral reorganisation of mossy fibres in the rat hippocampus after a unilateral intracerebroventricular kainic acid injection. *Brain Research*, **609**, 321–6.

Sutherland, R.J. and Rudy, J.W. (1989). Configural association theory: the role of the hippocampal formation in learning, memory and amnesia. *Psychobiology*, **17**, 129–44.

Sutula, T., He, X.X., Cavazos, J. and Scott, G. (1988). Synaptic reorganisation in the hippocampus induced by abnormal functional activity. *Science*, **239**, 1147–50.

Tauck, D.L. and Nadler, J.V. (1985). Evidence of functional mossy fiber sprouting in hippocampal formation of kainic acid-treated rats. *Journal of Neuroscience*, **5**, 1016–22.

Valenstein, E.S., Cox, V.C. and Kakolewski, J.W. (1969). The hypothalamus and motivated behaviour. In *Reinforcement and Behaviour* (ed. J.T. Tapp). London: Academic Press.

Walsh, R.N. and Cummins, R.A. (1976). The open field test: a critical review. *Psychological Bulletin*, **83**, 482–504.

Whittington, M.A. and Jefferys, J.G.R. (1994). Epileptic activity outlasts disinhibition after intrahippocampal tetanus toxin in the rat. *Journal of Physiology*, **481**, 593–604.

10

A neurobiological perspective of the behaviour disorders of epilepsy

MICHAEL R. TRIMBLE

Introduction

A full understanding of the development of psychoses in psychiatric practice can only be undertaken with knowledge of the underlying principles of brain organisation, and of the neurobehavioural consequences of CNS lesions. The former relates especially to those areas of the brain that modulate emotional behaviour, namely the limbic system and related tracts and pathways. The latter refer particularly to neurological diseases that have behavioural manifestations as an integral part of their clinical picture. Of these, epilepsy has been the most studied.

Some neuroanatomical principles

Recent advances in neuroanatomy that are of relevance to an understanding of links between epilepsy and behaviour include a better understanding of the role of the limbic system, and the delineation of the concepts of the extended amygdala, the ventral striatum, and the emotional motor system (EMS). Essentially, it is appreciated that the limbic system is far from being an independent grouping of neurones and tracts with few connections to adjacent structures. It has extensive inputs to the basal ganglia, influencing motor function directly (ventral striatum). Further, via the extended amygdala, it outputs directly to diencephalic and brain stem structures that 'set' emotional and motor tone (extended limbic system and the EMS). It thus becomes clear that CNS disorders that affect the limbic system are likely to have a profound effect on emotional behaviour, and epilepsy is a paradigm.

On the role of the limbic system

Although definitions of the limbic system vary, most agree that central components include the amygdala, hippocampus and their outflow pathways.

The latter include, importantly, the limbic forebrain structures such as the dopamine-rich nucleus accumbens and surrounding nuclei of the ventral striatum, and pathways to the hypothalamus, thalamus, and their connections down to the midbrain tegmentum and beyond.

It was Papez, in the 1930s, who first suggested that a limbic circuit, which comprised the hippocampus, the mammillary body of the thalamus, the anterior thalamus, the cingulate gyrus, and a loop back to the hippocampus, was a neural substrate for the emotions. The concept of the limbic system was developed further by MacLean (1990). Basing his ideas on comparative anatomy, he discussed the 'triune brain'. Essentially, he pointed out how human brains contain three main components, a neocortex, a paleocortex, and a reptilian brain. The basic concept was that the limbic system (the paleocortex) was only developed in a very rudimentary way prior to the rise of mammals, and is very poorly represented in reptiles. As MacLean noted:

> The history of the evolution of the limbic system is the history of the evolution of the mammals, while the history of the evolution of the mammals is the history of the development of a family way of life.

In other words, with the development of infant–maternal bonding, and the evolution of complex social behaviours, there has been a parallel development of the neuroanatomical arrangements of limbic structures.

There has been considerable work carried out on the hippocampus, and while its exact role remains controversial, it does play a prominent role in episodic memory, linking the present with the past, and information about the internal state of an organism with that about its immediate environment.

The extended amygdala and the ventral striatum

Much attention recently has been paid to the amygdala, and the delineation of the extended amygdala by Alheid and Heimer (1988). This refers to close anatomical connections between the amygdala and limbic forebrain structures. Thus, Nauta and colleagues repeatedly emphasised the extensive crosstalk between the limbic system and the basal ganglia (Nauta and Domesick, 1982). The extended amygdala is a broad range of cells connecting the basomedial and central amygdala to the bed nucleus of the stria terminalis and the connections between, including the sublenticular portion of the substantia innominata (see Figure 10.1). This is influenced by the afferents coming from the monoamine rich areas of the mesencephalon and brain stem, and in turn directly outputs to the ventral striatum, and the hypothalamus. The extended amygdala concept emphasises the importance

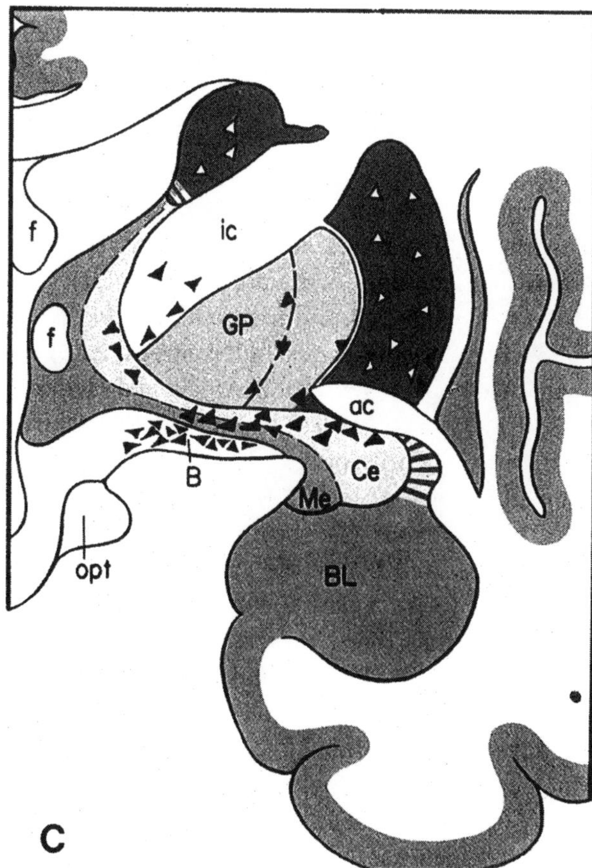

Figure 10.1. Showing schematically the connections of the extended amygdala. The medial and central amygdaloid nuclei (Me; Ce) connect with medially sited nuclei adjacent to the fornix (f) such as the bed nucleus of the stria terminalis. GP, globus pallidus; BL, basolateral amygdaloid nucleus; ic, internal capsule; ac, anterior commisure; opt, optic tract; B, basal nucleus of Meymert. (Reproduced with permission from Heimer *et al.*, 1991).

of the amygdala for the regulation of emotional behaviour, influencing autonomic and motoric function.

The extended amygdala is thus closely associated with the ventral striatum. The ventral striatum is contrasted with the dorsal striatum mainly by its limbic inputs, and output to the mediodorsal nucleus of the thalamus, as opposed to the ventrolateral, ventromedial and centromedial nucleus (Figure 10.2). The main components of the ventral striatum are the nucleus accumbens, the olfactory tubercle, and the anteroventral caudate-putamen.

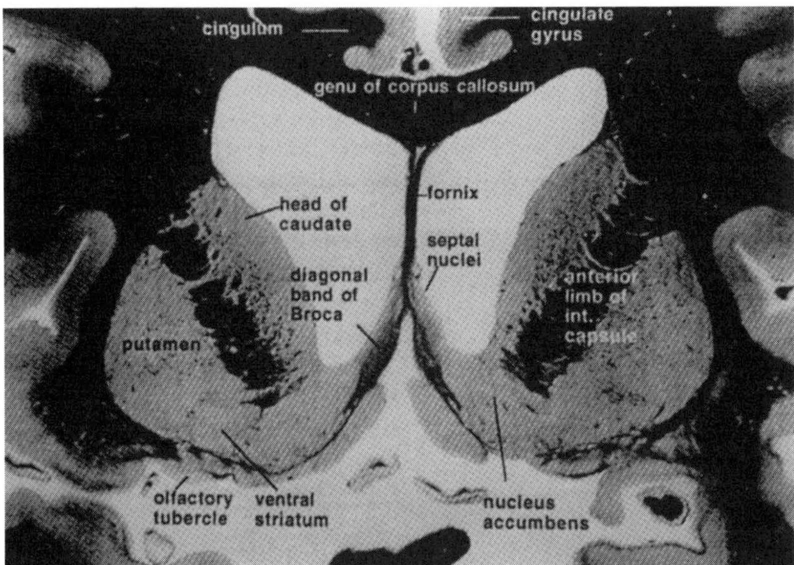

Figure 10.2. Showing the position of the nucleus accumbens, one of the main structures of the ventral striatum, in the human brain. It has parallel outputs to the ventral pallidum and thalamus, similar to the circuitry of the dorsal striatum. Reproduced with permission from Salloway and Cummings (1994).

The nucleus accumbens has a caudal boundary with the bed nucleus of the stria terminalis, which is difficult to establish anatomically, emphasising the interconnectedness with the extended amygdala. Anteriorly it extends into the ventromedial portion of the frontal lobe.

It has recently become appreciated that there are two components of the nucleus accumbens, a core and a shell (Heimer *et al.*, 1991). The core is striatal, projects to the ventral pallidum, and hence to the thalamus and back to cortex. The shell is essentially a part of the extended amygdala and projects both to the globus pallidus, but also to the hypothalamus and brain stem motor and autonomic nerves. Further, the core and the shell project directly to the ventral tegemental area (VTA) and the substantia nigra reticulata, directly setting motor tone in the basal ganglia circuitry.

Thus, the structures of the limbic system, especially the amygdala, so vital for emotional interpretation of sensory stimuli and emotional memory, have direct ways of influencing motor output through both somatomotor and autonomic pathways. The extended amygdala projects directly to the autonomic and endocrine systems, but also can modulate the circuitry of the motor loops and hence pyramidal outflow by influences on the VTA and substantia nigra (see Figure 10.3). A further direct pathway

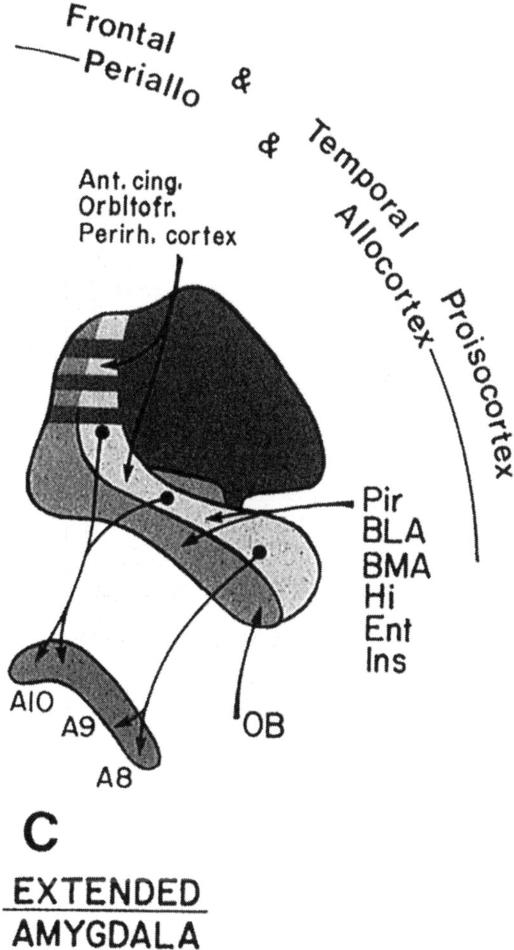

Figure 10.3. Showing some of the outputs of the extended amygdala. There are direct efferents to areas A 8, 9 and 10 (substantia nigra and ventral tegmental area), which exert a direct influence on the control of motor behaviour. Pir, piriform cortex; BLA, basolateral amygdala; BMA, basomedial amygdala; Hi, hippocampus; Ent, entorhinal cortex; Ins, insula.
(Reproduced with permission from Heimer *et al.*, 1991).

is from the extended amygdala to prefrontal cortex, and hence to the motor area of M3 and pyramidal tracts.

The extended limbic system

Nieuwenhuys (1997) has developed these concepts even further, referring to the greater limbic system. He emphasised the caudal projections to and from the rostral medulla, and then further connections with the spinal cord influencing autonomic function.

The final common pathway for emotional expression is through the autonomic nervous system, and the EMS. The latter includes key nuclear areas such as the periaqueductal grey matter (PAG), situated immediately below the superior colliculus, surrounding the aqueduct between the third and fourth ventricles. Stimulation leads to a variety of expressed emotions, especially threat and flight, and it is involved in pain perception (Bandler and Shipley, 1994). Also included are groups of neurones that seem to directly control autonomic function in the rostral medulla, and at the junction between the medulla and the pons. These include neurones regulating cardiac and respiratory function, and micturition. Some of the neurones (presympathetic cells) have direct monosynaptic inputs to the preganglionic sympathetic cells.

The neuropathology of epilepsy

The neuropathological changes in epilepsy are varied, but it has been known for a number of years that a specific form of pathology is found in many patients, particularly those with localisation-related temporal lobe epilepsy. Mesial temporal sclerosis is a specific pathological lesion, affecting largely hippocampal structures, particularly sub-fields within the hippocampus such as CA1. It is known to occur secondary to early anoxic brain damage. In some patients, the amygdala is also involved.

A key feature in many patients with this pathology is an early febrile convulsion, particularly one that has been prolonged or complicated. Patients may then be seizure free for several years, developing simple or complex partial seizures in their adolescence. Other pathologies found in the temporal lobes, that affect limbic system structures, often reflect developmental abnormalities. These include the hamartomas and dysembryoplastic neuronal tumours (DNT), reflecting an heterogenous group of mixed pathologies arising during fetal development. Again, patients with such pathologies often remain seizure free for many years, the first seizures erupting in late childhood or early adulthood.

It is common to speak loosely of 'temporal lobe epilepsy'. However, neuroanatomically, neurochemically, and neurophysiologically it is clear that there are a number of sub-divisions of the temporal lobes, as there are, for example, of the frontal lobes. It is suggested that one such subdivision involves the limbic portion (archicortex). Some authors distinguish a medial temporal epilepsy syndrome, which may be referred to as limbic

Table 10.1. *The medial temporal lobe epilepsy syndrome*

Complex partial seizures, often with secondary generalisation.
Difficult to control seizures.
Behaviour disorder, with personality change, affective symptoms, and occasionally psychosis.
A medical temporal lobe focus identified with EEG.
Pathology in these areas sometimes seen with MRI.

epilepsy, with the characteristics shown in Table 10.1. The importance of this distinction is that behaviour disorders appear to be an integral part of the medial temporal syndrome, reflecting on the central role that the limbic system and related structures play in the development of emotions and behaviours.

Limbic epilepsy may be defined as a form of seizure disorder, where pathology is found in limbic system structures, the latter usually arising during an early developmental period, in which patients have difficult to treat seizures, and present with behaviour disorders. If we consider the crucial role of the medial temporal structures in modulating emotional expression, it is hardly unlikely that a lesion in such structures, leading to dysfunction throughout crucial periods of psychosocial development, would leave the individual free from behavioural scars.

As will be noted (see below), the clinical phenomenology of the psychoses associated with temporal lobe epilepsy is often indistinguishable from paranoid states and schizophrenia in the absence of epilepsy. This may reflect the underlying anatomical similarities. Neuropathological studies of schizophrenia, of which there are now many, reveal that where abnormalities of the hippocampus, or parahippocampal gyrus, are looked for, they are often found (Trimble, 1995). Although the pathology differs from that of classic mesial temporal sclerosis, in particular by the absence of a gliosis, the frequently reported neuronal disarray, which probably reflects abnormal neuronal migration during foetal development, is thought to be interlinked with the development of the schizophrenia syndrome. The relevance of the limbic system, therefore, is that this neuronal circuitry that underlies the development of emotion and behaviour, is disrupted in patients who develop schizophrenia, but also in patients with one form of epilepsy, namely limbic epilepsy. As will be shown, it is those patients who are most susceptible to develop psychopathology, and the latter may resemble schizophrenia. Hence the use of the term 'the schizophrenia-like psychoses of epilepsy' adopted by Slater *et al.* (1963).

Personality change in epilepsy

A useful starting point is the work of Jaspers (1963), who made a clear distinction between psychogenic development and organic process – in other words, between personality and illness. He said 'We differentiate abnormal personality types that are anlage variants, from sick personalities in the narrower sense, where the change has been brought on by a process.' It is the change in the patient's habitual patterns of behaviour that indicates that a process has taken place, and that process may relate to underlying structural or functional changes within the central nervous system.

Although it is not here intended to outline the various forms of personality disorder that are described in such manuals as the DSM-IV (1994), two points need to be clarified. First, the kinds of personality changes that one sees with neurological disease do not necessarily conform to the personality disorders of diagnostic manuals of psychiatrists. Second, the personality change reported is usually a combination of both an exacerbation of the premorbid personality and, particularly if the burden of pathological change is on the frontal or temporal lobes, some new and distinctive feature that provides a clue to the possible cerebral localisation of the underlying process.

The association between temporal lobe epilepsy and personality disorders has been an issue of constant debate and confusion. The concept that there may be an interictal temporal lobe syndrome has been most strongly advocated by Geschwind and his colleagues. Thus, Waxman and Geschwind (1975) defined the interictal behaviour syndrome of temporal lobe epilepsy, emphasising alterations in sexual behaviour, hyperreligiosity, and hypergraphia – a tendency toward extensive and often compulsive writing. They suggested that in some patients, the syndrome appeared before any seizures; when present, even in the absence of further evidence, these features suggest dysfunction at this specific anatomical site. They contrasted this picture both with the frontal lobe syndrome and with the Kluver–Bucy syndrome. The latter occurs after bilateral extirpation of the medial temporal lobes, and has clinical features that contrast with those of the interictal syndrome (see below).

In the interictal syndrome the religiosity may be seen as sudden religious conversion or as a growing interest in mystical and religious themes, often with behaviour out of keeping with the patient's normal pattern. There may be compulsive church attendance, repetitive bible reading, or obsessive attachment to some unorthodox religious group. Alternatively, there may merely be an interest in the cosmic and supernatural or the conviction that the person has some special significance in the world, some messianic mission.

Meticulous attention to detail is another feature, as well as continual working over of an idea. Circumstantiality of speech and verbosity are also seen, with prolonged and tortuous explanations often being given for trivial events. To some extent this may be reflected in hypergraphia, with detailed and meticulous accounts of events being recorded, often with a moral or religious theme.

The disturbed sexuality is usually referred to as hyposexuality, with indifference to sexual contacts. However, in other patients it may manifest as a plasticity of responses, with development of unusual proclivities. It should be emphasised that the symptoms and signs that are associated with this syndrome are not necessarily maladaptive; some patients display remarkable talents and are productive members of society.

One interpretation of these findings was that an epileptic focus somehow leads to enhanced associations between affects and stimuli, a so-called functional hyperconnection between neocortical and limbic structures, possibly inhibiting events that normally prevent fortuitous sensory and affective connections developing (Bear and Fedio, 1977). To some extent this is the opposite of the Kluver–Bucy syndrome, in which limbic dysfunction leads to failure to attribute the appropriate emotional significance to stimuli, resulting in emotional blunting, diminished fear, aggression, inappropriate sexual behaviour and hypermetamorphosis – a limbic agnosia.

The personality changes associated with temporal lobe epilepsy are often not detected clinically unless specifically inquired about. Such features as hyperreligiosity, obsessionality, and circumstantiality are hardly the things that relatives or patients complain about to doctors. At times, these attributes flower into a psychosis, for example after loss of seizure control, or after a flurry of seizures. In some patients, an insidious development of psychosis is seen, the over-valued idea transforming into a fixed delusion.

Psychosis in epilepsy

In the middle of the 19th century, European psychiatrists noted the high incidence of psychotic episodes in institutionalised patients with epilepsy. Several authors described the specific psychopathology of psychiatric complications occurring in the context of epilepsy using terms like 'epilepsie larvée' (Morel, 1860), 'grand mal intellectuel' (Falret, 1860), 'epileptoid states' (Griesinger, 1868) and 'epileptic equivalents' (Hoffmann, 1872). Samt (1875) put forward the idea that the pathophysiology of certain psychoses occurring in the context of epilepsy, especially episodic twilight states, was identical to the pathophysiology of motor seizures. He suggested that in the absence of true seizures such epileptic equivalents were sufficient for a diagnosis of epilepsy.

With progress in diagnosis and treatment in epilepsy, epileptology shifted away from psychiatry to neurology. Psychiatric aspects were neglected until they were 'rediscovered' in the 1950s and 1960s (Landolt, 1953, Gastaut, 1956, Tellenbach, 1965). American and British authors reported an excess of schizophrenia-like psychoses in epilepsy patients, especially in those suffering from temporal lobe epilepsy (Gibbs, 1951; Pond, 1962; Slater and Beard, 1963).

Slater and his colleagues published a detailed analysis of 69 patients from two London hospitals who suffered from epilepsy and interictal psychoses. On the basis of this case series the authors challenged the antagonism theory, that schizophrenia and epilepsy were mutually exclusive, and postulated a positive link between them. Although Slater was criticised for drawing conclusions on the basis of insufficient statistics (Stevens, 1966), the temporal lobe hypothesis soon became broadly accepted and stimulated extensive research into the role of temporal lobe pathology in schizophrenia. The use of epileptic psychoses as a biological model or 'mock-up' of schizophrenia (Roberts *et al.*, 1990) is largely based on Gibbs' and Slater's work.

The possible impact of research into epileptic psychosis on the understanding of the pathophysiology of endogenous psychoses explains the bias in the literature towards study of interictal schizophrenia-like psychoses. The spectrum of psychotic syndromes in epilepsy is however much more complex and psychotic complications are not restricted to patients with temporal lobe epilepsy (Trimble, 1991).

Although to date no adequate epidemiological study of psychopathology in epilepsy has been carried out, clinical case series clearly indicate that psychosis is a significant problem in patients attending specialised centres. This suggests that there are risk factors for the development of psychosis related to complicated epilepsy and/or chronic illness.

Classification

There is no internationally accepted syndromic classification of psychoses in epilepsy. Psychiatric aspects are not considered in the international classification of epilepsies and the use of operational diagnostic systems for psychiatric disorders such as the DSM-IV is limited because, if applied strictly, a diagnosis of schizophrenia is not allowed in the context of epilepsy. For the time being it is suggested that patients with epilepsy and psychoses receive two separate diagnoses according to both the ICD and the DSM-IV. In addition, the relationship between onset of psychosis and seizure activity, antiepileptic therapy and changes of EEG findings, should be noted.

For pragmatic reasons, psychoses in epilepsy can be grouped according to their temporal relationship to seizures. It should be acknowledged that such a classification does not necessarily imply fundamental differences in terms of pathophysiology. Further consideration is given here only to the interictal psychoses.

Interictal psychoses

Interictal psychoses occur between seizures and cannot directly be linked to the ictus. Slater stated that, in the absence of epilepsy, the psychoses in their study group would have been diagnosed as schizophrenia (Slater and Beard, 1963). But they also mentioned distinct differences between process schizophrenia and the schizophrenia-like psychoses associated with epilepsy. They highlighted the preservation of warm affect and a high frequency of delusions and religious mystical experiences.

Other authors stressed the rarity of negative symptoms and the absence of formal thought disorder and catatonic states (Köhler, 1975). Tellenbach (1965) stated that delusions were less well organised and Sherwin (1984) remarked that neuroleptic treatment was less frequently necessary. There have been other authors however who denied any psychopathological differences between epileptic psychosis and schizophrenia (Helmchen, 1975; Kraft, Price and Peltier, 1984).

Using the Present State Examination and the CATEGO computer program, which is a semi-standardised and validated method for quantifying psychopathology, it has been possible to compare the presentation of psychosis in epilepsy with process schizophrenia. Very few significant differences emerged from such studies (Perez and Trimble, 1980; Toone, Garralda and Ron, 1982) which suggest that, assuming the patients were representative, a significant number will have a schizophrenia-like presentation indistinguishable from schizophrenia in the absence of epilepsy.

Phenomenology apart, Slater argued that the long-term prognosis of psychosis in epilepsy was better than in process schizophrenia. In a follow-up study on his patients he found that psychotic symptoms tended to remit and personality deterioration was rare (Glithero and Slater, 1963). Other authors also described outcome to be more favourable and long-term institutionalisation to be less frequent than in schizophrenia (Köhler, 1975; Sherwin, 1984). Unfortunately, there have been no longitudinal studies

Table 10.2. *Risk factors associated with interictal psychoses of epilepsy (Trimble, 1991)*

Sex	Bias to females
Age of onset of epilepsy	Early adolescence
Interval	Onset of seizures to onset of psychosis: 14 years (av.)
Epileptic syndrome	Temporal lobe epilepsy
Seizure type	Complex focal
Seizure frequency	Low, diminished
Neurological findings	Sinistrality
Pathology	Gangliogliomas, harmatomas
EEG	Mediobasal focus, especially left-sided

comparing the long-term outcome of psychosis in epilepsy and process schizophrenia.

Risk factors

The pathogenesis of psychotic episodes in epilepsy is likely to be heterogenous. In most patients a multitude of chronic and acute factors can be identified that are potentially responsible for the development of a psychiatric disorder. These factors are difficult to investigate in retrospect and the interpretation as either causally related or simply intercorrelated is arguable.

The literature on risk factors is highly controversial; studies are difficult to compare because of varying definitions of the epilepsy, the psychiatric disorder and the investigated risk factors. Most studies are restricted to interictal psychoses. Table 10.2 summarises factors that have frequently been described to be associated with psychosis in epilepsy (Trimble, 1991).

Genetic predisposition

With few exceptions (Jensen and Larsen, 1979), most authors do not find any evidence for an increased rate of psychiatric disorders in relatives of epilepsy patients with psychoses (Slater, Beard and Glithero, 1963; Flor-Henry, 1969; Perez and Trimble, 1980).

Sex distribution

There has been a bias towards female sex in several case series (Taylor, 1971), which has not been confirmed in controlled studies (Kristensen and Sindrup, 1978*a*,*b*; Bash and Mahnig, 1984).

Duration of epilepsy

The interval between age at onset of epilepsy and age at first manifestation of psychosis has been remarkably homogenous in many series, being in the region of 11 to 15 years (Trimble, 1991). This interval has been used to postulate the aetiological significance of the seizure disorder and a kindling-like mechanism. Some authors (Stevens, 1966; Bruens, 1974) have argued that the supposedly specific interval is an artifact. They noted a wide range of duration, being significantly shorter in patients with later onset of epilepsy. They also pointed out that anybody whose psychosis did not succeed their epilepsy was excluded in most series, and that there is a tendency in the general population for the age of onset of epilepsy to peak at an earlier age than that of schizophrenia.

Type of epilepsy

There is a clear excess of temporal lobe epilepsy in almost all case series of patients with epilepsy and psychosis. Summarising the data of 10 studies, 217 (or 76%) of 287 patients suffered from temporal lobe epilepsy (Trimble, 1991). The preponderance of this type of epilepsy is however not a uniform finding; in Gudmundsson's epidemiological study for example, only 7% suffered from 'psychomotor' epilepsy.

The nature of a possible link of psychoses to temporal lobe epilepsy is not entirely clear (Schmitz, 1992), partly due to ambiguities in the definition of TLE in the literature, either based on seizure symptomatology (psychomotor epilepsy), involvement of specific functional systems (limbic epilepsy) or on anatomical localisation as detected by depth EEG or neuroimaging (amygdalo-hippocampal epilepsy). Unfortunately, most authors have not sufficiently differentiated frontal and temporal lobe epilepsy.

The temporal lobe hypothesis, although widely accepted, has been criticised for being based on uncontrolled case series, such as in the studies by Gibbs (1951) and Slater and Beard (1963). It was argued that temporal lobe epilepsy is the most frequent type of epilepsy in the general population, and that there is an over-representation of this type of epilepsy in patients attending specialised centres. However, there is a general consensus that psychoses are very rare in patients with neocortical extratemporal epilepsies (Gibbs, 1951; Dongier, 1959; Stevens, 1966; Bruens, 1974; Onuma, 1983; Sengoku *et al.*, 1983; Schmitz, 1988).

Schneiderian first rank symptoms and chronicity are more frequent in patients with temporal lobe epilepsy (Schmitz, 1988; Trimble and Perez,

1982). This has considerable significance for psychiatrists attempting to unravel the underlying 'neurology' of the syndromes of schizophrenia.

Type of seizures

There is evidence from several studies that focal seizure symptoms that indicate ictal mesial temporal or limbic involvement are over-represented in patients with psychosis. Hermann and Chabria (1980) noted a relationship between ictal fear and high scores on paranoia and schizophrenia scales of the Minnesota Multiphasic Personality Inventory (MMPI). Kristensen and Sindrup (1978*a*,*b*) found an excess of dysmnesic and epigastric auras in their psychotic group. They also reported a higher rate of ictal amnesia. In another controlled study, ictal impairment of consciousness, indicating limbic involvement, was related to psychosis but simple seizure symptoms were not (Schmitz, 1988).

No seizure type is specifically related to psychosis in generalised epilepsies, but most patients with psychosis and generalised epilepsies have absence seizures (Schmitz, 1988).

Severity of epilepsy

The strongest risk factors for psychosis in epilepsy are those that indicate severity of epilepsy. These are long duration of active epilepsy (Slater and Beard, 1963), multiple seizure types (Ounsted, 1969; Bruens, 1974; Hermann *et al.*, 1982; Sengoku *et al.*, 1983; Rodin, Collomb and Pache, 1976; Lindsay, Ounsted and Richards, 1979; Schmitz, 1988), history of status epilepticus (Schmitz, 1988) and poor response to drug treatment (Lindsay *et al.*, 1979). Seizure frequency however is reported by most authors to be lower in psychotic epilepsy patients than in non-psychotic patients (Standage, 1973; Slater *et al.*, 1963; Flor-Henry, 1969; Sengoku *et al.*, 1983), but it has not been clarified whether seizure frequency was low before or during the psychotic episode.

Laterality

Left lateralisation of temporal lobe dysfunction or temporal lobe pathology as a risk factor for schizophreniform psychosis was originally suggested by Flor-Henry (1969). Studies supporting the laterality hypothesis have been made using surface EEG (Lindsay *et al.*, 1979), depth electrode recordings (Sherwin *et al.*, 1982), computed tomography (Toone *et al.*,

1982), neuropathology (Taylor, 1971), neuropsychology (Perez and Trimble, 1980), and PET (Trimble, 1986). The literature has been summarised by Trimble (1991). In a synopsis of 14 studies with 341 patients, 43% had left, 23% right and 34% bilateral abnormalities. This is a striking bias towards left lateralisation. However, lateralisation of epileptogenic foci was not confirmed in all controlled studies (Kristensen and Sindrup, 1978*a*,*b*; Dongier, 1959, Shukla *et al.*, 1979). Again, it has been suggested that certain symptoms, for example first rank psychotic symptoms, are associated with a specific side of focus (Trimble, 1986).

Structural lesions

The literature on brain damage and epileptic psychosis is very controversial. Some authors have suggested a higher rate of abnormal neurological examinations, diffuse slowing on the EEG and mental retardation (Kristensen and Sindrup, 1978*a*,*b*), whilst others could not find such an association with psychosis (Flor-Henry, 1969; Jensen and Larsen, 1979). Neuropathological studies from resected temporal lobes from patients with TLE have suggested a link between psychosis and the presence of cerebral malformations such as hamartomas and gangliogliomas as compared with mesial temporal sclerosis (Taylor, 1971). These findings have been seen as consistent with recent findings of structural abnormalities found in the brains of schizophrenic patients without epilepsy, which arise during fetal development.

Summary and conclusions

Behaviour changes are seen in people with epilepsy. These should be viewed as biologically interlinked with the epilepsy, several factors entwining to lead to the final common path. Thus epilepsy is not only seizures and its management requires more than just extinguishing seizures.

Patients with temporal lobe epilepsy, especially limbic seizures, are more susceptible to behaviour problems. These include personality changes and psychoses. However, many patients with temporal lobe epilepsy escape such complications. It is suggested here that crucial to their development is limbic system dysfunction, and in the patients described here medial temporal structures, especially the hippocampus and the amygdala, are involved. It is continuing abnormal activity, especially through developmental years, when the individual is becoming just that, namely the individual, that is so relevant. Maclean has emphasised the crucial role of limbic structures for mammalian, and therefore human social and emotional behaviours, and to disrupt their connectivity and continuity must distort the relationship between the inner and outer worlds, and the biological integrity of the individual.

It seems to be the case that small temporal lesions influence the brain widely, and the reciprocal cortical–limbic associations, and potential chaotic regulation of activity in and through the extended amygdala and beyond, allow for disruption of emotional development and the liability to develop behaviours that become accepted as psychopathological. We are just at the stage of being able to explore these clinically, but the hypotheses to be tested are often firmly bounded in data from neuroanatomical experimental work. Temporal lobe epilepsy provides a privileged inroad to the inner emotional world of the human mind, and its exploration from a neuroanatomical perspective.

References

Alheid, G.F. and Heimer, L. (1988). New perspectives in basal forebrain organisation of special relevance for neuropsychiatric disorders. *Neuroscience*, **27**, 1–39.

Bandler, R. and Shipley, M.T. (1994). Columnar organisation in the midbrain periaqueductal gray: modules for emotional expression? *Trends in the Neurosciences*, **17**, 379–89.

Bash, K.W. and Mahnig, P. (1984). Epileptiker in der psychiatrischen Klinik. Von der Daemmerattacke zur Psychose. *European Archives of Psychiatry and Neurological Science*, **234**, 237–49.

Bear, D.M. and Fedio, P. (1977). Quantitative analysis of interictal behaviour in temporal lobe epilepsy. *Archives of Neurology*, **34**, 454–67.

Bruens, J.H. (1971). Psychoses in epilepsy. *Psychiatria, Neurologia, Neurochirurgia*, **74**, 174–92.

Bruens, J.H. (1974). Psychoses in epilepsy. In *Handbook of Clinical Neurology*, (ed. P.J. Vinken and G.W. Bruyn), vol. 15, pp. 593–610. Amsterdam: North Holland.

Diagnostic and Statistical Manual of Mental Disorders, Fourth edition (DSM-IV) (1994). Washington DC: American Psychiatric Association.

Dongier, S. (1959/60). Statistical study of clinical and electroencephalographic manifestations of 536 psychotic episodes occuring in 516 epileptics between clinical seizures. *Epilepsia*, **1**, 117–42.

Falret, J. (1860), De l'état mental des épileptiques. *Archives Generales de Médecine*, **16**, 661–79.

Flor-Henry, P. (1969). Psychosis and temporal lobe epilepsy. A controlled investigation. *Epilepsia*, **10**, 363–95.

Gastaut, H. (1956). Colloque de Marseille. 15–19 Octobre 1956. Compte rendu du colloque sur l'étude électroclinique des épisodes psychotiques qui survennient chez les épileptiques en dehors des crises cliniques. *Revue Neurologique*, **95**, 587–616.

Gibbs, F.A. (1951). Ictal and non-ictal psychiatric disorders in temporal lobe epilepsy. *Journal of Nervous and Mental Disease*, **113**, 522–8.

Glithero, E. and Slater, E. (1963). The schizophrenia-like psychoses of epilepsy. IV Follow-up record and outcome. *British Journal of Psychiatry*, **109**, 134–42.

Griesinger, W. (1868). Über einige epileptoide Zustände. *Archiv für Psychiatrie und Nervenkrankheiten*, **1**, 320–33.

Heimer, L., Olmos, J., Alheid, G.F. and Zaborszky, L. (1991). Perestroika in the basal forebrain: opening the border between neurology and psychiatry. In *Progress in Brain Research*, vol. 87 (ed. G. Holstege), pp. 109–62. Holland: Elsevier Science Publishers.

Helmchen, H. (1975). Zerebrale Bedingungkonstellationen psychopathologischer Syndrome bei Epileptikern. In *Entwicklungstendenzen biologischer Psychiatrie* (ed. H. Helmchen and H. Hippius), pp. 125–48. Stuttgart: Thieme.

Hermann, B.P. and Chabria, S. (1980). Interictal psychopathology in patients with ictal fear. *Archives of Neurology*, **37**, 667–8.

Hermann, B.P., Dikmen, S., Schwartz, M.S. and Karnes, W.E. (1982). Psychopathology in patients with ictal fear: a quantitative investigation. *Neurology*, **32**, 7–11.

Hoffmann, F. (1872). Über die Eintheilung der Nervenkrankheiten in Siegburg. *Allgemeine Zeitschrift für Psychiatrie*, **19**, 367–91.

Jaspers, K. (1963). *Psychopathology* (trans. J. Hoenig and M.W. Hamilton). Manchester, England: Manchester University Press.

Jensen, I. and Larsen, J.K. (1979). Mental aspects of temporal lobe epilepsy. *Journal of Neurology, Neurosurgery and Psychiatry*, **42**, 256–65.

Köhler, G.K. (1975). Epileptische Psychosen – Klassifikationsversuche und EEG-Verlaufsbeobachtungen. *Fortschritte der Neurologie und Psychiatrie*, **43**, 99–153.

Köhler, G.K. (1980). Zur Einteilung der Psychosen bei Epilepsie. Zum Begriff 'Psychosen bei Epilepsie' bzw. 'epileptische Psychosen'. In *Psychopathologische und Pathogenetische Probleme Psychotischer Syndrome bei Epilepsie* (ed. P. Wolf and G.K. Köhler), pp. 11–18. Bern: Huber.

Kraft, A.M., Price, T.R.P. and Peltier, D. (1984). Complex partial seizures and schizophrenia. *Comprehensive Psychiatry*, **25**, 113–24.

Kristensen, O. and Sindrup, H.H. (1978*a*). Psychomotor epilepsy and psychosis. I. Physical aspects. *Acta Neurologica Scandinavica*, **57**, 361–9.

Kristensen, O. and Sindrup, H.H. (1978*b*). Psychomotor epilepsy and psychosis. II. Electroencephalographic findings. *Acta Neurologica Scandinavica*, **57**, 370–9.

Landolt, H. (1953). Serial electroencephalographic investigations during psychotic episodes in epileptic patients and during schizophrenic attacks. In *Lectures on Epilepsy* (ed. A.M. Lorentz), pp. 91–133. Amsterdam: Elsevier.

Lindsay, J., Ounsted, C. and Richards, P. (1979). Long-term outcome in children with temporal lobe seizures. II. Psychiatric aspects in childhood and adult life. *Developmental Medicine Child Neurology*, **21**, 630–6.

MacLean, P. (1990). *The Triune Brain*. New York: Plenum Press.

Morel, B. (1860). D'une forme de délire, suite d'une surexcitation nerveuse se rattachent a une varieté non encore d'écrite d'épilepsie. *Gazette Hebdomadaire de Médicine et de Chirugie*, **7**, 773–5.

Nauta, W.T.H. and Domesick, V.B. (1982). Neural associations of the limbic system. In *The Neural Basis of Behaviour* (ed. A. Beckman), pp. 175–206. New York: Spectrum.

Niewenhuys, R. (1996). The greater limbic system, the emotional motor system and the brain. In *The Emotional Motor System* (ed. G. Holstege, R. Bandler and C.B. Saper), pp. 551–82. Amsterdam: Elsevier.
Onuma, T. (1983). Limbic lobe epilepsy with paranoid symptoms: analysis of clinical features and psychological tests. *Folia Psychiat. Neurol. Jpn*, **37**, 253–8.
Ounsted, C. (1969). Aggression and epilepsy. Rage in children with temporal lobe epilepsy. *Journal of Psychosomatic Research*, **13**, 237–42.
Papez, J.W. (1937). A proposed mechanism of emotion. *Archives of Neurology and Psychiatry*, **38**, 725–33.
Perez, M.M. and Trimble, M.R. (1980). Epileptic psychosis – diagnostic comparison with process schizophrenia. *British Journal of Psychiatry*, **137**, 245–9.
Pond, D.A. (1962). Discussion Remark. *Proceedings of the Royal Society of Medicine*, **55**, 316.
Roberts, G.W., Done, D.J., Bruton, C. and Crow, T.J. (1990). A 'mock up' of schizophrenia: temporal lobe epilepsy and schizophrenia-like psychosis. *Biological Psychiatry*, **28**, 127–43.
Rodin, E.A., Collomb, H. and Pache, D. (1976). Differences between patients with temporal lobe seizures and those with other forms of epileptic attacks. *Epilepsia*, **17**, 313–20.
Salloway, S. and Cummings, J. (1994). Subcortical disease and neuropsychiatric illness. *Journal of Neuropsychiatry*, **6**, 93–9.
Samt, P. (1875). Epileptische Irreseinsformen. *Archiv für Psychiatrie und Nervenkrankheiten*, **5**, 393–444.
Samt, P. (1876). Epileptische Irreseinsformen. *Archiv für Psychiatrie und Nervenkrankheiten*, **6**, 110–216.
Schmitz, B. (1988). Psychosen bei Epilepsie. Eine epidemiologische Untersuchung. Thesis, FU Berlin.
Schmitz, B. (1992). Psychosis and epilepsy. The link to the temporal lobe. In *The Temporal Lobes and the Limbic System* (ed. M.R. Trimble and T.G. Bolwig), pp. 149–67. Wrightson Biomedical Publishing Ltd.
Sengoku, A., Yagi, K., Seino, M. and Wada, T. (1983). Risks of occurrence of psychoses in relation to the types of epilepsies and epileptic seizures. *Folia Psychiat. Neurol. Jpn.*, **37**, 221–6.
Sherwin, I. (1984). Differential psychiatric features in epilepsy; relationship to lesion laterality. *Acta Psychiatrica Scandinavica*, (Suppl 313) **69**, 92–103.
Sherwin, I., Peron Magnan, P., Bancaud, J. *et al.* (1982). Prevalence of psychosis in epilepsy as a function of the laterality of the epileptogenic lesion. *Archives of Neurology*, **39**, 621–5.
Shukla, G.D., Srivastava, O.N., Katiyar, B.C. *et al.* (1979). Psychiatric manifestations in temporal lobe epilepsy. A controlled study. *British Journal of Psychiatry*, **135**, 411–17.
Slater, E. and Beard, A.W. (1963). The schizophrenia-like psychoses of epilepsy V. Discussion and conclusions. *British Journal of Psychiatry*, **109**, 143–50.
Slater, E., Beard, A.W. and Glithero, E. (1963). The schizophrenia-like psychoses of epilepsy. V. Discussion and conclusions. *British Journal of Psychiatry*, **109**, 95–150.
Standage, K.F. (1973). Schizophreniform psychosis among epileptics in a mental hospital. *British Journal of Psychiatry*, **123**, 231–2.
Stevens, J.R. (1966). Psychiatric implications of psychomotor epilepsy. *Archives of General Psychiatry*, **14**, 461–71.

Taylor, D.C. (1971). Ontogenesis of chronic epileptic psychoses: a reanalysis. *Psychological Medicine*, **1**, 247–53.

Tellenbach, H. (1965). Epilepsie als Anfallsleiden und als Psychose. Uber alternative Psychosen paranoider prägung bei 'forcierter Normalisierung' (Landolt) des Elektroencephalogramms Epileptischer. *Nervenarzt*, **36**, 190–202.

Toone, B., Dawson, J. and Driver, M.V. (1982*a*). Psychoses of epilepsy. A radiological evaluation. *British Journal of Psychiatry*, **140**, 244–8.

Toone, B., Garralda, M.E. and Ron, M.A. (1982*b*). The psychoses of epilepsy and the functional psychoses: a clinical and phenomenological comparison. *British Journal of Psychology*, **141**, 256–61.

Trimble, M.R. (1986*a*). PET-scanning in epilepsy. In *Aspects of Epilepsy and Psychiatry* (ed. M.R. Trimble and T.G. Bolwig), pp. 147–62. Chichester: John Wiley & Sons.

Trimble, M.R. (1986*b*). Positive and negative symptoms in psychiatry. *British Journal of Psychiatry*, **148**, 587–9.

Trimble, M. (1991). *The Psychoses of Epilepsy*. New York: Raven Press.

Trimble, M.R. (1995). *Biological Psychiatry*, 2nd Edition. Chichester: John Wiley & Sons.

Trimble, M.R. and Perez, M.M. (1982). The phenomenology of the chronic psychoses of epilepsy. In *Temporal Lobe Epilepsy, Mania and Schizophrenia and the Limbic System* (ed. W.P. Koella and M.R Trimble), pp. 98–105. Basel: Karger.

Waxman, S.G. and Geschwind, N. (1975). The interictal behaviour syndromes of temporal lobe epilepsy. *Archives of General Psychiatry*, **32**, 1580–6.

Section VI

Perspectives on neurodevelopment: the case of schizophrenia

11

Early disorders and later schizophrenia: a developmental neuropsychiatric perspective

ERIC TAYLOR

Introduction

Developmental neuropsychiatry is concerned with the pathways through which brain dysfunction is expressed in psychological problems at different ages. I have reviewed its scope and findings elsewhere (Taylor, 1991*a*). The subject has recently acquired particular relevance to adult psychiatrists. First, there was the finding, from studying the natural history of child psychiatric disorders, that delays in development are antecedents of schizophrenia and also of a wide variety of adult disability, including personality disorders and other psychoses (Zeitlin, 1986). Second, there were findings from the study of schizophrenia that abnormal birth histories and developmental disorders in childhood are present in a higher proportion of the childhoods of people with schizophrenia than in those of normal controls (Werry and Taylor, 1994). Third, animal experiments gave a most interesting model of how developmental effects might appear. Goldman-Rakic *et al.* (1983) described a series of experiments on rhesus monkeys in which bilateral damage to parts of the frontal cortex in infancy produced no immediate effect, yet the same animals in adult life developed a deficit in delayed learning very similar to that which appeared in animals given the same lesions in adult life. The implication was that there may be 'sleeper' effects. Early damage may not become manifest until the developmental stage is reached at which the damaged part of the brain would normally be taking up the function being tested. The immature brain may use quite different strategies from the mature one in achieving the same goal.

These links between the concerns of child and adult psychiatry should eventually enrich both fields greatly. At present, however, they are giving rise to some confusion because the underlying assumptions and approaches of the two disciplines are in many ways very different. At a simple level, perinatal brain damage has been used less and less by paediatricians and child psychiatrists to explain developmental problems (Gaffney *et al.*, 1994) so the emphasis on birth trauma from the clinical work on schizophrenia and the animal experiments has seemed like an anachronism. At a more theoretical level, the interpretation of how problems develop is different for those concerned primarily with children and those with adults. From the perspective of an adult psychiatrist looking at the early history of patients with schizophrenia it seems natural to suppose that the high rate of developmental disorders is explained either by their being early signs of schizophrenia or by their being evidence of a brain pathology that is a direct cause of schizophrenia. From the perspective of a child psychiatrist considering the adult outcome of child patients, it seems equally natural to consider neurodevelopmental delays as indicators of nonspecific vulnerability, whose adult consequences cannot be foreseen in childhood because they are dependent upon circumstances arising later in development. Yet these two notions are incompatible, and which one is correct will have strong implications for what sort of preventive strategy is likely to be worthwhile.

The tension between these views is the theme for this chapter. I shall discuss some possible causes in early development that have been implicated by schizophrenia researchers: perinatal trauma, foetal exposure to pathogenic agents, and genes affecting early development of the brain. For each of these, their impact on child development will be considered as well as their suggested roles in the pathogenesis of schizophrenia. The issue for each is the extent to which their suggested role in schizophrenia is compatible with conclusions already drawn in the developmental literature, or suggests a unique developmental mechanism.

Birth trauma

Physical and chemical traumata in the perinatal period have long been regarded as causes of psychiatric disorders in childhood. Obstetric complications (OCs) are more common in the histories of people who subsequently show intellectual retardation (Scott, 1994), autism (Lord and Rutter, 1994) and hyperkinetic disorder (Taylor *et al.*, 1991). Anorexia nervosa, obsessive-compulsive disorder, and hysteria have been associated with perinatal abnormalities in at least some studies. The mechanisms involved have been unclear. Most studies on intellectual retardation have considered that the association arises because obstetric complications are commoner in, and markers to, other forms of environmental deprivation. A genetic study of autism has made it clear that obstetric complications are more frequent because they result from a genetically abnormal foetus, not because they cause autism (Bailey *et al.*, 1995).

Until recently, perinatal damage usually had to be inferred from a history of potentially damaging events such as toxaemia of pregnancy, birth asphyxia, premature gestational age, or low birth weight. Most babies exposed to such events will not develop structural pathology of the brain. Investigators have therefore been trying to detect putative consequences of damage in populations heavily diluted with normal individuals. The task was all the harder because the physical risk factors are quite strongly associated with psychosocial adversity. Pregnancy and childbirth are more hazardous for deprived mothers, and in most countries their obstetric care is worse. Perinatal mortality is much increased in the most disadvantaged. The same social factors would have placed the children at risk even if their births had been entirely normal. Indeed, reviewers such as Gottfried (1973) found it impossible to be clear that neonatal asphyxia had a direct effect upon later intelligence. Sameroff and Chandler (1975) argued that failures of caretaking were the overwhelmingly strong influence on the bulk of psychological problems in children at risk.

Subsequent multivariate studies of the deveopment of children with perinatal risk factors tended to confirm the strong predictive power of the psychosocial environment and the weak influence of biological perinatal factors once family adversity was allowed for (Nichols and Chen, 1981; Neligan *et al.*, 1976; Werner and Smith, 1977). Increasing knowledge of cerebral palsy made it clear that many forms of motor disability were not due to abnormal deliveries, but reflected prenatal abnormalities that could themselves give rise to an abnormal delivery (Nelson and Ellenberg, 1986).

It remained possible that the perinatal events might exert a more powerful force for ill on the smaller number of children whose brains were abnormal. It was essential to move from 'exposure to risk' to 'markers of damage': from the presence of a potentially harmful agent to the evidence that it had indeed caused harm to that individual child. This is an important step in methodology. The lack of a marker to individual damage (such as a neurochemical change or imaging evidence of tissue destruction) has seriously handicapped the study of many other potential risks, such as lead exposure.

A simple, clinical index of damage is whether the child at risk shows neurological signs of poor coordination. This strategy has been vigorously exploited. It has allowed, for example, a follow-up into adult life (Shaffer *et al.*, 1983). Children whose perinatal course was recorded as part of the Perinatal Collaborative Survey, and whose neurological status was noted at age seven as part of the same study, were identified again at age 16–18. Those who had soft signs at seven were more likely to be diagnosed as having an affective disorder in adolescence; their IQs were lower, and they were rated as more deviant on a scale of dependency/withdrawal.

Motor incoordination, however, is a poor marker to brain injury. It may be a part of the disorder to be explained rather than a sign of the damage that could explain it. Better measures of brain damage were therefore needed. Autopsy findings on neonates had already shown the presence of intraventricular haemorrhages in preterm babies who died. Computerised axial tomography and ultrasound scans quickly showed that intraventricular haemorrhages were common in very low birth weight (VLBW) infants and that many survived. Many of these bleeds happen in the germinal matrix at the head of the caudate nucleus, and can extend into the ventricles or other areas of the brain.

Follow-up of children with evidence of haemorrhage has emphasised that they are much more strongly at risk for developmental delays. The apparent risk may increase as children get older, as more types of dysfunction can be detected (Costello *et al.*, 1988). It is still rather early for final conclusions on this. One has to wait until groups of systematically scanned infants have grown to an age where subtle developmental delays can be detected – in practice, seven years and onwards. Many such series are now being followed up.

Other types of neuropathology are important too. Ultrasound scans quickly evolved to the point where they could detect leukomalacia: either transient areas of increased density to echo or persistent cystic lesions round the ventricles and in subcortical white matter. These, too, compromise the infant's neurological development: tone is reduced in the early weeks of life and extensive lesions very often lead on to cerebral palsy. Frontoparietal cysts often lead to better neurological outcome, but are associated with hyperactivity at the age of two years (Casaer *et al.*, 1991).

Neonatal hypoxia in full-term infants is a much more controversial cause of neurodevelopmental problems. Like other obstetric factors, it has been given great importance in medico-legal decisions. However, a truer perspective comes when one appreciates the frequency with which prenatal disorder of the foetus causes delay in resuscitation and the infrequency with which birth asphyxia causes cerebral palsy (Hall, 1989). Asphyxia is at most a weak risk factor, not an indication that the brain has been damaged. The occurrence of actual damage may be witnessed by persistent seizure activity in the EEG, or magnetic resonance or ultrasound evidence of a low pulsatility index. If a full-term infant has no neurological deficit, then birth asphyxia is unlikely to be the cause of any later problem.

By contrast with hypoxia, other treatable complications of the neonatal period seem to have quite direct results on later development. Lucas, Morley and Cole (1988) found that moderate hypoglycaemia in preterm infants showed a strong dose–response relationship with developmental delay. Hypoglycaemia on five or more separate days predicted a three-fold increase in neurodevelopmental impairment at 18 months.

These advances make it possible to reinterpret the older controversy about social as against neurological determinants of developmental disorders. It now seems very likely that, when perinatal risk factors cause actual damage to the substance of the brain, the result is often an abnormality in the control of movements during early postnatal life. It is probable that they also give rise directly to cognitive impairments in later childhood; but the extent of this will not be clear until well-imaged series reach school age. So, reproductive casualty causes later psychological dysfunction.

These findings also call for reopening the issue of a continuum of reproductive casualty. For many forms of stress – including prematurity and hypoxia – the threshold for damage is quite high. For other kinds of injury – such as hypoglycaemia – there is a low threshold and a continuum of damage. The question needs to shift to the factors that determine thresholds for harmful effects.

The existence of direct neurological effects does not mean that they are the only factors operating. Later psychiatric dysfunction may also reflect the way that family relationships are deeply influenced by the anxiety about a critically ill neonate (Corter and Minde, 1987). This will need much more study. Psychiatric disorders are not influenced by the same processes as learning delays. Factors such as parental education, intelligence and occupation are all indices to the psychosocial processes that determine IQ. For the determination of psychiatric disorders, the details of interpersonal processes are much more important. They will have to be taken into account by the new generation of longitudinal research that can now be done.

Birth trauma and schizophrenia

The main implication of the developmental studies considered above is to cast doubt on a direct and simple causal account of how OCs cause schizophrenia. It may well be true that OCs are specific to schizophrenia in that they are more common than in mixed groups of adult psychiatric patients (Lewis and Murray, 1987). However, this high rate of OCs may be a marker to poverty and low social class rather than to causative brain damage; or OCs may be more probable because they result from a pre-existing abnormality of the foetus (Goodman, 1988).

The causative role of OCs would be clearer if they were less common in schizophrenics with a family history of schizophrenia, for this would suggest that they constitute an alternative aetiology. At present, however, the evidence is somewhat contradictory (Lewis, 1990) and no clear conclusion is possible. It might seem that clear evidence would come from the study of twins who are discordant for schizophrenia; and indeed the schizophrenic twin in a discordant pair of identical twins is more likely to show OCs and to have enlarged cerebral ventricles and diminished temporal lobes (Suddath *et al.*, 1989). However, the interpretation of this is not obvious. Discordance in monozygotic twin pairs does not imply an environmental cause. In fact, there is evidence against it: nonschizophrenic monozygotic twins of schizophrenic patients are at the same high risk of having a child who develops schizophrenia as are the probands themselves (Gottesman and Bertelson, 1989). There is therefore a range of genetic expression, and the presence of OCs is just as likely to be a manifestation of the factors determining expression as the cause of the disorder.

Neuropathological findings might reveal the nature of any brain alteration. Hollister and Cannon (Chapter 12) review a substantial literature that has shown many brain abnormalities in schizophrenia, 'no one unique feature of schizophrenia', and no clear pathogenesis. Post-mortem studies in the last decade have found that some structural brain abnormalities are more common in schizophrenia. Schizophrenic brains are, for example, a little lighter than those of normal controls, and have smaller temporal lobe structures; but they do not usually show the gliosis that might be expected in a degenerative disorder (Bogerts, Meerts and Schonfeldt-Bausch, 1985; Brown *et al.*, 1986; Bruton *et al.*, 1990). Jakob and Beckmann (1986) found that schizophrenic brains are more likely to show heterotopic pre-alpha cells in the entorhinal cortex, suggesting an abnormality of neuronal migration (which would be expected to date from the first years of life).

In vivo studies by neuroimaging obviously give less pathological detail, but are consistent in finding an increased rate of many abnormalities in schizophrenia. Cerebral ventricular enlargement has been found repeatedly in subgroups of people with schizophrenia; it is present very early in the evolution of the disorder (Nyback *et al.*, 1982; Weinberger *et al.*, 1982); and it is not related to the extent of treatment with neuroleptics (Williams *et al.*, 1985). Indeed, the study by Williams *et al.* (1985) suggested that larger ventricles were more probable in those with a poor social adjustment before the illness started. All the pathological findings seem to be particularly marked in early-onset schizophrenia.

Both histological and neuroimaging data are therefore suggestive – but not definitely confirmatory – of an early-onset and non-progressive abnormality of the brain in some cases of schizophrenia. The findings come from group studies, and neuroimaging is not yet a routine investigation for schizophrenia because the precision of findings is not yet good enough for individual diagnosis.

The aetiology of these findings is not yet known. They could be determined genetically, or they could result from damage to the developing brain. It has been claimed that they bear witness to an aetiology in brain damage, on the grounds that they may be more common in sporadic than in familial schizophrenia. The best evidence here is a replicated finding from neuroimaging studies of monozygotic twins who are discordant for schizophrenia. The affected twin is more likely to have enlarged ventricles and a decreased volume of the temporal lobe (Murray *et al.*, 1985; Reveley *et al.*, 1982; Suddath *et al.*, 1989). However, discordance in monozygotic twin pairs does not imply that the basic cause was environmental. As already described above, an unaffected co-twin is still very likely to transmit the disorder. Any cerebral changes in the affected twin therefore imply an effect of brain abnormalities upon the expression of an inherited tendency, or an effect of whatever factors lead to expression of the genotype upon cerebral structure.

It would be important to know if there is anything distinctive about the neurodevelopmental disorders of preschizophrenia. Not only would this help to clarify the possible mechanisms; it is also important in interpreting the above evidence. If there is nothing distinctive, then the likely story must be that the effect of perinatal abnormalities in the development of schizophrenia is similar to that of perinatal abnormalities generally: a weak effect, present only above a high threshold of injury, and accounting for less of the outcome than the psychosocial abnormalities that often coexist. If there is a specific pattern, then the lessons from neurodevelopmental psychiatry generally may not apply. The question is further considered below, as part of the issue of whether childhood syndromes have particular links with specific adult syndromes of disorder.

Genetic factors

Genetic inheritance is implicated in most of the neurodevelopmental disorders. The evidence is clearest for autism, where twin and family studies have shown a very strong and highly expressed genetic risk. They have also made it clear that the phenotype is in fact very much broader than the classical picture of autism – co-twins are at risk for a wide range of learning difficulties.

It seems to be common for characteristic syndromes to have a much broader phenotype. In autism, for instance, the phenotype includes isolated and subtle disturbances of language, cognition and social relating. There are also some striking counter-instances, in which the expression of a distinctive syndrome is precisely determined by the structure of DNA. The behavioural phenotypes of single genes include some very specific syndromes such as Lesch–Nyhan; and quite subtle details of DNA can have very specific consequences (such as the development of Prader–Willi or Angelman syndromes). No doubt many more instances will be found as the human genome is mapped. There are rare individual pedigrees where all affected family members have a specific neuropsychological abnormality.

Such specificities are, however, exceptional. It is much more commonly found that the genetic risk is for a wide variety of differing types of cognitive and/or behavioural impairment. How should we understand it? First, the genes could be rather nonspecific risks for brain development; other factors then determine whether a specific syndrome will develop. This would not suffice as an explanation of most disorders. In autism, the rare and characteristic syndrome accounts for a higher proportion of cases in those at genetic risk than it would in those with other neurological risk factors. A second possibility is that there is a spectrum of genetic constitutions, each of which has a very characteristic outcome but in the aggregate produce an apparently very broad phenotype: the explanation from multiple conditions. This is improbable because it predicts what is seldom found – a constant form of disorder within a single pedigree (allowing for complicating factors such as assortative mating). The third, and most likely explanation is that a genetic risk exerts its effects on brain development in complex and variable ways – for instance, if the absence of an organising gene led to a chaotic pattern of neuronal migration resulting in any of several types of dysfunction; or if the route from neuropsychological dysfunction to psychiatric syndromes depended upon the psychological environment.

Genetic findings in schizophrenia

Many types of research have given evidence that there is a substantial genetic component. *Family studies* leave little doubt that schizophrenia manifests as a familial disorder (Tsuang, Gilbertson and Faraone, 1991). The risk is about 8% if one has a sibling with the disorder, 12% if a parent is affected, 40% if both parents, 55% if an identical twin.

The risk rates in early-onset schizophrenia are probably higher though there is little good research (Hanson and Gottesman, 1976; Werry and Taylor, 1994). Recent work generally confirms that, in males at least, onset before the age of 17 is associated with an increased risk for other relatives (Pulver *et al.*, 1990). The elevated risk applies chiefly to schizophrenic and schizotypal disorders. It has been suggested that the traditional, strict genetic separation from affective disorder needs to be qualified, since bipolar affective disorder is twice as common among the relatives of people with schizophrenia as is found in a control group (Kendler, Gruenberg and Tsuang, 1985; McGuffin, Murray and Reveley, 1987). This led Crow (1986) to argue for a genetic continuum of the psychoses – though the lack of an elevated risk for schizophrenia in those with affective disorder has restrained most psychiatrists from following suit. It is perhaps more probable that an inherited affective disorder can sometimes manifest with symptoms close enough to schizophrenia to meet the criteria for the latter diagnosis. In keeping with this view is the better prognosis for people with schizophrenia who have a family history of affective disorder (Kendler and Tsuang, 1988).

Adoption studies have been able to estimate genetic heritability at between 0.6 and 0.7 and environmental familial factors to account for less than 20% of the variance in liability (Kendler, 1988). From these studies, one should note especially the biological paternal half-siblings of schizophrenic adoptees, who are at greater risk than those of control adoptees even though they do not share a common pre- or peri-natal background. If their rates are as high as those of maternal half-siblings, as it appears, then the influence of the foetal environment is probably small.

Twin studies also very strongly support a genetic component, through the difference between concordance rates for monozygotic twins (about 55%) and same-sex dizygotic twins (about 12%) (Gottesman and Shields, 1982). They have also made it clear that there is a range of genetic expression, as in most of the neuropsychiatric disorders with early onset. The non-schizophrenic monozygotic twins of people with schizophrenia are at increased risk of schizotypal and schizoid personality, and of other forms of personality disorder; they can even carry the genetic liability without showing the disorder.

There is, in short, little doubt about the existence of a genetic diathesis. The further questions are about the interaction of genetic with environmental factors; and the extent to which genetic mechanisms account for the association between schizophrenia and neurodevelopmental delays. There are several models of how causes might interact. Genetic inheritance and early brain trauma might be alternative routes to the same disorders. In current evidence this idea is unsupported because it predicts that, within a group of people with disorder, there will be an inverse relationship between the two classes of cause. Genetic inheritance might be a necessary condition, but not sufficient, brain trauma leading to the expression of the tendency. Genetic inheritance might be a relatively nonspecific risk factor; with brain trauma acting as a pathoplastic factor to make it more probable that schizophrenia – rather than another form of disorder – will appear. Brain trauma might be a nonspecific risk, raising the probability of all forms of psychiatric disorder: it would only be a risk for schizophrenia in those who already have a specific (e.g. genetic) predisposition. Finally, it is still possible that brain trauma is seldom a risk factor for schizophrenia; the association could come about because trauma is a marker to the real risk factors such as a genetically abnormal foetus.

Fetal abnormalities

The developing embryo is protected against many environmental hazards, but not against all. One of the clearest demonstrations of neurological vulnerability came in the after-effects of the atomic bomb explosions at Hiroshima and Nagasaki. The rate of mental retardation was very strongly related to the gestational stage at which the embryos had been irradiated (Otake and Schull, 1984). Neurodevelopmental delays are more frequent in the development of children who were exposed as foetuses to a maternal intake of alcohol (Taylor, 1991*b*) or benzodiazepines (Viggedal *et al.*, 1993). The neuropsychological effects do not seem to be very specific but include disturbances of behaviour and activity control as well as various alterations of learning. Schizophrenia is not yet implicated as an outcome, but this could be because cohort studies have not yet been able to extend their period of follow-up to the age by which schizophrenia is likely to have announced itself.

It is well known that some viruses can cross the placenta and cause damage to the developing brain. Rubella, cytomegalovirus and human immunodeficiency virus are outstanding examples. Between them, however, they account for a very small percentage of cases of neurodevelopmental delay and investigation of people with schizophrenia has not suggested that any of these viruses is likely to have a substantial aetiological effect. The current evidence for the involvement of other viruses therefore has to come from more indirect sources and especially from histories of exposure as indexed by season of birth effects or immigration.

Seasonality and virus infection

Disproportionate numbers of births in some seasons of the year are known to characterise early-onset problems such as autism (Bolton *et al.*, 1992). The reasons are not known, but viral infections are frequently invoked as the cause. There appear to be season-of-birth effects in schizophrenia. More than 40 articles (reviewed by Bradbury and Miller, 1985), taken together, yield a strong case for an increased rate of winter births among schizophrenic patients who are known to therapeutic services. The effect varies with geographical location: for example, it is stronger in the northern than in the southern states of the USA. The reasons are not known with any certainty; they are often taken to point to a seasonally varying pathogen such as an infective agent, but are not known to be accounted for by any such agent.

Mednick, Parnos and Shulsinger (1987) were able to relate the clinical diagnosis of schizophrenia to birth information in a cohort of young adults in Copenhagen. An A2 influenza epidemic occurred in 1957 and could be timed from records of hospital admissions. The later development of schizophrenia was more common in those who had been in the second trimester of gestation during the epidemic. Accordingly, efforts have been made to link the dates of birth of people with known schizophrenia to historical records of influenza rates. Maternal infection with influenza during the second trimester of gestation has been associated epidemiologically with the later development of schizophrenia in some studies, but not others (Eaton, 1991). Sham *et al.* (1992) reported national data from England and Wales in 1938–1960 and estimated that between 1 and 2% of schizophrenic births could be explained by the number of influenza deaths in the previous months. This is obviously circumstantial evidence; though persuasive, it does not amount to a known pathogenesis. One of the research problems is the unsatisfactory nature of the nationally and routinely gathered data about schizophrenia admissions.

Immigration

In early-onset disorders such as autism, a high rate in immigrants has been described for some time (Gillberg, 1990). The reasons are not known with confidence, but are often attributed to a reduced immunity to viral infections in the host country – a conclusion gathering a little support from the suggestion that the risk is higher when immigration has taken place over a greater distance. In the case of schizophrenia, it has been apparent for 20 years, from routinely gathered admission data, that first-admission rates among first-generation Afro-Caribbean migrants to Britain are markedly raised (Glover, 1989). The reasons for this have attracted much controversy. Racial stereotyping by psychiatrists is probably not sufficient to explain the increase: a case vignette study by Lewis, Croft-Jeffreys and David (1990) examined the diagnostic practices of British psychiatrists directly, and concluded that psychiatrists underdiagnosed schizophrenia in patients identified as West Indian by comparison with white patients. Elective migration of those with early signs of disorder is not the reason either (Harrison *et al.*, 1988). The difference is so great that it seems to point to an environmental cause: but it does not by itself favour any one of the major aetiological theories. The difference is present both for males and female, and both for those migrants born in the West Indies and those born in the UK. Exposure to unfamiliar viruses is one possibility among many.

Postnatal brain damage

Neurological disorders are frequent causes of chronic ill health in childhood. It has long been known that brain diseases are especially likely to be associated with psychiatric complications. The epidemiological studies of the Isle of Wight established the great increase of prevalence of psychiatric disorder in those with disorders affecting the brain, even by comparison with other chronic physical illnesses of childhood (Rutter, 1989). Follow-up studies of head injury during childhood have contributed another useful piece of basic knowledge, that the brain injury is indeed the cause of the increased rate of psychopathology (Rutter, Chadwick and Shaffer, 1983). The mechanisms through which brain abnormality leads to psychological disorder are the major topic for most investigators now.

General conclusions about brain damage should be relevant to the study of schizophrenia, but are not yet well founded. Knowledge is still at the level where much has to be done in the basic charting of the psychological development of children with different types of abnormal brain function. Too many investigations in the past have relied upon convenient populations rather than seeking a representative series; too many have sought the consequences of brain damage as though they expected to find a static deficit, modified only in degree by later recovery and experience. This simple view clearly does scant justice to the complexity of neurological and psychological development. Researchers are beginning to evolve schemes of neurological assessment in infancy that assess patterns of change rather than disabilities at just a single point in time (e.g. Amiel-Tison and Stewart, 1989). Psychological assessment of older children over extended time periods has shown that different sorts of cerebral pathology may give rise to different types of course: for instance, the falling IQ of children with Down's syndrome and those with the fragile-X syndrome, by contrast with the stable or rising IQ of children with intellectual retardation associated with cerebral palsy (Burack, Hodapp and Zigler, 1988).

The course of development after the brain is damaged is likely to be influenced by many neurological factors. The brain lesions themselves may persist, or wane (as for many of the children who have encountered neonatal adversity or later head trauma), or intensify (when, for instance, uncontrolled seizures bring about further deterioration of brain function), or be complicated by other lesions (as the structural defects due to phenylketonuria's effects upon myelination are compounded by its effects on neurotransmitter metabolism). The lesions may have a variety of effects upon the rest of the brain. Other parts of the brain may take over the function of a damaged area, either using the same strategies as were used by the original part or substituting a different strategy for achieving the same end. The neurones involved by damage may – depending upon their developmental stage – regenerate new terminals, and connecting neurones may produce new ones. This process of growth within the central nervous system may be harmful as well as helpful, for anomalous connections may impair the processing of information (Goodman, 1987). A brain that has suffered damage does not just display a deficit: it has adapted to the abnormality. Indeed, this process of compensation may be a major determinant of the outcome. Lesions of early onset tend to have less specific psychological consequences and, often, more diffuse ones. This may reflect the greater power of compensatory mechanisms in the early life of the brain.

However, we have already noted considerable limits to plasticity: especially in the case of genetically and chromosomally determined disorders, where there may be striking and even pathognomonic specificities of psychological presentation such as the self-biting of the Lesch–Nyhan syndrome. It may simply be that, where there are such specific presentations, they arise because the particular regions of the brain concerned are excluded from the operation of compensatory mechanisms. The striking overeating of the Prader–Willi syndrome can be reproduced by focal lesions in later childhood such as those that follow surgical excision of craniopharyngiomata (Skorzewska *et al.*, 1989). It may also be that a genetically determined abnormality does not trigger the processes of compensation; or that the genetic abnormality includes an abnormality of the triggering processes. There is therefore nothing implausible about the suggestion that schizophrenia is the consequence of a single specific developmental abnormality; nor anything incompatible between this and the wide range of developmental outcomes seen in those at risk for schizophrenia.

Specific and nonspecific causes

So far we have found little contradiction between the neurodevelopmental and the schizophrenic literatures. Rather similar types of association with environmental stressors are being reported. The main problem of interpretation is whether the neurodevelopmental associations are specifically a part of the pathogenesis of schizophrenia or a nonspecific risk factor. Genetic strategies should be a strong way of attacking the question, to examine the possibility of cosegregation of neurodevelopmental disorders with schizophrenia. Such evidence, however, is lacking. For the moment, the specificity can be considered in three ways. (1) Are the neurodevelopmental antecedents of schizophrenia different from other forms of neurodevelopmental association? (2) If so, do the specific associations only, or all kinds of neurodevelopmental abnormality, raise the risk for schizophrenia? (3) Are the neurodevelopmental anomalies risks only for schizophrenia or for a wider range of adult psychiatric disorders?

The first question has usually been addressed with retrospective methodology – which has not indicated anything very distinctive, and probably would not have the strength to do so. Archival studies of the school careers of identified adult patients have indicated only a somewhat poorer school performance than that of controls. A case record study of people who had been patients of the same hospital both as children and as adults suggested one possibly distinctive feature in childhood – a description of 'bizarre' personal relationships (Zeitlin, 1986). It is difficult to know what to make of this, which was an impression of the investigator who read the notes. Even if it can be reproduced with reliable methods, it might still point to the beginning of the schizophrenia itself rather than to specific neurodevelopmental anomalies. More recently, it has been possible to link adult records of mental illness to research measures in childhood by analysing birth cohorts followed up for many years. The people who later developed schizophrenia were marked in childhood by higher rates of 'hyperactive' and other problematic behaviour. This is a much stronger source of evidence for the earlier conclusion that psychological problems can antedate schizophrenia by many years. Obviously, most children with these behavioural abnormalities did not develop schizophrenia and the specificity of the association is still in some doubt.

Specific or nonspecific neuropsychological impairments?

What can be concluded from neuropsychological analyses of people with schizophrenia by comparison with neurodevelopmental delays? There have been strikingly few such studies, but the paradigm could be fruitful. If those who develop schizophrenia have the same types of problem – in cognition, decision and motor control – as people with other types of neurodevelopmental abnormality, then it would be reasonable to conclude that those problems are a general risk rather than markers to a specific vulnerability to schizophrenia.

The evidence is circumstantial. First, there seems to be a very high rate of language disorders in clinical studies of early-onset schizophrenia. This is not as compelling as it might be if the control groups were of people who had develomental problems: it may simply bear witness to the frequency with which language is involved in many types of childhood brain dysfunction.

The next source of evidence is the analyses that have been carried out of information processing in schizophrenia and (separately) in other disorders. Very many studies have found changes in psychological and physiological tests in schizophrenia (reviewed by Holzman, 1987). For example, the Continuous Performance Test (CPT) is performed poorly by nearly half of patients with schizophrenia – even after the acute episode is over (Wohlberg and Kornetsky, 1973). Reaction time has long been known to be prolonged in schizophrenia and used as an index of impaired set (Rodnick and Shakow, 1940). Irrelevant, distracting information impairs performance on simple tests of memory in schizophrenia (Lawson, McGhie and Chapman, 1964). The amplitude of the P300 component of the evoked potential is reduced (Baribeau-Brown, Picton and Gosselin, 1983).

The clearest line of development to be involved is that of *selective attention*. The CPT impairment is not the result of poor vigilance, for it is not a function of the length of time for which the test is given. Rather, it depends upon the load that is placed on the early stages of information processing. Perceptual sensitivity, as assessed from signal-to-noise discrimination, is the measure that is impaired; populations at risk for schizophrenia show a deficit when the perceptual difficulty is increased by presenting a very blurred image to be detected (Nuechterlein, 1983). Rather similarly a 'span of apprehension' task showed a difference between people with schizophrenia and normal controls (Asarnow and MacCrimmon, 1981). Superficially this is a memory task, requiring recognition of very briefly presented letters. However, the deficit only appears when irrelevant letters are presented at the same time, and is worse when there is more irrelevant information.

The interpretation of these findings in terms of a selective attention breakdown is not certain. They could also (like many of the developmental experiments supposed to be about selective attention) result from a reduction of the capacity to process information. However, a failure of selective attention has also been implicated in analyses of the problems people with schizophrenia (and depression) have in memory for dichotic listening (Hemsley and Zawada, 1976). Their difficulty came especially in distinguishing between relevant and irrelevant digits, read out loud by different voices.

Latent inhibition experiments are also relevant: they depend upon the usual tendency for the learning of a response to a stimulus to be slower if the stimulus has previously been made familiar by presentation as a redundant piece of information. A new task based upon it is learned less efficiently and reaction time is longer. One can argue that the person originally learned that it was irrelevant, so does not pay much attention to it. People with acute schizophrenia show less of this inhibition of responsiveness (Baruch, Hemsley and Gray, 1988). This is not to be explained by filter breakdown and increased incidental learning, for then people with schizophrenia would have to have learned more about the stimulus during its initial presentations – including that it is irrelevant. Rather it implies that schizophrenia is associated with a diminished ability to form or use knowledge about the previous importance of stimuli.

This breakdown of selective attention in schizophrenia has little parallel, as far as we know, in other types of information processing deficit. This statement needs some expansion, for the evidence is admittedly strong that children with 'attention deficit disorder' (ADHD) get poor scores when they perform on tests that are supposed to measure attention. These tests include the Continuous Performance Test (Ross and Ross, 1976; Whalen and Henker, 1976; Rosenthal and Allen, 1978; Hoy *et al.*, 1978; Loiselle *et al.*, 1980), the Matching Familiar Figures Test (Fuhrman and Kendall, 1986; Messer, 1976), visual memory tests where there is a high demand upon information-processing resources (Douglas, 1983; Sprague and Sleator, 1977), repetitive reaction time tests and speeded classification tests

(Sykes, Douglas and Morgenstern, 1973), the allocation of processing capacity in line with changing task demands (Sergeant and Scholten, 1985), and the maintenance of readiness to respond in reaction time tests with varying delays after a preparatory signal (Sonuga-Barke and Taylor, 1992). However, a selective attention deficit does not account for these difficulties, and the addition of irrelevant distracting information does not lead to impairment of performance in ADHD any more than it does in normal children.

Inhibitory control has a much stronger claim to being a process that is impaired in ADHD. The best-known way of testing the idea of impulsiveness is through Kagan's Matching Familiar Figures test (cited above). In conditions of uncertainty, impulsive children make rapid and inaccurate responses; in the theory, they are inaccurate because they are too rapid. The analysis applies well in some epidemiological research. Not only are hyperactive children unduly quick in their response, but accuracy falls as they take less time to do it (Fuhrman and Kendall, 1986; Taylor *et al.*, 1991). Schachar and Logan (1990) have directly tested the idea that children with hyperactivity are less able to inhibit a response than others, and found that the prediction holds for children with the serious problem of hyperkinetic disorder (not for those with ADHD). Rapport *et al.* (1986) tied this more closely to the obtaining of reward with the finding that children with hyperactivity were more likely to respond for a small immediate reward than for a large delayed one. One result of this impulsiveness is that children choose to take less time over tasks they are given. If the task needs more time to be completed accurately, then their accuracy will suffer. If this is so, then their performance should increase to normal levels when the time taken is controlled experimentally, and indeed in one experiment involving new learning this has proved to be the case (Sonuga-Barke, Heptinstall and Taylor, 1992). Nothing resembling this pattern has been found when people with schizophrenia are tested.

These arguments convey the strongest case available that the neurodevelopmental deficits that precede schizophrenia are unique. The case is not at all conclusive. There has been very little direct comparison of different groups. Nuechterlein *et al.* (1986) reported a signal detection analysis of a CPT in which children at high risk for schizophrenia showed a difference in signal detection while children with ADHD showed an 'impulsive' lowering of their threshold for signal recognition. Unfortunately, attempts at replication of these results led to quite different patterns of findings. Case definition and the tests used could all be more sophisticated now, and a return to the question would be timely.

What is the picture when neurodevelopmental problems are followed prospectively? Uncertain. Practical and conceptual obstacles to this type of research are formidable. Sample sizes have to be much larger than are normally used to assess psychological outcome, because of the need for large numbers of subjects if one is to detect differences between groups in a relatively rare outcome such as schizophrenia. The follow-up has to be sufficiently long that a reasonable number of at-risk individuals have lived through the period of greatest risk for developing schizophrenia. It is noteworthy that the various follow-up studies of children with reading disabilities have not reported any of their subjects developing schizophrenia. It is also of interest that the longitudinal studies of children with ADHD into early adult life have not detected psychotic illness as an outcome. On the other hand, many of these outcome studies have been unlikely to find psychoses because low compliance rates may well mean that the illest subjects are missed; and the widespread practice of excluding subjects with neurological signs or low IQ may well have led to overlooking the most neurodevelopmentally disabled children.

In two longitudinal studies there have been hints that schizophrenia spectrum disorders may be seen in a few cases. Receptive language disorders were followed up by Rutter and Mahwood (1991); three out of 25 children had psychotic symptoms when re-evaluated, by contrast with none of the children who had showed the full syndrome of autism. Children with pervasive hyperactivity were followed up by Taylor *et al.* (1996); three young men at the age of 17 had schizotypal problems. These numbers are clearly too small to calculate rates or to test for significance. They can only be taken to suggest that there may be something to study and to add to the justification for large follow-up studies of those with neurodevelopmental disorders.

What about the outcome when children with schizophrenia-specific abnormalities are followed up? Are they at risk only for schizophrenia or for other types of disorder? The main strategy has been to follow those at risk because they are the offspring of one or both parents with a schizophrenic illness. Long-term evidence comes from the findings of the New York High-Risk Project (Erlenmeyer-Kimling and Cornblatt, 1987). They found, like others, that children who were at risk because they had a schizophrenic illness, had deficits on a range of 'attention tests' (CPT, span of apprehension, and digit span). The study was able to follow the children to their early adult life, by which time a few had undergone psychiatric hospitalisation. Their breakdown could be predicted from childhood status by their score on these attention tests.

It is tempting to conclude that the impairment of attention is in itself the risk factor for schizophrenia. This, however, would go too far. For one thing, many children in the general population (around 5%) will show comparable impairment of attention and it is not at all clear that they are also at risk. If it is only a risk in those with a schizophrenic inheritance, then perhaps it is an indirect marker rather than a specific vulnerability. Another query arises from a report by the same study that those who later broke down had also had a lower IQ in childhood (Erlenmeyer-Kimling and Cornblatt, 1987). Perhaps the risk factor was not specifically a failure of selective attention, but a more general cognitive problem. Further, the uncertainty over the types of breakdown that had led to hospitalisation make it doubtful whether the risk was for a specific psychosis or for an increased chance of any type of adverse outcome.

The follow-up of children with diagnosed schizophrenia should be informative for the specificity of outcome (Werry and Taylor, 1994). It appears that negative symptoms are strongly associated with neurodevelopmental problems. It also appears that negative symptoms are strongly persistent, and account for much of the poor outcome in young people with schizophrenia. If these observations prove to be correct, then the most important developmental track may not be that of schizophrenia at all. Rather, an early-onset neurodevelomental delay may have a direct continuity with negative symptoms, disturbances of language and attention, and a poor social adjustment in adult life. Children on this track do not necessarily develop any formal mental illness; but they are at risk for several. Schizophrenia is most commonly diagnosed when positive symptoms develop; but the occurrence of an acute schizophrenic illness does not alter the developmental track. Other types of illness, such as affective disorder, may also appear: the neurodevelopmental impairment should have the same prognostic significance in them as in those with schizophrenia. These predictions, like those of the other developmental models considered above, could be tested by longitudinal studies of course.

Conclusion

Abnormalities of neuropsychological development in childhood are common. They are antecedents of a wide range of psychiatric disability in adult life, including many forms of cognitive impairment and emotional disturbance and, through hyperactivity, antisocial disturbances of personality. Similar early abnormalities are antecedents of schizophrenia. It is not clear whether the antecedents of schizophrenia are different from those that lead to other types of adult problem, and this should be an issue for future research. At present the suggestions are that attention and language problems may be the most specific predictors; and if this is the case the mechanism might well be through the development of disorganised thought processes. The childhood problems are known to have genetic contributions to their aetiology; in many cases (such as autism and specific reading retardation) the genetic influences are very strong. Early insults to the developing brain are not very often causative, and their effects are usually mediated through complex pathways, so the presence of neurodevelopmental antecedents of schizophrenia does not imply that acquired causes are likely to exert their influence by causing schizophrenogenic brain damage. Early insults may have high thresholds for causing damage (e.g. closed head injury where only severe trauma should be included in aetiological formulations) or low thresholds (e.g. neonatal hypoglycaemia, whose presence may well have gone undetected at the time). Their effects are usually modified greatly by the resilience of the developing brain – for instance, lateralised brain injury in early life does not have the same localising implications for language and visuospatial abnormalities as in adults (Taylor, 1991*a*). The developmental contributions to schizophrenia need longitudinal study.

References

Amiel-Tison, C. and Stewart, A. (1989). Follow-up studies during the first five years of life: a pervasive assessment of neurological function. *Archives of Disease in Childhood*, **64**, 496–502.

Asarnow, R.F. and MacCrimmon, D.J. (1981). Span of apprehension deficits during postpsychotic stages of schizophrenia: a replication and extension. *Archives of General Psychiatry*, **38**, 1006–11.

Bailey, A.J., Le Couteur, A., Gottesman, I.I. *et al.* (1995). Autism as a strongly genetic disorder: evidence from a British twin study. *Psychological Medicine*, **25**, 63–77.

Baribeau-Brown, J., Picton, T.W. and Gosselin, J.Y. (1983). Schizophrenia: a neurophysiological evaluation of abnormal information processing. *Science*, **219**, 874–6.

Baruch, I., Hemsley, D.R. and Gray, J.A. (1988). Differential performance of acute and chronic schizophrenics in a latent inhibition task. *Journal of Nervous and Mental Disease*, **176**, 598–606.

Bogerts, B., Meerts, E. and Schonfeldt-Bausch, R. (1985). Basal ganglia and limbic system pathology in schizophrenia. *Archives of General Psychiatry*, **42**, 784–91.

Bolton, P., Pickles, A., Harrington, R. *et al.* (1992). Season of birth: issues, approaches and findings for autism. *Journal of Child Psychology and Psychiatry*, **3**, 509–31.

Bradbury, T.N. and Miller, G.A. (1985). Season of birth in schizophrenia: a review of evidence, methodology and etiology. *Psychological Bulletin*, **98**, 569–94.

Brown, R., Colter, N., Corsellis, J.A.N. *et al.* (1986). Postmortem evidence of structural brain changes in schizophrenia: differences in brain weight, temporal horn area and parahippocampal gyrus compared with affective disorder. *Archives of General Psychiatry*, **43**, 36–42.

Bruton, C.J., Crow, T.J., Firth, C.D. *et al.* (1990). Schizophrenia and the brain. *Psychological Medicine*, **20**, 285–304.

Burack, J.A., Hodapp, R.M. and Zigler, E. (1988). Issues in the classification of mental retardation: differentiating among organic etiologies. *Journal of Child Psychology and Psychiatry*, **29**, 765–79.

Casaer, P., de Vries, L. and Marlow, N. (1991). Prenatal and perinatal risk factors for psychosocial development. In *Biological Risk Factors for Psychosocial Disorders* (ed. M. Rutter and P. Casaer), pp. 139–74. Cambridge: Cambridge University Press.

Corter, C.M. and Minde, K.K. (1987). Impact of infant prematurity on family systems. *Advances in Developmental and Behavioral Pediatrics*, **8**, 1–48.

Costello, A.M. de L., Hamilton, P.A., Baudin, J. *et al.* (1988). Prediction of neurodevelopmental impairment at four years from brain ultrasound appearance of very preterm infants. *Developmental Medicine and Child Neurology*, **30**, 711–22.

Crow, T.J. (1986). The continuum of psychosis and its implication for the structure of the gene. *British Journal of Psychiatry*, **149**, 419–29.

Douglas, V.I. (1983). Attentional and cognitive problems. In *Developmental Neuropsychiatry* (ed. M. Rutter), pp. 280–329. New York: Guilford.

Eaton, W.W. (1991). Update on the epidemiology of schizophrenia. *Epidemiological Review*, **13**, 302–38.

Erlenmeyer-Kimling, L. and Cornblatt, B. (1987). The New York High-Risk Project: a follow-up report. *Schizophrenia Bulletin*, **13**, 451–61.

Fuhrman, M.J. and Kendall, P.C. (1986). Cognitive tempo and behavioural adjustment in children. *Cognitive Therapy and Research*, **10**, 45–50.

Gaffney, G., Sellers, S., Flavell, V. *et al.* (1994). Case-control study of intrapartum care, cerebral palsy, and perinatal death. *British Medical Journal*, **308**, 743–50.

Gillberg, C. (1990). Autism and pervasive developmental disorders. *Journal of Child Psychology and Psychiatry*, **31**, 99–119.

Glover, E.R. (1989). Differences in psychiatric admission patterns between Caribbeans from different islands. *Social Psychiatry and Psychiatric Epidemiology*, **24**, 209–11.

Goldman-Rakic, P.S., Isseroff, A., Schwartz, M.L. and Bugbee, N.M. (1983). The neurobiology of cognitive development. In *Mussen's Handbook of Child Psychology*, 4th edition, vol. 2, (ed. M.M. Haith and J.J. Campos), pp. 281–344. New York: Wiley.

Goodman, R. (1987). The developmental neurobiology of language. In *Language Development and Disorders* (ed. W. Yule and M. Rutter), pp. 129–45. London: MacKeith Press.

Goodman, R. (1988). Are complications of pregnancy and birth causes of schizophrenia? *Developmental Medicine and Child Neurology*, **30**, 391–5.

Gottesman, I. and Bertelson, A. (1989). Confirming unexpressed genotypes for schizophrenia. *Archives of General Psychiatry*, **46**, 867–72.

Gottesman, I.I. and Shields, J. (1982). *Schizophrenia: The Epigenetic Puzzle.* Cambridge: Cambridge University Press.

Gottfried, A.W. (1973). Intellectual consequences of perinatal anoxia. *Psychopharmacology Bulletin*, **14**, 39–40.

Hall, D. (1989). Birth asphyxia and cerebral palsy. *British Medical Journal*, **299**, 279–82.

Hanson, D.R. and Gottesman, I.I. (1976). The genetics, if any, of infantile autism and childhood schizophrenia. *Journal of Autism and Childhood Schizophrenia*, **6**, 209–34.

Harrison, G., Owens, D., Holton, T. *et al.* (1988). A prospective study of severe mental disorder in Afro-Caribbean patients. *Psychological Medicine*, **18**, 643–57.

Hemsley, D.R. and Zawada, S.L. (1976). Filtering and the cognitive deficits in schizophrenia. *British Journal of Psychiatry*, **128**, 456–61.

Holzman, P.S. (1987). Recent studies of psychophysiology in schizophrenia. *Schizophrenia Bulletin*, **13**, 49–75.

Hoy, E., Weiss, G., Minde, K. and Cohen, N. (1978). The hyperactive child at adolescence: cognitive, emotional and social functioning. *Journal of Abnormal Child Psychology*, **6**, 311–24.

Jakob, H. and Beckmann, H. (1986). Prenatal development disturbances in the limbic allocortex in schizophrenics. *Journal of Neural Transmission*, **65**, 303–26.

Kendler, K.S. (1988). The genetics of schizophrenia: an overview. In *Handbook of Schizophrenia*, vol. 3 (ed. M.T. Tsuang and J.C. Simpson), pp. 437–62. New York: Elsevier.

Kendler, K.S. and Tsuang, M.T. (1988). Outcome and familial psychopathology in schizophrenia. *Archives of General Psychiatry*, **45**, 338–46.

Kendler, K.S., Gruenberg, A.M. and Tsuang, M.T. (1985). Psychiatric illness in first degree relatives of schizophrenic and surgical control patients. *Archives of General Psychiatry*, **42**, 770–9.

Lawson, J.S., McGhie, A. and Chapman, J. (1964). Perception of speech in schizophrenia. *British Journal of Psychiatry*, **110**, 375–80.

Lewis, S.W. (1990). Computerized tomography in schizophrenia 15 years on. *British Journal of Psychiatry*, **157** (suppl. 9), 16–24.

Lewis, S.W. and Murray, R.W. (1987). Obstetric complications, neurodevelopmental deviance and risk of schizophrenia. *Journal of Psychiatric Research*, **21**, 413–21.

Lewis, G., Croft-Jeffreys, C. and David, A. (1990). Are British psychiatrists racist? *British Journal of Psychiatry*, **157**, 410–15.

Loiselle, D.L., Stamm, J.S., Maitinsky, S. and Whipple, S.C. (1980). Evoked potential and behavioural signs of attentive dysfunctions in hyperactive boys. *Psychophysiology*, **17**, 193–201.

Lord, C. and Rutter, M. (1994). Autism and pervasive developmental disorders. In *Child and Adolescent Psychiatry: Modern Approaches*, 3rd edition, (ed. M. Rutter, E. Taylor and L. Hersov), pp. 569–93. Oxford: Blackwell Scientific Publications.

Lucas, A., Morley, R. and Cole, T.J. (1988). Adverse neurodevelopmental outcome of moderate neonatal hypoglycaemia. *British Medical Journal*, **297**, 1304–8.

McGuffin, P., Murray, R.M. and Reveley, A.M. (1987). Genetic influence on the psychoses. *British Medical Bulletin*, **43**, 531–56.

Mednick, S., Parnos, J. and Shulsinger, F. (1987). The Copenhagen High Risk Project 1962–1986. *Schizophrenia Bulletin*, **13**, 485–95.

Messer, S. (1976), Reflection–impulsivity: a review. *Psychological Bulletin*, **83**, 1026–52.

Murray, R.M., Reveley, A.M., Reveley, M.A. *et al.* (1985). Genes and environment in schizophrenia. In *Genetic Aspects of Human Behaviour* (ed. T. Sakai and T. Tsuboi), pp. 63–74. Tokyo and New York: Igakushoin.

Neligan, G.A., Kolvin, I., Scott, D. McL. and Garside, R.F. (1976). *Born Too Soon or Born Too Small.* Clinics in Developmental Medicine, No. 61. London: SIMP/Heinemann; Philadelphia, PA: Lippincott.

Nelson, K.B. and Ellenberg, J.H. (1986). Antecedents of cerebral palsy: multivariate analysis of risk. *New England Journal of Medicine*, **315**, 81–6.

Nichols, P.L. and Chen, T.-C. (1981). *Minimal Brain Dysfunction: A Prospective Study*. Hillsdale, NJ: Erlbaum.

Nuechterlein, K.H. (1983). Signal detection in vigilance tasks and behavioral attributes among offspring of schizophrenic mothers and among hyperactive children. *Journal of Abnormal Psychology*, **92**, 4–28.

Nuechterlein, K.H., Edell, W.S., Norris, M. and Dawson, M.E. (1986). Attention vulnerability indicators, thought disorder, and negative symptoms. *Schizophrenia Bulletin*, **12**, 408–26.

Nyback, H., Weisel, R.A., Berggren, B.K. and Hindmarsh, T. (1982). Computer tomography of the brain in patients with acute psychosis and healthy volunteers. *Acta Psychiatrica Scandinavica*, **65**, 403–14.

Otake, M. and Schull, W.J. (1984). In utero exposure to A-bomb radiation and mental retardation: a reassessment. *British Journal of Radiology*, **57**, 409–14.

Pulver, A.E., Brown, C.H., Wolyntec, P. *et al.* (1990). Schizophrenia: age at onset, gender and familial risk. *Acta Psychiatrica Scandinavica*, **82**, 344–51.

Rapport, M.D., Tucker, S.B., DuPaul, G.J. *et al.* (1986). Hyperactivity and frustration: the influence of control over and size of rewards in delaying gratification. *Journal of Abnormal Child Psychology*, **14**, 191–204.

Reveley, A.M., Reveley, M.A., Clifford, C. and Murray, R.M. (1982). Cerebral ventricular size in twins discordant for schizophrenia. *Lancet*, **1**, 540–1.

Rodnick, E.H. and Shakow, D. (1940). Set in the schizophrenic as measured by a composite reaction time index. *American Journal of Psychiatry*, **97**, 214–25.

Rosenthal, R.H. and Allen, T.W. (1978). An examination of attention, arousal and learning dysfunctions of hyperkinetic children. *Psychological Bulletin*, **85**, 689–715.

Ross, D.M. and Ross, S.A. (1976). *Hyperactivity: Research, Theory and Action.* New York: Wiley.

Rutter, M. (1989). Child psychiatric disorders in ICD-10. *Journal of Child Psychology and Psychiatry*, **30**, 499–514.

Rutter, M., Chadwick, O. and Shaffer, D. (1983). Head injury. In *Developmental Neuropsychiatry* (ed. M. Rutter), pp. 83–111. New York: Guilford.

Rutter, M. and Mahwood, L. (1991). The long-term psychological sequelae of specific developmental disorders of speech and language. In *Biological Risk Factors for Psychological Disorders* (ed. M. Rutter and P. Casaer), pp. 233–59. Cambridge: Cambridge University Press.

Sameroff, A.J. and Chandler, M.J. (1975). Reproductive risk and the continuum of caretaking casualty. In *Review of Child Development Research*, vol. 4 (ed. F.D. Horowitz), pp. 187–244. Chicago: University of Chicago Press.

Schacher, R. and Logan, G.D. (1990). Impulsivity and inhibitory control in development and psychopathology. *Developmental Psychology*, **26**, 1–11.

Scott, S. (1994). Mental retardation. In *Child and Adolescent Psychiatry: Modern Approaches*, 3rd edition (ed. M. Rutter, E. Taylor and L. Hersov), pp. 616–46. Oxford: Blackwell Scientific Publications.

Sergeant, J.A. and Scholten, C.A. (1985). On data limitations in hyperactivity. *Journal of Child Psychology and Psychiatry*, **26**, 111–24.

Shaffer, D., O'Connor, P.A., Shafer, S.Q. and Prupis, S. (1983). Neurological 'soft signs': their origins and significance for behavior. In *Developmental Neuropsychiatry* (ed. M. Rutter), pp. 144–80. New York: Guilford.

Sham, P.C., O'Callaghan, E., Takei, N. *et al.* (1992). Schizophrenia following prenatal exposure to influenza epidemics between 1939 and 1960. *British Journal of Psychiatry*, **160**, 461–6.

Skorzewska, A., Lall, S., Waserman, J. and Guyda, H. (1989). Abnormal food-seeking behaviour after surgery for craniopharyngioma. *Neuropsychobiology*, **21**, 17–20.

Sonuga-Barke, E. and Taylor, E. (1992). The effect of delay on hyperactive and non-hyperactive children's response times: Research note. *Journal of Child Psychology and Psychiatry*, **33**, 1091–6.

Sonuga-Barke, E.J.S., Heptinstall, E. and Taylor, E. (1992). Hyperactivity and delay aversion: II. The effects of self versus externally imposed stimulus presentation periods on memory. *Journal of Child Psychology and Psychiatry*, **33**, 399–410.

Sprague, R.L. and Sleator, E.K. (1977). Methylphenidate in hyperkinetic children: Differences in dose effects on learning and social behaviour. *Science*, **198**, 1274–76.

Suddath, R.L., Casanova, M.D., Goldberg, T.E. *et al.* (1989). Temporal lobe pathology in schizophrenia: a quantitative magnetic resonance imaging study. *American Journal of Psychiatry*, **146**, 464–72.

Sykes, D.H., Douglas, V.I. and Morgenstern, G. (1973). Sustained attention in hyperactive children. *Journal of Child Psychology and Psychiatry*, **14**, 213–20.

Taylor, E.A. (1991*a*). Toxins and allergens. In *Biological Risk Factors for Psychosocial Disorders* (ed. M. Rutter and P. Casaer), pp. 19–232. Cambridge: Cambridge University Press.

Taylor, E. (1991*b*). Developmental neuropsychiatry. *Journal of Child Psychology and Psychiatry Annual Research Review*, **1**, 3–47.

Taylor, E., Sandberg, S., Thorley, G. and Giles, S. (1991). *The Epidemiology of Childhood Hyperactivity*. Maudsley Monograph No. 33. Oxford: Oxford University Press.

Taylor, E., Chadwick, O., Heptinstall, E. and Danckaerts, M. (1996). Hyperactivity and conduct problems as risk factors for adolescent development. *Journal of the American Academy of Child and Adolescent Psychiatry*, **35**, 1213–26.

Tsuang, M.T., Gilbertson, M.W. and Faraone, S.V. (1991). The genetics of schizophrenia: current knowledge and future directions. *Schizophrenia Research*, **4**, 157–71.

Viggedal, G., Hagberg, B.S., Laegreid, L. and Aronsson, M. (1993). Mental development in late infancy after prenatal exposure to benzodiazepines – a prospective study. *Journal of Child Psychology and Psychiatry*, **34**, 295–305.

Weinberger, D.R., Delisi, L.E., Perman, G.P. *et al.* (1982). Computed tomography in schizophreniform disorder and other acute psychiatric disorders. *Archives of General Psychiatry*, **39**, 778–83.

Werner, E. and Smith, E. (1977). *Kauai's Children Come of Age*. Honolulu: University of Hawaii Press.

Werry, J.S. and Taylor, E. (1994). Schizophrenic and allied disorders. In *Child and Adolescent Psychiatry: Modern Approaches*, 3rd edition (ed. M. Rutter, E. Taylor and L. Hersov), pp. 594–615. Oxford: Blackwell Scientific Publications.

Whalen, C.K. and Henker, B. (1976). Psychostimulants and children: a review and analysis. *Psychological Bulletin*, **83**, 1113–30.

Williams, A.O., Reveley, M.A., Kolakowska, T. *et al.* (1985). Schizophrenia with good and poor outcome: II. Cerebral ventricular size and its clinical significance. *British Journal of Psychiatry*, **146**, 239–46.

Wohlberg, G.W. and Kornetsky, C. (1973). Sustained attention in remitted schizophrenia. *Archives of General Psychiatry*, **28**, 533–7.

Zeitlin, H. (1986). *The Natural History of Psychiatric Disorders in Children.* Maudsley Monograph No. 29. Oxford: Oxford University Press.

12

Neurodevelopmental disturbances in the aetiology of schizophrenia

J. MEGGINSON HOLLISTER & TYRONE D. CANNON

Introduction

Recent efforts to unravel the mystery of schizophrenia have suggested a central role of structural and functional abnormalities of the brain in the disorder's aetiology and pathophysiology. One formulation that has gained some popularity in the past decade is that schizophrenia is a neurodevelopmental condition whose origins can be traced to the earliest phases of brain development *in utero*. Indeed, a vast body of post-mortem and neuroimaging research has demonstrated that the brains of these patients are deviant at both the microscopic and gross levels compared to those of healthy individuals. Several post-mortem studies have found evidence of cellular positioning abnormalities consistent with genetic or teratogenic disturbances during gestation. In neuroimaging studies, structural abnormalities such as ventricular enlargement and reduced temporal lobe volumes have been observed in both first-episode and chronic patients, indicating that these abnormalities are present at least as early as the beginning stages of psychosis. In addition, neurobehavioural and neuromotor abnormalities have been observed among preschizophrenia children and among those at high genetic risk. There is also accumulating evidence that obstetric complications such as perinatal hypoxia, viral infection, and rhesus incompatibility may adversely impact fetal neurodevelopment leading to an increased risk for schizophrenia later in life.

Despite these interesting leads, there is as yet no direct proof that the brain abnormalities critical for the expression of schizophrenia are in fact neurodevelopmental in origin. An alternative formulation is that such abnormalities accrue in severity over time as a secondary consequence of a more basic (but as yet unidentified) component of the disease process in schizophrenia, a process that could be at least partially active long before the first overt manifestations of psychosis. In the latter case, it would seem more appropriate to view schizophrenia as a neurodegenerative condition, as Kraepelin (1919) hypothesised nearly a century ago.

Any comprehensive account of schizophrenia must confront not only the different possible meanings of the brain abnormalities observed in these patients, but also the multifactorial nature of the risk factors for schizophrenia, the considerable heterogeneity in the clinical manifestations of the syndrome, and the fact that onset of formal diagnostic symptoms and signs typically occurs in late adolescence and early adulthood. In this chapter we will present a summary of the current work pertaining to neurodevelopmental models of schizophrenia by briefly reviewing evidence addressing the following issues: (1) To what extent can the brain abnormalities in schizophrenia be traced to neurodevelopmental versus neurodegenerative or iatrogenic processes? (2) Are the brain abnormalities in schizophrenia ubiquitous or, rather, confined to subgroup(s) of patients with possibly different etiologies? (3) If at least some of the abnormalities are likely to originate during brain development, what factors account for the latency of onset of formal diagnostic symptoms and signs?

Neurodevelopmental versus neurodegenerative processes

Post-mortem findings

Post-mortem studies provide a unique window into the origins of the brain abnormalities in schizophrenia, since developmental and atrophic or degenerative processes have different characteristic influences on cytoarchitecture. Findings of cellular disarray and reduced cell densities in the absence of substantial gliosis are thought to indicate perturbed fetal neurodevelopment, whereas findings of cell loss with substantial gliosis and other signs of cellular degeneration are thought to indicate either a discrete insult (likely postnatal in origin) or a neurodegenerative process. Post-mortem studies of schizophrenia can be divided into: (1) those reporting evidence consistent with cellular migratory disturbances during gestation, (2) those reporting evidence of cell loss without significant gliosis, and (3) those reporting cell loss with substantial glial scarring.

Cellular migration

A number of neuropathology studies have reported findings in the brains of schizophrenics consistent with disturbances of neuronal migration. Cellular anomalies consistent with perturbed migration include reduced thickness of the granule cell layer in the hippocampal formation (McLardy, 1974), disorientation and disarray of hippocampal pyramidal cells (Scheibel and Kovelman, 1981; Kovelman and Scheibel, 1984; Altschuler *et al.*, 1987; Jeste and Lohr, 1989; Benes, Davidson and Bird, 1991*b*; Conrad *et al.*, 1991), and cytoarchitectural disturbances in the prefrontal cortex, anterior cingulate, primary motor cortex (Benes, Davidson and Bird, 1986; Benes, 1987), and entorhinal cortex (Jakob and Beckman, 1986; Falkai, Bogerts, and Rozumek, 1988*a*; Falkai and Bogerts, 1989; Casanova, Stevens and Kleinman, 1990; Arnold *et al.*, 1991; Beckmann and Jakob, 1991). Recently, abnormal neuronal distribution in the dorsolateral prefrontal cortex and lateral and medial temporal lobes of deceased schizophrenics were reported (Akbarian *et al.*, 1993*a*,*b*).

These cytoarchitectural anomalies implicate disruptions in neuronal migration during intrauterine life. Such anomalies could result from genetic or teratogenic influences or their interaction. For instance, Nowakowski (1991) presented several models of perturbed neurodevelopment of the hippocampal formation in mice that result from autosomal recessive gene mutations. The ectopias (abnormal positioning of neurones) characteristic of these mouse strains reflect disruptions of one or more of the basic cellular processes in neurodevelopment: cell proliferation, cell migration and cell differentiation. For example, one strain of mice shows a disruption of migration of late-generated pyramidal cells that are destined for CA3c; the lesion in this case is characterised by cells that follow the proper migratory path but stop short of the proper destination (Hippocampal Lamination Defect Mutation). A second type of ectopia resulting from a genetic mutation is one in which the proliferation and migration of granule cells of the dentate gyrus and pyramidal cells of the hippocampus are disturbed (Dreher Mutant); the lesion in this case is characterised by either too few or too many of these cell types in their proper location, as well as abnormal positioning. Nowakowski (1991) emphasised the striking similarities between the neuropathology observed in these mice strains and that observed in the brains of deceased schizophrenics.

Environmental causes of such ectopias are also possible. In view of the fact that obstetric complications are associated with an increased risk for schizophrenia among offspring of schizophrenic mothers but not of control mothers (Parnas *et al.*, 1982*b*; Cannon, Mednick and Parnas, 1990), such environmental influences are unlikely to play a major role in the neuropathology that predisposes to schizophrenia without the participation of genetic factors. For this reason, most neurodevelopmental theories of schizophrenia posit some form of a two-hit hypothesis or diathesis–stress interaction. In the models to be discussed below, the neurodevelopmental aberrations are not directly genetically determined but result from a secondary genetic process. All three of these models suggest that genetically determined aspects of the maternal or fetal system (first hit) combine with endogenous or exogenous factors (second hit) leading to perturbed fetal neurodevelopment through the consequences of that interaction.

First, pointing to the evidence indicating that prenatal infection with influenza is associated with increased risk for schizophrenia in adulthood (e.g. Mednick *et al.*, 1988), Conrad and Scheibel (1987) have proposed that fetal infection by influenza virus may be responsible for the perturbed neurodevelopment observed in some types of schizophrenia. Fetal infection by the influenza virus in mice is known to impair the adhesive properties of nuclear cell adhesion molecules (NCAMs), which are necessary for proper neuronal migration. Conrad and Scheibel have noted parallels between the disorientation of the pyramidal cells of the hippocampus observed in some schizophrenics and the cellular disarray observed in reeler and staggerer mice (Conrad and Scheibel, 1987). The cellular disarray observed in these mice is thought to result from defects in the regulation of the adhesive properties of NCAMs and related molecules (Edelman, 1982; Pinto-Lord, Evrard and Caviness, 1982; Nowakowski, 1988) secondary to the toxic effect of virus on these molecules (Conrad and Scheibel, 1987). Therefore, in this model, the placental barrier of the fetus is somehow compromised (first hit) leading to exposure of the developing fetal brain to virus (second hit). The virus crosses the immature fetal blood–brain barrier, impairs the action of NCAMs and related molecules, disrupting fetal neurodevelopment in regions of the brain developing at that time.

An alternative model that also stems from the finding that prenatal exposure to influenza virus increases the risk for schizophrenia later in life is that perturbations in fetal neurodevelopment are the consequence of atypical maternal immune response to influenza during pregnancy. Some suggest that a pregnant woman develops autoantibodies to the influenza virus in an atypical immune response (first hit) (Wright, Gill and Murray, 1993; Laing *et al.*, 1995). These autoantibodies then cross the placenta and the immature fetal blood–brain barrier and cause neurodevelopmental damage to the unborn child by cross-reacting with fetal brain tissue antigens (second hit).

We have recently proposed another model associated with atypical maternal immune response (Hollister, Laing and Mednick, 1996). In this model, a woman develops alloantibodies against paternally inherited alloantigens in the fetus (first hit), such as is observed in rhesus incompatibility. These alloantibodies then cross the placenta, causing haemolytic disease of the fetus and newborn. This condition can cause chronic hypoxia *in utero* and/or hyperbilirubinaemia, both of which are capable of perturbing fetal neurodevelopment (second hit). Chronic hypoxia is known to be neurotoxic to specific regions of the brain including the hippocampus and can also lead to intraventricular hemorrhage (Larroche, 1984; Rorke, 1992). Bilirubin, at elevated levels, is particularly toxic to the pallidum, subthalamic nucleus, cranial nerve nuclei, brain stem, dentate and roof nuclei, inferior olivary nuclei, nuclei gracilis and cuneatus, and less often in the putamen, lateral geniculate bodies, lateral nuclei of thalamus and spinal grey in developing fetus (Rorke, 1992).

Volume and cellular density

The second type of post-mortem finding in schizophrenia is abnormal regional brain volume and altered cell density. Reduced volumes of the internal pallidum, hippocampus, parahippocampal gyrus and amygdala (Bogerts, Meertz and Schonfeldt-Bausch, 1985; Falkai and Bogerts, 1986; Bogerts *et al.*, 1990*a*; Suddath *et al.*, 1990; Heckers *et al.*, 1991*a*), lowered volume and cell densities in the entorhinal cortex (Falkai *et al.*, 1988*a*), reduced total neurone and glial cell number in mediodorsal thalamic nucleus and nucleus accumbens (Pakkenberg *et al.*, 1990, 1992*a,b*), reduced neuronal density without gliosis in the prefrontal cortex, anterior cingulate and primary motor cortex (Benes *et al.*, 1986, 1991*a*; Benes, 1987) have all been reported. By contrast, Selemon, Rajkowska and Goldman-Rakic (1993) have presented preliminary data showing increases in pyramidal cell density in regions of the dorsolateral prefrontal cortex. Likewise, Dagg *et al.* (1994) reported increases in pyramidal cell density in the cingulate cortex of schizophrenic brains, and Heckers *et al.* (1991*b*) reported increase in striatal volume on the left side and pallidal volume on the right side for schizophrenia patients, but no differences from controls in cortical or white matter volume. Others report no change in cellular density in the brains of schizophrenics (Akbarian *et al.*, 1993*a*).

The significance of altered density and volumes in various regions of the schizophrenic brain is less clearly associated with neurodevelopmental aberration than in the case of cytoarchitectural abnormalities. However, altered cell densities and volumes in these regions may reflect disturbances. of proliferation/migration or excessive neuronal dropout early in life, possibly during fetal or neonatal development (Cannon and Mednick, 1991). Evidence supporting this perspective is found in studies of the hippocampal formation in schizophrenics, where the same cell groups that show ectopia are also shown to be reduced in density (Falkai *et al.*, 1988*a*; Jakob and Beckmann, 1986). Of course, altered cell density and regional brain volumes could also reflect excessive postnatal neuronal pruning, since developmental elimination of cells and their processes continues into adolescence and young adulthood (see 'Neural Pruning' below). Finally, it is important that many of the regions showing volume reductions in the post-mortem studies have also been implicated as deviant *in vivo* imaging studies of schizophrenics (see '*In Vivo* Findings' below).

Gliosis

Progressive degenerative or inflammatory brain disease is suggested when increased densities or absolute numbers of reactive glial cells, especially astrocytes, are present (Bogerts and Falkai, 1991). In addition, pathological events occurring after the second trimester of pregnancy such as viral infections, hypoxia, or atrophic processes can cause increased glial cell densities (Bogerts and Falkai, 1991).

Gliosis has been described as occurring in several areas of the schizophrenic brain. Nasrallah *et al.* (1983) reported gliosis, anteriorly and posteriorly, in the corpus callosum of late onset schizophrenics as compared to early onset schizophrenics. Periventricular gliosis was reported by Nieto and Escobar (1972), and gliosis in the midbrain tegmentum, bed nucleus of the stria terminalis, basal nucleus, medial thalamus, amygdala and hippocampus was reported by Stevens (1982). Bruton *et al.* (1990) reported periventricular fibrous gliosis in half of the schizophrenic brains studied. Fisman (1975) reported glial knots and perivascular infiltrations in the brainstem. Finally, Averback (1981) found evidence of cellular degeneration in the nucleus of the ansa lenticularis in a sample of schizophrenics.

On the other hand, several researchers found no evidence of gliosis in the medial temporal lobe, cingulate gyrus or hypothalamic periventricular regions of schizophrenic brains (Falkai and Bogerts, 1986; Roberts, Kleinman and Weinberger, 1986, 1987; Casonova, 1988; Falkai *et al.*, 1988*a*; Benes, 1987; Stevens and Casonova, 1988). It is important to note that these negative studies have been criticised for methodology not sensitive enough to detect moderate degrees of gliosis and for small sample size (Bogerts and Falkai, 1991).

Neural pruning

Neural pruning is a controlled, regulated, physiological process that is considered a normal part of neurodevelopment (Margolis, Chung and

Post, 1994), and refers to the reduction of neural elements of any type, including nerve tissue, neurones, synapses or dendrites (Keshavan, Anderson and Pettegrew, 1994). In 1982, Feinberg proposed that an abnormality in synaptic pruning may play a fundamental role in the aetiology of schizophrenia (Feinberg, 1982). The suggestion that faulty neural pruning is part of the neuromal development in schizophrenia may help explain some of the mysteries of the illness such as latency of onset, gender differences, and clinical features. For instance, the fact that neural pruning occurs postnatally in humans from childhood to adolescence may help explain why overt psychotic thought process in schizophrenia is most usually not observed until adolescence or later. With respect to gender differences in schizophrenia, sex hormones have been indicated in the function of neural and synaptic pruning (as well as proliferation) and may therefore impact the manifestation of the disorder in the two sexes differently (Keshavan *et al.*, 1994). Finally, computer simulations of neural information processing systems that were subjected to hyperpruning produced cognitive pathology that could conceivably lead to the positive type symptomatology observed in schizophrenia (Hoffman and Dobscha, 1989). Keshavan *et al.* (1994) rightly pointed out that the computer-derived models of Hoffman and Dobscha need to be empirically tested using a human model.

Keshavan *et al.* (1994) noted that Feinberg's hypothesis leaves several questions unanswered. These questions include: Is the postulated abnormality one of too much pruning, too little, or in the wrong neural elements? Is the defective pruning caused by early intranatal or perinatal lesions or by postnatal events? What is the relationship between synaptic pruning and the neurochemical abnormalities thought to underlie schizophrenia? These authors suggested that schizophrenia may result from more than one neurodevelopmental trajectory, and this might explain the heterogeneity of the disorder. For instance, one type of schizophrenia may result from an 'early' neurodevelopmental abnormality like those described previously in this chapter, while another type of schizophrenia may result from a 'late' neurodevelopmental abnormality such as excessive neural pruning, and another type of schizophrenia from an interaction of faulty 'early' development and faulty (or not) 'late' development. The advantage of including neural pruning into the neurodevelopmental model of schizophrenia is its temporal association with the illness onset, and the fact that this process is also genetically mediated (Keshavan *et al.*, 1994).

Analysis of post-mortem findings

There is no question that post-mortem studies of the brains of schizophrenics reveal certain abnormalities consistent with very early developmental aberrations, and possibly also consistent with 'late' developmental anomalies. The wide range of abnormalities described is probably directly related to the heterogeneity of the syndrome. Until such a time that better methods of subgrouping individuals with schizophrenia exists, studies such as those described above will probably be limited by patient samples that include a 'mixed bag' of at least partially aetiologically distinct illnesses.

Although some evidence of gliosis exists, whether such findings indicate a neurodegenerative process in schizophrenia is questionable. One possible cause of gliosis is teratogenic influences in the late stages of pregnancy and the birth process, and therefore the scarring may represent residue of a static insult that followed earlier neurodevelopmental aberrations. In other words, the glial scarring might be evidence of the 'second hit', and not indicative of a primary neurodegenerative process. Moreover, the gliosis observed in schizophrenic brains is not as extensive as that observed in degenerative diseases such as Huntington's chorea and Alzheimer's disease. Still, autopsy studies can go only so far in addressing the issue of whether there is neurodegeneration in schizophrenia. To get a more definitive view of this issue, we require longitudinal investigation of brain structure within the same individuals over time. Such studies are possible using *in vivo* brain imaging techniques, to which we turn next.

In vivo *findings*

Neuroimaging studies

The most consistently replicated findings in neuroimaging studies of schizophrenic brains are enlargement of the third and lateral ventricles and increased prominence of the cortical sulci and fissures. Ventriculomegaly and cortical sulcal prominence are general, nonspecific signs of brain pathology (Cannon and Marco, 1994). Studies that examine whether these changes reflect proximal or distal tissue reductions find evidence that ventricular enlargement is associated with cell loss in periventricular regions (Cannon and Marco, 1994). More recent work with magnetic resonance imaging (MRI), which permits evaluation of regional grey matter volume, has found volume reductions of temporal lobe structures and of the hippocampus in particular (Suddath *et al.*, 1989; Bogerts *et al.*, 1990*b*). Reductions in frontal lobe size have not been consistently replicated

(Andreasen *et al.*, 1986, 1990; DeMyer *et al.*, 1988). In addition, Raine *et al.* (1992) and Klausner *et al.* (1992) reported increased frontal horn size, while Rubin *et al.* (1993) reported greater sulcal size in the frontal regions. A recent study by Kikinis *et al.* (1994) found abnormal sulco-gyral patterns in schizophrenics using MRI. They suggested that the anomalous surface patterns of the schizophrenics may have neurodevelopmental origins.

We have previously reviewed studies investigating ventricular enlargement and sulcal prominence in an attempt to elucidate the significance of these abnormalities to the schizophrenia illness (i.e. is there a causal, consequential, or spurious relationship between schizophrenia and these structural brain abnormalities?) (Cannon, 1991*a*). We found that neither gender nor race were found to be significantly related to third and lateral ventricular enlargement or cortical sulcal prominence in most studies. Nor were history of head injury, substance abuse, or past neuroleptic treatment found to be related to structural brain abnormalities. In the case of treatment effects, a few studies that did find correlations between brain abnormalities and treatment factors also found evidence of abnormalities in the never treated subjects (Johnstone *et al.*, 1976, 1978; Weinberger *et al.*, 1979).

In our review, age and duration of illness were the only factors that showed a trend toward correlation with ventricular and sulcal enlargement (Cannon, 1991*a*). Even so, a majority of these studies found no relationship between the two factors and the three indices of brain pathology. Furthermore, if duration of illness and age were the cause of the observed brain abnormalities, then the brain pathology should not be present among very young patients with schizophrenia. Also, ten studies of teenage psychotics, first episode schizophreniform patients, and schizophrenics within one or two years of onset, found ventricular enlargement in these samples despite the younger age of subjects and shorter duration of illness. Our conclusion was that the structural brain pathology observed in schizophrenia is probably not a consequence of the illness or its treatment, and that ventricular enlargement in schizophrenia is probably not progressive beyond that associated with normal aging (Cannon, 1991*a*).

The only illness history variable that appears to be related to ventricular size in schizophrenia is severity of illness as indexed by cumulative length of hospitalisation (Pandurangi *et al.*, 1986; Cannon, 1991*a*). This relationship is independent of age of subjects, exposure to neuroleptic treatment and electroconvulsive therapy (Cannon and Marco, 1994), and may indicate that the severity of the observed brain pathology varies along a continuum associated with the severity of the schizophrenia illness (Eyler-Zorrilla and Cannon, 1995).

If the brain pathology in schizophrenia is not a consequence of the illness, then the second possibility is that it is associated with the aetiology of schizophrenia. The strongest evidence for an aetiological role of ventricular enlargement in the development of schizophrenia is in its relationship to genetic and perinatal factors. Two main perspectives exist on how these two factors may contribute to the brain pathology of schizophrenia. First, genetic and perinatal factors may interact in a two-hit model as discussed earlier, or secondly, perinatal factors may cause structural brain abnormalities that mimic the genetically determined brain pathology of schizophrenia resulting in a 'teratogenic' form of the illness. Two types of study design exist to examine the importance of genetic and perinatal factors to brain abnormalities in schizophrenia: (1) comparisons among schizophrenics, their non-ill relatives, and unrelated normal controls, and (2) comparisons of unrelated samples of schizophrenics and controls in terms of family history of schizophrenia and history of obstetric complications.

Comparison of schizophrenics with their unaffected relatives and unrelated normal controls suggest that there is a significant genetic contribution to the brain abnormalities related to schizophrenia. The conclusion from four studies examining ventricular size and schizophrenia in families and twins is that a genetic component in increased ventricular size exists, but that environmental factors such as obstetric complications, head injury or drug use may also play a role (Cannon, 1991*a*). In these comparisons, schizophrenics show the greatest ventricular enlargement, followed by their non-ill siblings, followed by unrelated, psychiatrically normal controls (Weinberger *et al.*, 1981; DeLisi *et al.*, 1986; Cannon *et al.*, 1993).

Comparisons of individuals at low, high and super high risk for schizophrenia support the contention that a large component of these structural brain abnormalities derive from mechanisms associated with genotypic predisposition for schizophrenia. We have found that individuals who were at super high risk for schizophrenia (i.e. both parents with schizophrenia spectrum disorders), and who had sustained delivery complications, are at greatest risk for schizophrenia and the most likely to evidence ventriculomegaly, whereas as genetic risk for schizophrenia decreases, the weaker the relationship between schizophrenia, delivery complications, and ventriculomegaly. This suggested to us that a part of the expression of the genetic predisposition for schizophrenia is a vulnerability of the fetal brain, especially to birth trauma. Therefore, the phenotypic expression of the pro-schizophrenia genotype appears some time prior to delivery and takes the form of a fragile fetal brain that is more easily compromised by teratogenic influences (Mednick and Cannon, 1991; Eyler-Zorrilla and Cannon, 1995). In contrast, the cortical abnormalities in schizophrenia appear to be more dependent on genetic factors than environmental ones, as these abnormalities were found to vary in severity with degree of genetic risk for schizophrenia but were unrelated to the environmental factors examined, including delivery complications, pregnancy complications and low birth weight (Cannon *et al.*, 1993).

An alternative method for assessing the genetic contribution to brain abnormalities in schizophrenia is the familial-sporadic design. In this approach, individuals with schizophrenia who have a history of familial schizophrenia (FH+) are compared to individuals with schizophrenia who do not have a familial history for the illness (FH−). The results from these studies are quite varied. Some studies find ventricular enlargement only in FH− patients; some studies find ventricular enlargement only in FH+ patients; while still others find no relationship (Cannon and Marco, 1994). The methodologic weaknesses inherent in the familial-sporadic design probably explain these equivocal findings. These weaknesses include, first and foremost, that because the genetic contribution to the aetiology of schizophrenia is partial and requires an environmental contribution to result in the illness, many family members who have the necessary genotype will not manifest the phenotype. Secondly, small family size or attrition of affected family members may occur, resulting in a sample that is not representative of the true incidence of familial schizophrenia. And, lastly, some FH studies defined familial risk as the presence of any major psychiatric illness, which is a dubious basis from which to infer genetic risk for schizophrenia (Cannon and Marco, 1994).

Neurobehavioural studies

Neurobehavioural and neuromotor abnormalities have been reported in studies of infants and children at high risk for schizophrenia and in those infants and children who develop the illness later in life, suggesting that these abnormalities may be premorbid signs of the illness. In addition, movement abnormalities have long been reported among schizophrenia patients, but their aetiological importance has been obscured by the known side-effects of neuroleptic medications on motor systems. The following discussion will provide a brief review of this literature, and discuss whether neuromotor abnormalities in schizophrenics are a clue to the aetiology of the illness, a consequence of it, or an unrelated phenomenon.

Neuromotor anomalies have been reported among infants and toddlers who later develop schizophrenia showing that these abnormalities precede the onset of schizophrenia by many years (Fish *et al.*, 1992). Mednick and Silverton (1987) reported neuromotor abnormalities among individuals who later developed schizophrenia. Jones, Murray and Rodgers (1995), in a comprehensive study of childhood risk factors for adult schizophrenia, found two premorbid neurobehavioural signs that predicted schizophrenia: a delay to reach the motor milestone of walking and an excess of twitches and grimaces at age 15. Poorer motor skills and neuromotor abnormalities in preschizophrenia infants between birth and two years of age were reported by Walker, Savolie and Davis (1994) in a study that reviewed home videos of families in which one of the children developed schizophrenia later in life. Walker states that the abnormal movements seen most commonly in the children who later developed schizophrenia included prolonged fisting, hyperextension of the fingers, wrist hyper flexion and pronation of the hand.

Reports of movement abnormalities in adolescent and adult schizophrenics are similar in quality to those observed in preschizophrenia infants (Walker, 1994). Because of the side-effects of neuroleptic medications, the most informative studies of neuromotor abnormalities in schizophrenia are those of never-medicated patients. Postural and movement abnormalities were observed in patients with dementia praecox prior to the use of neuroleptic medication (Reiter, 1926 as cited in Walker, 1994). In addition, there was an association of movement abnormalities with advancing age, especially in the months preceding death. Casey and Hansen (1984) reviewed 28 studies published between 1959 and 1984 that suggested an increase in movement disorders among nonmedicated schizophrenics, with a tendency for increased abnormalities among the older patients.

Additionally, movement abnormalities in schizophrenia may be associated with earthly onset of the illness and severity of symptoms (Walker, 1994). Investigators in a few studies reported that abnormal neuromotor behaviours were more common among adolescent psychiatric patients (Kennard, 1960; Hertzig and Birch, 1966, 1968). Also other investigators find neuromotor abnormalities to be negatively correlated with age at onset of illness (Hertzig and Birch, 1966; Yarden and Discipio, 1971) and positively correlated with premorbid impairment (Rochford *et al.*, 1970), severity of symptoms (Manshreck *et al.*, 1981), and poor outcome (Rochford *et al.*, 1970; Johnstone *et al.*, 1990).

Psychosocial and cognitive deficits have also been reported among children at high risk and those destined to develop schizophrenia.

Emotional instability (Watt, 1972, 1978; Watt and Lubensky, 1976; Watt, Grubb and Erlenmeyer-Kimling, 1982; John, Mednick and Schulsinger, 1982; Janes, Weeks and Worland, 1983; Schwartzman, Ledingham and Serbin, 1985; Olin, John and Mednick, 1995), poor affective control (Parnas and Jorgensen, 1989; Parnas *et al.*, 1982*a*), social anxiety, withdrawn, aloof, disruptive (Jones *et al.*, 1995), less motivation and more verbal negativity (Janes *et al.*, 1983; Watt *et al.*, 1982) have all been reported in children at high risk for schizophrenia and in those who later developed the illness. Impaired premorbid intellectual functioning as well as cognitive abnormalities after the illness onset have also been reported (Jones *et al.*, 1995; Fenton, Wyatt and McGlashan, 1994; Cannon *et al.*, 1994).

In summary, the appearance of neurobehavioural and neuromotor abnormalities before the onset of the psychotic symptomatology in schizophrenia provides strong support for those advocating a neurodevelopmental disease model. These behavioural precursors to the schizophrenic illness demonstrate that the brains of these individuals are at some level abnormally functioning even prior to overt expression of thought disorder and hallucinations.

Distribution of abnormalities

Two competing models exist to explain the distribution of structural brain abnormalities in schizophrenia. These models are the subtype model and the continuum-severity model. The subtype model predicts that the distribution of the brain abnormalities in schizophrenia should be multimodal, with the number of modes dependent on the number of clinical subtypes of the illness. Under this model, if a bimodal distribution of abnormalities was found, then schizophrenics with abnormalities should present a qualitatively distinct clinical picture from the schizophrenics without brain abnormalities. The continuum-severity model predicts a unimodal distribution of structural brain abnormalities, with patients at the upper and lower ends of the distribution differing in severity but not type of schizophrenic symptomatology.

Evidence for subtype model

Crow (1989) proposed that structural brain abnormalities may characterise an aetiologically distinct subgroup of schizophrenia patients with poor premorbid history, cognitive impairment, poor response to neuroleptics, and prominent negative symptoms. The notion that ventricular enlargement may mark such a distinct subgroup is supported by the fact that about half of these patients have ventricular brain ratios outside the range of the control distribution. However, two main problems exist with Crow's tenet. First, robust clinical differences between schizophrenia patients with larger and smaller ventricles do not exist. In a review of studies examining this question, only seven of 20 studies reported more negative symptoms among patients with enlarged ventricles, although the discrepant findings may be the result of methodological weaknesses (Cannon, 1991*b*). Second, a bimodal distribution of ventricular enlargement and other structural measures in schizophrenia is not observed, as would be expected if the measures defined aetiologically distinct subgroups (Cannon and Marco, 1994).

With respect to diagnostic subtypes, no consistent pattern of correlation between brain abnormalities and traditional classifications emerges. Some studies found a relationship between 'Kraepelinian' categories (i.e. residual, hebephrenic, undifferentiated) and ventricular enlargement, but not between paranoid or acute subtype categories. Several other studies found no relationship, and two other studies found larger ventricles in the patients with paranoid or 'positive' subtype diagnoses (see Cannon, 1991*b*).

Evidence for continuum-severity model

Weinberger (1987) noted that the most well-studied brain measure in schizophrenia research, the ventricle to brain ratio (VBR), has a unimodal and not bimodal distribution with a significant positive skew. Such a distribution is clearly more easily explained by the continuum-severity model than by the subtype model. In addition, severity of illness as indexed by cumulative length of hospitalisation has been shown to be a significant predictor of mean VBR and mean effect size (Cannon, 1991*b*; Raz and Raz, 1990). On the other hand, if the continuum model were correct, then every schizophrenic should have structural brain abnormalities to some degree, and thus there should not be overlap between the schizophrenic and normal control distributions on these measures. This, however, is not the case. Indeed, fully 57% of subjects in these two groups overlap on ventricular size (Raz and Raz, 1990).

Eyler-Zorrilla and Cannon (1995) argue that the 57% overlap between schizophrenics and normal controls on brain measures may be the result primarily of random genetic factors that influence brain morphology. For instance, Reveley *et al.* (1982) found that 90% of variance in ventricular size in normal twins was accounted for by between-family variance. Therefore, the ideal comparison group in a study of brain abnormalities in schizophrenia consists of first degree relatives, especially healthy siblings or co-twin. Four studies (Weinberger *et al.*, 1981; Reveley *et al.*, 1982; DeLisi *et al.*, 1986; Suddath *et al.*, 1990) have used healthy siblings or co-twins of schizophrenics as controls. There was a large increase in sensitivity of these studies (i.e. on average 80%) in discriminating between schizophrenics and non-schizophrenics (Eyler-Zorrilla and Cannon, 1995) as compared to studies that use unrelated control samples (i.e. on average 43%). In conclusion, given appropriate biological controls, all or nearly all individuals with schizophrenia show significant structural brain abnormalities, and this pathology is probably distributed on a continuum associated with increasing severity of the disorder.

Latency of onset and neurodevelopment

The neurodevelopment model can also help explain the latency of onset of schizophrenia. For instance, Weinberger (1987) proposed that the effects of an early neurodevelopmental disturbance may only become apparent following normal neurodevelopmental events that occur in late adolescence or early adulthood, when brain regions reach functional maturity. Alternatively, faulty pruning of neural elements or faulty myelination during 'late' stage neurodevelopment may interact with neurodevelopmental abberations that have prenatal and/or perinatal origins. The presence of neuromotor and neurobehavioural abnormalities in infancy and childhood may be the phenotypic representation of 'early' stage neurodevelopmental anomalies, with psychotic symptomatology manifesting as the 'late' stages of neurodevelopment are passed. Walker (1994) described a course of neurodevelopmental events that might lead to this presentation in some types of schizophrenia. She pointed out that the motor region is more myelinated and metabolically active than other areas of the cerebral cortex such as the frontal or limbic cortex during infancy, and so if an abnormality of cortical–subcortical circuitry exists, it is more likely to be manifested in motor dysfunction (at this time). However, with development, the sensorimotor cortex becomes less metabolically active relative to other regions and cortical–subcortical interconnections become more complex. And, in fact, by young adulthood, the sensorimotor cortex becomes the least metabolically active region of the cortex, while the frontal and limbic regions are among the most active and myelination of neural pathways is completed. One would thus expect the emergence of the psychotic symptomatology to occur after the last stages of neurodevelopment are passed.

Bogerts (1989) suggested that hormonal factors during puberty may be related to the latency of onset. During puberty, limbic structures are main targets of stress- and age-related hormones such as corticosteroids and gonadosteroids. Bogerts suggested that the influence of these hormones on already compromised limbic structures results in psychotic symptomatology.

Conclusions

We have briefly reviewed findings from post-mortem, neuroimaging, and neurobehavioural studies that unequivocally demonstrate that individuals with schizophrenia evidence abnormalities in all these areas. A question that arises when considering these reports is whether or not a single pathogenic process that affects a delimited range of structures can be described, and whether the dysfunction that results has general or discrete effects on behaviour and cognition in these individuals? The evidence is more consistent with the involvement of many developmental processes affecting many different regions, and manifesting in many different ways (Cannon and Mednick, 1991). Early neurodevelopmental disturbances can cascade and interact with each other and with other later neurodevelopmental processes, producing a variety of phenotypic structural deviations with diverse clinical manifestations.

A neurodevelopmental approach to schizophrenia is useful in explaining the failure of science in identifying any one unique feature of schizophrenia despite decades of research. As we have attempted to convey, neurodevelopment follows a complex and precise set of events, and is vulnerable to any number of insults both endogenous and exogenous. In addition, the timing and the severity of these hypothesised insults will directly affect the nature of the resulting neuropathology. Furthermore, each individual is exposed to a unique environment and set of life events that may interact with their specific neuropathology, contributing further to the differential presentation of the illness. With all these variables going into the mix, it is no wonder that the formula creating schizophrenia remains elusive. It is our belief, however, that with increasing knowledge of how normal neurodevelopment proceeds we may better understand the causes and consequences of faulty neurodevelopment and the role that they play in schizophrenia. With this knowledge, improvement in treatment for those already afflicted with schizophrenia might be achieved, and better yet, preventive measures could be taken to avoid the neurodevelopmental aberrations that may lead to schizophrenia in future generations.

References

Akbarian, S., Bunney, W.E., Potkin, S.G. *et al.* (1993*a*). Altered distribution of nicotinamide-adenine dinucleotide phosphate-diaphorase cells in frontal lobe of schizophrenics implies disturbances in cortical development. *Archives of General Psychiatry*, **50**, 169–87.

Akbarian, S., Vinuela, A., Kim, J.J. *et al.* (1993*b*). Distorted distribution of nicotinamide-adenine dinucleotide phosphate-diaphorase neurons in temporal lobe of schizophrenics implies anomalous cortical development. *Archives of General Psychiatry*, **50**, 178–87.

Altshuler, L.L., Conrad, A., Kovelman, J.A. and Scheibel, A. (1987). Hippocampal pyramidal cell orientation in schizophrenia. *Archives of General Psychiatry*, **44**, 1094–8.

Andreasen, N.C., Nasrallah, H.A., Dunn, V. *et al.* (1986). Structural abnormalities in the frontal system in schizophrenia. *Archives of General Psychiatry*, **43**, 136–44.

Andreasen, N.C., Ehrhardt, J.C., Swayze, V.W. *et al.* (1990). Magnetic resonance imaging of the brain in schizophrenia: the pathophysiological significance of structural abnormalities. *Archives of General Psychiatry*, **47**, 35–44.

Arnold, S.E., Hyman, B.T., Van Hosesen, G.W. and Damasio, A.R. (1991). Some cytoarchitectural abnormalities in the entorhinal cortex in schizophrenia. *Archives of General Psychiatry*, **48**, 625–32.

Averback, P. (1981). Structural lesions of the brain in young schizophrenics, *Le Journal Canadien des Sciences Neurologiques*, **8**, 73–8.

Beckmann, H. and Jakob, H. (1991). Prenatal disturbances of nerve cell migration in the entorhinal region: a common vulnerability factor in functional psychoses? *Journal of Neural Transmission*, **84**, 155–64.

Benes, F.M. (1987). An analysis of the arrangement of neurons in the cingulate cortex of schizophrenic patients. *Archives of General Psychiatry*, **44**, 608–16.

Benes, F.M., Davidson, B. and Bird, E.D. (1986). Quantitative cytoarchitectural studies of the cerebral cortex of schizophrenics. *Archives of General Psychiatry*, **43**, 31–5.

Benes, F.M., McSparren, J., Bird, E.D. *et al.* (1991*a*). Deficits in small interneurons in prefrontal and cingulate cortices of schizophrenic and schizoaffective patients. *Archives of General Psychiatry*, **48**, 996–1001.

Benes, F.M., Sorensen, I. and Bird, E.D. (1991*b*). Reduced neuronal size in posterior hippocampus of schizophrenic patients. *Schizophrenia Bulletin*, **17**, 597–608.

Bogerts, B. (1989). Limbic and paralimbic pathology in schizophrenia: interaction with age and stress related factors. In *Schizophrenia: Scientific Progress* (ed. S.C. Schulz and C.A. Tamminga), pp. 216–26. Oxford: Oxford University Press.

Bogerts, B. and Falkai, P. (1991). Clinical and neurodevelopmental aspects of brain pathology in schizophrenia. In *Developmental Neuropathology of Schizophrenia* (ed. S.A. Mednick, T.D. Cannon, C.E. Barr and J.M. LaFosse), pp. 93–120. New York: Plenum Press.

Bogerts, B., Meertz, E. and Schonfeldt-Bausch, R. (1985). Basal ganglia and limbic system pathology in schizophrenia: a morphometric study of brain volume and shrinkage. *Archives of General Psychiatry*, **42**, 784–91.

Bogerts, B., Falkai, P., Haupts, M. *et al.* (1990*a*). Postmortem volume measurements of limbic systems and basal ganglia structures in chronic schizophrenics. Initial results from a new brain collection. *Schizophrenia Research*, **3**, 295–301.

Bogerts, B., Ashtari, M., Degreef, G. *et al.* (1990*b*). Reduced temporal limbic structure volumes on magnetic resonance images in first episode schizophrenia. *Psychiatry Research*, **35**, 1–13.

Bruton, C.J., Crow, T.J., Frith, C.D. *et al.* (1990). Schizophrenia and the brain: a prospective clinico-neuropathological study. *Psychological Medicine*, **20**, 285–304.

Cannon, T.D. (1991*a*). The possible neurodevelopmental significance of structural imaging findings in schizophrenia. In *Developmental Neuropathology of Schizophrenia* (ed. S.A. Mednick, T.D. Cannon, C.E. Barr and J.M. LaFosse) pp. 149–66. New York: Plenum Press.

Cannon, T.D. (1991*b*). Genetic and perinatal sources of structural brain abnormalities in schizophrenia. In *Fetal Neural Development and Adult Schizophrenia* (ed. S.A. Mednick, T.D. Cannon, C.E. Barr and M. Lyon), pp. 174–98. Cambridge: Cambridge University Press.

Cannon, T.D. and Marco, E.J. (1994). Structural brain abnormalities as indicators of vulnerability to schizophrenia. *Schizophrenia Bulletin*, **20**, 89–102.

Cannon, T.D. and Mednick, S.A. (1991). Fetal neural development and adult schizophrenia: an elaboration of the paradigm. In *Fetal Neural Development and Adult Schizophrenia* (ed. S.A. Mednick, T.D. Cannon, C.E. Barr and M. Lyon), pp. 227–37. Cambridge: Cambridge University Press.

Cannon, T.D., Mednick, S.A. and Parnas, J. (1990). Antecedents of predominantly negative and predominantly positive-symptom schizophrenia in a high-risk population. *Archives of General Psychiatry*, **47**, 622–32.

Cannon, T.D., Mednick, S.A., Parnas, J. *et al.* (1993). Developmental brain abnormalities in the offspring of schizophrenic mothers. I. Contributions of genetic and perinatal factors. *Archives of General Psychiatry*, **50**, 551–63.

Cannon, T.D., Eyler Zorrilla, L., Shtasel, D. *et al.* (1994). Neuropsychological functioning in siblings discordant for schizophrenia and healthy volunteers. *Archives of General Psychiatry*, **51**, 651–61.

Casanova, M.F., Kleinman, J.E. and Weinberger, D.R. (1988). Neuropathological studies on the limbic system of schizophrenics. *ACNP* Abstract Number 1988.

Casonova, M.F., Stevens, J.R. and Kleinman, J.E. (1990). Astrocytosis in the molecular layer of the dentate gyrus: a study in Alzheimer's disease and schizophrenia. *Psychiatry Research*, **35**, 149–66.

Casey, D.E. and Hansen, T.E. (1984). Spontaneous dyskinesias. In *Neuropsychiatric Movement Disorders* (ed. D.V. Jeste and R.J. Wyatt), pp. 68–95. Washington DC: American Psychiatric Press, Inc.

Conrad, A.J. and Scheibel, A.B. (1987). Schizophrenia and the hippocampus: the embryological hypothesis extended. *Schizophrenia Bulletin*, **13**, 577–88.

Conrad, A.J., Abebe, T., Austin, R. *et al.* (1991). Hippocampal pyramidal cell disarray in schizophrenia as a bilateral phenomenon. *Archives of General Psychiatry*, **48**, 413–17.

Crow, T.J. (1989). A current view of the Type II syndrome: age of onset, intellectual impairment, and the meaning of structural changes in the brain. *British Journal of Psychiatry*, **7**, 15–20.

Dagg, B.M., Booth, J.D., McLaughlin, J.E. and Dolan, R.J. (1994). A morphometric study of the cingulate cortex in mood disorder and schizophrenia. *Schizophrenia Research*, **11**, 137.

DeLisi, L.E., Goldin, L.R., Hamovit, J.R. *et al.* (1986). A family study of the association of increased ventricular size with schizophrenia. *Archives of General Psychiatry*, **43**, 148–53.

DeMyer, M.K., Gilmer, R.L., Hendrie, H.C. *et al.* (1988). Magnetic resonance brain images in schizophrenic and normal subjects: influence of diagnosis and education. *Schizophrenia Bulletin*, **14**, 21–37.

Edelman, G. (1982). Embryonic to adult conversion of neural cell adhesion molecules in normal and staggerer mice. *Proceedings National Academy of Science USA*, **79**, 703–6.

Eyler-Zorrilla, L.T. and Cannon, T.D. (1995). Structural brain abnormalities in schizophrenia: distribution, etiology, and implications. In *Neural Development and Schizophrenia: Theory and Research* (ed. S.A. Mednick and J.M. Hollister) pp. 57–69. New York: Plenum Press.

Falkai, P. and Bogerts, B. (1989). Cell loss in the hippocampus of schizophrenics. *European Archives of Psychiatry and Neurological Science*, **106**, 505–17.

Falkai, P., Bogerts, B. and Rozumek, M. (1988*a*). Cell loss and volume reduction in the entorhinal cortex of schizophrenics. *Biological Psychiatry*, **24**, 515–21.

Falkai, P., Bogerts, B., Roberts, G.W. and Crow, T.J. (1988*b*). Measurement of the alpha-cell-migration in the entorhinal region: a marker for developmental disturbances in schizophrenia? *Schizophrenia Research*, **1**, 157–8.

Feinberg, I. (1982). Schizophrenia: caused by a fault in programmed synaptic elimination during adolescence? *Journal of Psychiatry Research*, **17**, 319–30.

Fenton, W.S., Wyatt, R.J. and McGlashan, T.H. (1994). Risk factors for spontaneous dyskinesia in schizophrenia. *Archives of General Psychiatry*, **51**, 643–50.

Fish, B., Marcus, J., Hans, S.L. *et al.* (1992). Infants at risk for schizophrenia: sequelae of a genetic neurointegrative defect. *Archives of General Psychiatry*, **49**, 221–35.

Fisman, M. (1975). The brain stem in psychosis. *British Journal of Psychiatry*, **126**, 414–22.

Heckers, S., Heinsen, H., Geiger, B. and Beckman, H. (1991*a*). Hippocampal neuron number in schizophrenia: a stereological study. *Archives of General Psychiatry*, **48**, 1002–8.

Heckers, S., Heinsen, H., Heinsen, Y. and Beckmann, H. (1991*b*). Cortex, white matter, and basal ganglia in schizophrenia: a volumetric postmortem study. *Biological Psychiatry*, **29**, 556–66.

Hertzig, M.E. and Birch, H.G. (1966). Neurologic organization in psychiatrically disturbed adolescent girls. *Archives of General Psychiatry*, **15**, 590–8.

Hertzig, M.E. and Birch, H.G. (1968). Neurologic organization in psychiatrically disturbed adolescents: a comparative consideration of sex differences. *Archives of General Psychiatry*, **19**, 528–37.

Hoffman, R.E. and Dobscha, S.K. (1989). Cortical pruning and the development of schizophrenia: a computer model. *Schizophrenia Bulletin*, **15**, 477–90.

Hollister, J.M., Laing, P. and Mednick, S.A. (1996). Rhesus incompatibility as a risk factor for schizophrenia in male adults. *Archives of General Psychiatry*, **53**, 19–24.

Jakob, J. and Beckmann, H. (1986). Prenatal developmental disturbances in the limbic allocortex in schizophrenics. *Journal of Neural Transmission*, **65**, 303–26.

Janes, C.L., Weeks, D.G. and Worland, J. (1983). School behavior in adolescent children of parents with mental disorder. *Journal of Nervous and Mental Disease*, **171**, 234–40.

Jeste, D.V. and Lohr, J.B. (1989). Hippocampal pathologic findings in schizophrenia: a morphometric study. *Archives of General Psychiatry*, **46**, 1019–24.

John, R.S., Mednick, S.A. and Schulsinger, F. (1982). Teacher reports as a predictor of schizophrenia and borderline schizophrenia: a Bayesian decision analysis. *Journal of Abnormal Psychology*, **91**, 399–413.

Johnstone, E.C., Crow, T.J., Frith, C.D. *et al.* (1976). Cerebral ventricular size and cognitive impairment in chronic schizophrenia. *Lancet*, 924–6.

Johnstone, E.C., Crow, T.J., Frith, C.D. *et al.* (1978). The dementia of dementia praecox. *Acta Psychiatrica Scandinavica*, **57**, 305–24.

Johnstone, E.C., MacMillan, J.F., Frith, C.D. *et al.* (1990). Further investigation of outcome following first schizophrenic episodes. *British Journal of Psychiatry*, **157**, 182–9.

Jones, P., Murray, R. and Rodgers, B. (1995). Childhood risk factors for adult schizophrenia in a general population birth cohort at age 43 years. In *Neural Development of Schizophrenia: Theory and Research* (ed. S.A. Mednick and J.M. Hollister), pp. 151–76. New York: Plenum Press.

Kennard, M.A. (1960). Value of equivocal signs in neurologic diagnosis. *Neurology*, **10**, 753–64.

Keshavan, M.S., Anderson, S. and Pettegrew, J.W. (1994). Is schizophrenia due to excessive synaptic pruning in the prefrontal cortex? The Feinberg Hypothesis revisited. *Journal of Psychiatric Research*, **28**, 239–65.

Kikinis, R., Shenton, M.E., Gerig, G. *et al.* (1994). Temporal lobe sulci-gyral pattern anomalies in schizophrenia: an in vivo MR three-dimensional surface rendering study. *Neuroscience Letters*, **182**, 7–12.

Klausner, J.D., Sweeney, J.P., Deck, M.D. *et al.* (1992). Clinical correlates of cerebral ventricular enlargement in schizophrenia. *Journal of Nervous and Mental Disorders*, **180**, 407.

Kovelman, J.A. and Scheibel, A.B. (1984). A neurohistological correlate of schizophrenia. *Biological Psychiatry*, **19**, 1601–21.

Kraepelin, E. (1919). *Dementia Praecox and Paraphrenia*. Edinburgh: Livingstone.

Laing, P., Knight, J.G., Wright, P. and Irving, W.L. (1995). Disruption of fetal brain development by maternal antibodies as an etiological factor in schizophrenia. In *Neural Development of Schizophrenia: Theory and Research* (ed. S.A. Mednick and J.M. Hollister), pp. 215–46. New York: Plenum Press.

Larroche, J.-C. (1984). Perinatal brain damage. In *Greenfield's Neuropathology*, 4th edition (ed. J.H. Adams, J.A.N. Corsellis and L.W. Duchen), pp. 458–80. New York: John Wiley & Sons.

Manshreck, T.C., Maher, B.A., Rucklos, M.E. *et al.* (1981). Deficient motor synchrony in schizophrenia. *Journal of Abnormal Psychology*, **90**, 321–8.

Margolis, R.L., Chang, D.-M. and Post, R.M. (1994). Programmed cell death: implications for neuropsychiatric disorders. *Biological Psychiatry*, **35**, 946–56.

McLardy, T. (1974). Hippocampal zinc and structural deficits in brains from chronic alcoholics and some schizophrenics. *Journal of Orthomolecular Psychiatry*, **4**, 32–6.

Mednick, S.A. and Cannon, T.D. (1991). Fetal development, birth and the syndromes of adult schizophrenia. In *Fetal Neural Development and Adult Schizophrenia* (ed. S.A. Mednick, T.D. Cannon, C.E. Barr, M. Lyon) pp. 3–13. Cambridge: Cambridge University Press.

Mednick, S.A., Machon, R.A., Huttunen, M.O. and Bonett, D. (1988). Adult schizophrenia following prenatal exposure to an influenza epidemic. *Archives of General Psychiatry*, **45**, 189–92.

Mednick, S.A. and Silverton, L. (1987). High risk studies of the etiology of schizophrenia. In *Handbok of Schizophrenia, Vol. 3: Nosology, Epidemiology and Genetics* (ed. M.T. Tsuang and J.C. Simpson), pp. 543–62. Amsterdam: Elsevier.

Nasrallah, H.A., McCalley-Whitters, M., Rauscher, F.P. *et al.* (1983). A histological study of the corpus callosum in chronic schizophrenia. *Psychiatry Research*, **8**, 151–60.

Nieto, D. and Escobar, A. (1972). Major psychoses. In *Pathology of the Nervous System* (ed. J. Minkler), pp. 2654–65. New York: McGraw-Hill.

Nowakowski, R.S. (1988). Development of the hippocampal formation in mutant mice. *Drug Development Research*, **15**, 315.

Nowakowski, R.S. (1991). Neuronal migration and differentiation during normal and genetically perturbed development of the hippocampal formation. In *Developmental Neuropathology of Schizophrenia* (ed. S.A. Mednick, T.D. Cannon, C.E. Barr and J.M. LaFosse), pp. 29–60. New York: Plenum Press.

Olin, S.S., John, R.S. and Mednick, S.A. (1995). Assessing the predictive value of teacher reports in a high risk sample for schizophrenia: a ROC analysis. *Schizophrenia Research*, **16**, 53–66.

Pakkenberg, B. (1990). Pronounced reduction of total neuron number in mediodorsal thalamic nucleus and nucleus accumbens in schizophrenics. *Archives of General Psychiatry*, **47**, 1023–8.

Pakkenberg, B. (1992*a*). Stereological quantitation of human brains from normal and schizophrenic individuals. *Acta Neurologica Scandinavica*, **137** (suppl), 20–33.

Pakkenberg, B. (1992*b*). The volume of the mediodorsal thalamic nucleus in treated and untreated schizophrenics. *Schizophrenia Research*, **7**, 95–100.

Pandurangi, A.K., Dewan, M.J., Boucher, M. *et al.* (1986). A comprehensive study of chronic schizophrenic patients: II Biological, neuropsychological, and clinical correlates of CT abnormality. *Acta Psychiatrica Scandinavica*, **73**, 161–71.

Parnas, J. and Jorgensen, A. (1989). Premorbid psychopathology in schizophrenia spectrum. *British Journal of Psychiatry*, **155**, 623–7.

Parnas, J., Schulsinger, F., Schulsinger, H. and Mednick, S.A. (1982*a*). Behavioral precursors of schizophrenia spectrum: a prospective study. *Archives of General Psychiatry*, **39**, 658–64.

Parnas, J., Schulsinger, F., Teasedale, T.W. *et al.* (1982*b*). Perinatal complications and clinical outcome within the schizophrenia spectrum. *British Journal of Psychiatry*, **140**, 416–20.

Pinto-Lord, M.C., Evrard, P. and Caviness, V.S. (1982). Obstructed neuronal migration along radial glial fibres in the neocortex of the Reeler mouse: a golgi-EM analysis. *Developmental Brain Research*, **4**, 379.

Raine, A., Lencz, T., Reynolds, G.P. *et al.* (1992). An evaluation of structural and functional prefrontal deficits in schizophrenia: MRI and neuropsychological measures. *Psychiatry Research: Neuroimaging*, **45**, 123–37.

Raz, S. and Raz, N. (1990). Structural brain abnormalities in the major psychoses: a quantitative review of the evidence from computerized imaging. *Psychological Bulletin*, **108**, 93–108.

Reiter, P.J. (1926). Extrapyramidal motor disturbances in dementia praecox. *Acta Psychiatrica et Neurologica Scandinavica*, **1**, 287–309.

Reveley, M.A., Reveley, M.A., Clifford, C.A. and Murray, R.M. (1982). Cerebral ventricular size in twins discordant for schizophrenia. *Lancet*, **1**, 540–1.
Roberts, G.W., Colter, N., Lofthouse, R. *et al.* (1986). Gliosis in schizophrenia: a survey. *Biological Psychiatry*, **21**, 1043–50.
Roberts, G.W., Colter, N., Lofthouse, R. *et al.* (1987). Is there gliosis in schizophrenia? Investigation of the temporal lobe. *Biological Psychiatry*, **22**, 1459–68.
Rochford, J.M., Detre, T., Tucker, G.J. and Harrow, M. (1970). Neuropsychological impairments in functional psychiatric diseases. *Archives of General Psychiatry*, **22**, 114–19.
Rorke, L.B. (1992). Perinatal brain damage. In *Greenfield's Neuropathology*, 5th edition (ed. J.H. Adams and L.W. Duchen), pp. 639–708. New York: Oxford University Press.
Rubin, P., Karle, A., Moller-Madsen, S. *et al.* (1993). Computerized tomography in newly diagnosed schizophrenia and schizophreniform disorder: a controlled blind study. *British Journal of Psychiatry*, **163**, 604–12.
Scheibel, A.B. and Kovelman, J.A. (1981). Disorientation of the hippocampal pyramidal cells and its processes in the schizophrenic patient. *Biological Psychiatry*, **16**, 101–2.
Schwartzman, A.E., Ledingham, J.E. and Serbin, L.A. (1985). Identification of children at risk for adult schizophrenia: a longitudinal study. *International Review of Applied Psychology*, **34**, 363–80.
Selemon, L.D., Rajkowska, G. and Goldman-Rakic, P.S. (1993). A morphometric analysis of the prefrontal areas 9 and 46 in the schizophrenic and normal human brain. *Schizophrenia Research*, **9**, 151.
Stevens, J.R. (1982). Neuropathology of schizophrenia. *Archives of General Psychiatry*, **39**, 1131–9.
Stevens, J.R. and Casanova, M.F. (1988). Is there a neuropathology of schizophrenia? *Biological Psychiatry*, **24**, 123–8.
Suddath, R.L., Christison, G., Torrey, E.F. *et al.* (1989). Quantitative magnetic resonance imaging in twin pairs discordant for schizophrenia. *Schizophrenia Research*, **2**, 129.
Suddath, R.L., Christison, G.W., Torrey, E.F. *et al.* (1990). Anatomical abnormalities in the brains of monozygotic twins discordant for schizophrenia. *New England Journal of Medicine*, **322**, 789–94.
Walker, E.F. (1994). Developmentally moderated expressions of the neuropathology underlying schizophrenia. *Schizophrenia Bulletin*, **20**, 453–80.
Walker, E.F., Savoie, T. and Davis, D. (1994). Neuromotor precursors of schizophrenia. *Schizophrenia Bulletin*, **20**, 441–51.
Watt, N.F. (1972). Longitudinal changes in the social behavior of children hospitalized for schizophrenia as adults. *Journal of Nervous and Mental Disease*, **155**, 42–54.
Watt, N.F. (1978). Patterns of childhood social development in adult schizophrenics. *Archives of General Psychiatry*, **35**, 160–5.
Watt, N.F. and Lubensky, A.W. (1976). Childhood roots of schizophrenia. *Journal of Counseling and Clinical Psychology*, **44**, 363–75.
Watt, N.F., Grubb, T.W. and Erlenmeyer-Kimling, L. (1982). Social, emotional and intellectual behavior at school among children at high risk for schizophrenia. *Journal of Counseling and Clinical Psychology*, **50**, 171–81.
Weinberger, D.R. (1987). Implications of normal brain development for the pathogenesis of schizophrenia. *Archives of General Psychiatry*, **44**, 660–9.

Weinberger, D.R., Torrey, E.F., Neophytides, A.N. and Wyatt, R.J. (1979). Lateral cerebral ventricular enlargement in schizophrenia. *Archives of General Psychiatry*, **36**, 735–9.

Weinberger, D.R., DeLisi, L.E., Neophytides, A.N. and Wyatt, R.J. (1981). Familial aspects of CT scan abnormalities in chronic schizophrenic patients. *Psychiatric Research*, **4**, 65–71.

Wright, P., Gill, M. and Murray, R.M. (1993). Schizophrenia: genetics and the maternal immune response to viral infection. *American Journal of Genetics (Neuropsychiatric Genetics)*, **48**, 40–6.

Yarden, P.E. and Discipio, W.J. (1971). Abnormal movements and prognosis in schizophrenia. *American Journal of Psychiatry*, **128**, 317–23.

Section VII

Imaging brain and mind: new approaches

13

Magnetic resonance spectroscopy in neuropsychiatry

MICHAEL MAIER

Introduction

Significant advances in the study of the human brain have been made possible with the use of nuclear magnetic resonance (NMR) technology. Magnetic resonance imaging (MRI), magnetic resonance spectroscopy (MRS), and more recently functional MRI (fMRI) have been important developments.

MRI provides high resolution spatial images and is able to demonstrate alterations in anatomy that accompany disease processes, and fMRI demonstrates regional blood flow changes within the brain. These two applications of NMR have become a familiar concept for most clinicians. Only MRS, however, is able to provide a means of looking at the biochemical parameters in brain disease by detecting, non-invasively, the major brain metabolites.

NMR was developed around 1945 as a tool to study the magnetic properties of atomic nuclei, and the first NMR experiment was performed simultaneously, but independently, by Purcell, Torrey and Pound (1946) and Bloch, Hansen and Packard (1946) in the USA, and Bloch and Purcell were awarded the Nobel Prize in 1952 for their discovery.

It was with the advent of powerful computers that tomographic techniques became possible and in 1973 Lauterbur reported the first reconstruction of a proton spin density map using nuclear magnetic resonance. In the same year Mansfield and Grannell independently demonstrated the Fourier relationship between the spin density and the NMR signal acquired in the presence of a magnetic field gradient.

Initially, NMR spectroscopy experiments were done *in vitro* on biological samples and in 1973 Moon and Richards obtained a Phosphorus-31 spectrum of a suspension of erythrocytes. As larger and more stable magnets became available larger parts of the human body were studied.

Table 13.1. *A selection of biologically interesting nuclei that can be studied by NMR, together with their relative sensitivities and natural abundance of the isotopes*

Atomic nucleus	Sensitivity	Natural abundance (%)
^{1}H	100	100
^{31}P	6.6	100
^{19}F	83.4	100
^{7}Li	29	93
^{23}Na	9.2	100
^{13}C	1.6	1.1
^{39}K	5.1	93

Hoult *et al.* (1974) obtained NMR spectra from non-perfused muscle and initial human *in vivo* studies of the brain using proton MRS were done by Bottomley *et al.* (1985) and Luyten *et al.* (1986). Today it is possible to do *in vivo* NMR, not only of protons (^{1}H) and phosphorous (^{31}P), but studies of ^{13}C, ^{19}F, and ^{7}Li have also been reported. Reviews of MR techniques, applied to the brain, have appeared in the literature (Keshavan, Kapur and Pettegrew, 1991*a*; de Certaines *et al.*, 1992; Shulman *et al.*, 1993; Vion-Dury *et al.*, 1994; Maier, 1995).

In this chapter the principles and application of MRS to the investigations of neuropsychiatric conditions will be reviewed.

The principles of nuclear magnetic resonance

Various names are used to describe this technology, and their origins are mainly historical. The phenomenon was initially called nuclear induction in the 1940s. Later in the 1950s it was called nuclear paramagnetic resonance, and only since the 1950s has the term nuclear magnetic resonance been preferred to describe the physical process. When clinical imaging methods were developed the nuclear term was dropped partly because of patients' concern about the danger of radioactivity. MR imaging and spectroscopy have become the preferred names for the radiological techniques, although the term NMR is still preferable when describing the physical phenomenon itself.

Some atomic nuclei possess angular momentum, a property also called spin in quantum mechanics. Only nuclei with a spin value greater than zero can be detected by NMR and Table 13.1 shows some biologically interesting nuclei together with their natural abundance and their relative sensitivity in the NMR experiment.

Nuclear spin is a quantum mechanical concept and for the proton the spin value is quantised i.e. it can only take on certain values in a magnetic field. The NMR experiment measures the sum of all the individual spins present in the sample being studied and the bulk magnetisation from all the spins in the sample can be represented by a vector. In addition all NMR active atomic nuclei possess a magnetic dipole moment, and they behave as if they were small bar magnets and they will tend to align with a magnetic field. These two properties of angular momentum and a magnetic dipole cause the atomic nucleus, and the magnetisation vector, to move in a precessional way (like a gyroscope) in the magnetic field. The precessional frequency (ω), also called the Larmor frequency, is determined by a property of the nucleus called the magnetogyric ratio (γ) and the strength of the magnetic field (B_0), on which it is linearly dependent. The relationship between these three constants is;

$$\omega = \gamma \times B_0$$

Thus a proton which has a resonant frequency of 64 MHz at 1.5 T will have a resonant frequency of 128 MHz at 3 T.

The role of the magnet of the scanner is to align the individual spins along the direction of the field, thereby producing a net magnetic moment, and consequently the person in the magnet becomes magnetised but the magnetisation is very small. The magnetisation vector can then be perturbed by a brief pulse of energy, at the Larmor frequency, and the nuclei are forced away from their orientation along the direction of the static magnetic field. Once the perturbing pulse is switched off the nuclei will reorientate themselves along the static field in a time called the spin-lattice relaxation time (T_1). There will be loss of phase coherence in the x–y plane with a relaxation time called the spin-spin relaxation time (T_2). T_1 and T_2 are also called the longitudinal and transverse relaxation times respectively. The precessional motion of the net magnetisation vector as it reorientates itself with the magnetic field can induce an alternating voltage signal in a coil of wire, with an axis orthogonal to the magnetic field, that constitutes the receiver coil of the typical MR imaging machine. This signal is called the free induction decay (shown in Figure 13.1a). When a Fourier transformation is applied to this FID it yields a spectrum like the one seen in Figure 13.1b.

Because individual nuclei find themselves in various different magnetic fields caused by differing chemical and molecular environments they give rise to a spectrum of signals, also known as chemical shift.

Whilst the concentration of protons in the brain, due to water, is around

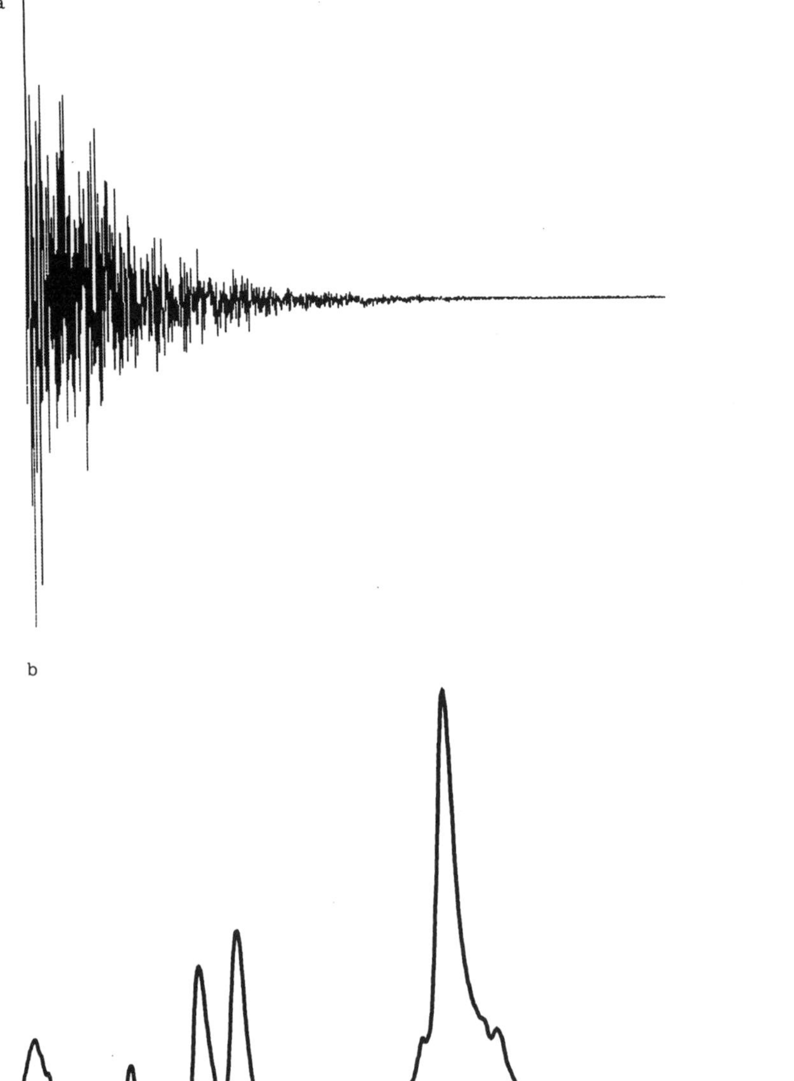

Figure 13.1. (a). The decay of the NMR signal over time, also called the Free Induction Decay (FID).
(b) The FID can be transformed to display the component frequencies of the decaying signal and thus produce a spectrum.

80–100 molar, making the acquisition of MR images relatively simple, MRS has been a more challenging technique. The concentration of brain metabolites is in the millimolar range and lower (some 10 000-fold smaller than proton concentrations of water). The current lower level of detectability by MRS is around the millimolar range, and many interesting metabolites in the brain are consequently at concentrations much lower than can be detected by MRS. Imaging can be done on machines that have relatively low magnetic fields (0.1–1.0 T), whereas MRS is difficult at low magnetic fields because the separation of spectral lines (chemical shift) depends on the magnitude of the field. It is accepted that the minimum field strength necessary for proton spectroscopy is 1.5 T, and machines with fields of up to 4 T are now available. For comparison the earth's magnetic field is between 30 and 70 μT depending on the latitude, and large electromagnets that pick up scrap metal and cars have fields of 1.5–2.0 T but their fields are extremely inhomogeneous.

Because of the low concentration of metabolites the smallest volume of interest routinely used in proton MRS is around 1 cm^3. For nuclei that are less sensitive than protons larger volumes of interest need to be selected; for ^{31}P, where the signal is only 1/20 as strong (Table 13.1) as that obtained from protons, volumes of interest need to be about 27 cm^3 in order to give a sufficient signal. In contrast to localised single voxel spectroscopy chemical shift imaging is a combination of both spectroscopic and imaging techniques to produce images of individual metabolites (Brown, Kincaid and Ugurbil, 1982), which allows large areas of the brain to be studied simultaneously. These images show distributions of metabolites and have been used to locate epileptic foci in epilepsy and in future may be used to identify regions of metabolite abnormality in the brain that demand further investigation.

Hydrogen, phosphorous and carbon are the commonest building blocks of molecules in the body and it is fortunate that these atomic nuclei are NMR active and MRS has already been used in medical research in a variety of fields such as the study of brain pathology and metabolism, cancer diagnosis, cardiac metabolism, the liver, kidney and the musculoskeletal system.

(a) Proton magnetic resonance spectroscopy (^1H-MRS)

Proton spectroscopy is perhaps the most powerful MRS modality as most molecules in the body contain hydrogen and the technique is only limited by the concentration of the metabolite being studied (Frahm *et al.*, 1989).

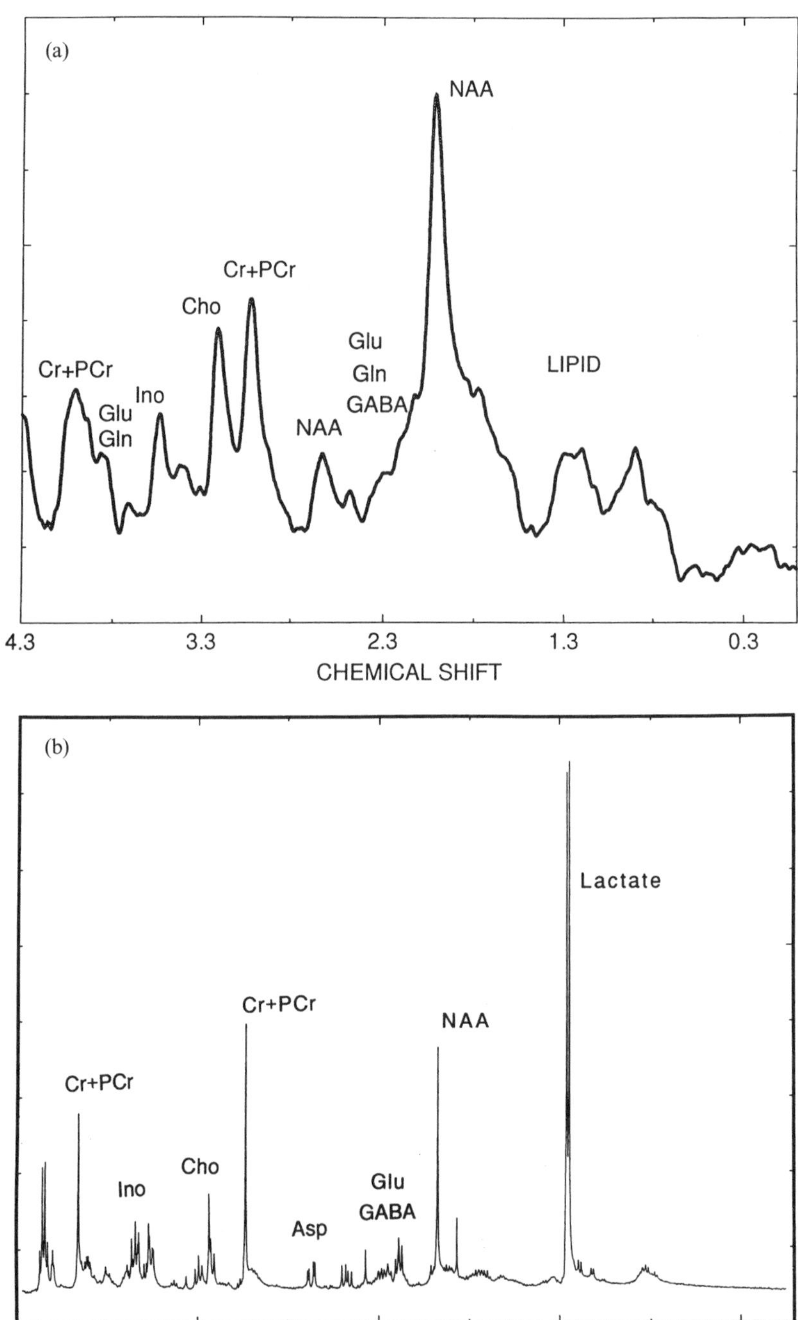
(a)
NAA
Cr+PCr
Cho
Glu
Gln
GABA
LIPID
Cr+PCr
Ino
Glu
Gln
NAA
4.3
3.3
2.3
1.3
0.3
CHEMICAL SHIFT
(b)
Lactate
Cr+PCr
NAA
Cr+PCr
Cho
Ino
Glu
GABA
Asp
4.3
3.3
2.3
1.3
0.3
CHEMICAL SHIFT

Figures 13.2(a,b) show an *in vitro* and an *in vivo* spectrum of human brain for comparison. The *in vivo* spectrum has been collected from a volume of interest of around 4 cm^3, whereas the *in vitro* spectrum is from a prepared homogenate of a few milligrams of cerebral tissue. In the *in vivo* spectrum one can see the inherently poorer resolution of spectral lines, and larger line widths, compared to *in vitro* spectroscopy. Because the *in vitro* experiment is inherently more sensitive many more peaks can be seen in the *in vitro* sample than *in vivo*.

The peak due to *N*-acetyl aspartate (NAA) is often the largest signal in the *in vivo* spectrum. In addition a signal due to the combined sum of creatine and phosphocreatine (Cr+PCr) is also strong, as is that due to the sum of the choline-containing compounds (Cho).

The exact biochemical role of these compounds has not been established and is a current area of research. The relevance of these metabolites in ^{1}H-MRS has been discussed by Vion-Dury *et al.* (1994). NAA is an intra-neuronal chemical, synthesised in the mitochondria and exported into the neural cytosol but its role in neuronal function is not fully understood (Birken and Oldendorf, 1989; Koller, Zaczek and Coyle, 1984; Miller, 1991). However, it has been shown that it is not present in non-neuronal tumours such as gliomas (Gill *et al.*, 1990), and animal experiments have shown NAA to decline following selective neuronal death after kainate injection (Koller *et al.*, 1984). Reduced levels of NAA *in vivo* have been reported in a variety of conditions leading to neuronal or axonal loss such as in acute and chronic multiple sclerosis (Arnold *et al.*, 1990; Miller *et al.*, 1991), acute cerebral infarction (Bruhn *et al.*, 1989; Fisher *et al.*, 1992), hypoxic-ischaemic encephalopathy (Graham *et al.*, 1994), Creutzfeldt–Jakob disease (Bruhn *et al.*, 1991), HIV (Chong *et al.*, 1993; Meyerhoff *et al.*, 1994), and seizure disorders (Breiter *et al.*, 1994).

Evidence suggests that reversible changes in NAA can also occur, but that the extent of reversibility depends on whether neuronal or axonal death has occurred. Thus complete normalisation of NAA has been reported in successfully treated diabetic ketoacidosis in rats (Brenner *et al.*,

Figure 13.2. Proton NMR spectra of (a) *in vivo* human brain obtained at 1.5 T, and (b) *in vitro* perchloric acid extract of human brain at 11.5 T, demonstrating the higher resolution of spectral resonances obtained at high magnetic fields *in vitro*. Peak assignments are shown for *N*-acetyl aspartate (NAA); glutamate (Glu); glutamine (Gln); gamma-amino butyric acid (GABA); aspartate (Asp); creatine and phosphocreatine (Cr+PCr); choline (Cho); and inositol (Ino). Chemical shifts in parts per million.

1993), whilst only modest recoveries have been observed in evolving MS lesions (Davie *et al.*, 1994; De Stefano *et al.*, 1993) and following acute ischaemia (Arnold, 1992; Espanol *et al.*, 1992). Conversely, raised levels of NAA have been reported in Canavan's disease, a rare demyelinating autosomal recessive disorder linked with abnormally high concentrations of NAA in the brain as a result of aspartoacylase deficiency (Grodd *et al.*, 1990; Austin *et al.*, 1991).

The signal ascribed to Cho is due to quarternary ammonium methyl groups which are a part of choline, as well as other compounds such as glycerophosphocholine and phosphocholine and these also contribute to the signal. Choline is also present as part of membrane-associated molecules such as phosphatidylcholine and sphingomyelin and thus represents a major component of the myelin in the brain. It is unclear, however, how much these important molecules contribute to the Cho signal in MRS because of their restricted movement in the lipid membrane, and consequent short relaxation times.

Creatine and phosphocreatine both contribute to the Cr+PCr signal and they represent the storage form of high energy phosphate in the brain and are linked via the ATP/ADP equilibrium.

Peaks that can be seen in an *in vivo* proton spectrum are:

1. *N*-acetyl residues; of which *N*-acetyl aspartate (NAA) is the largest contributor, but there are also contributions from *N*-acetyl aspartate glutamate (NAAG), glutamate and sialic acid.
2. Creatine/phosphocreatine (Cr+PCr).
3. Quaternary ammonium methyl groups containing contributions from choline (Cho), phosphorylcholine, glycerylphosphorylcholine, taurine and inositols.
4. Myo-inositol (including myo-inositol monophosphate and glycine).
5. Glutamine, glutamate, alanine, aspartate, gamma aminobutyric acid.
6. Glucose.
7. Lactate.

Normal adult brain has been studied both by single voxel methods and by spectroscopic imaging (Michaelis *et al.*, 1993; Tedeschi *et al.*, 1995). A couple of general conclusions have been made by Tedeschi *et al.*; these are that in the normal brain there are no left/right asymmetries in the nine regions they studied, and that statistically significant patterns of signal distribution of metabolites can be identified.

The developmental changes in the brain between the immediate postnatal period and adolescence have been investigated by Toft *et al.* (1994 *a,b*) and Kreis *et al.* (1993) and in adulthood and the senium by Christiansen *et al.* (1993). It was found that in adulthood the concentration of NAA was significantly higher in the occipital lobe than in the basal ganglia, temporal and frontal lobes, and that there was also a significantly higher concentration of NAA in the occipital part of the brain in the younger age group than in the older one. There was no significant regional or age dependent variation in T_1 and T_2 relaxation times.

(b) Phosphorus magnetic resonance spectroscopy (^{31}P-MRS)

After hydrogen, phosphorous is the most important naturally occurring element in biological MRS studies, and phosphorous spectroscopy allows the direct measurement of brain membrane phospholipids and high energy phosphate metabolism. An *in vivo* phosphorus spectrum of brain is shown in Figure 13.3.

The *in vivo* phosphorus spectrum typically shows the following peaks.

1. Three peaks from adenosine triphosphate (α-ATP, β-ATP and γ-ATP)
2. Phosphocreatine (PCr)
3. Phosphodiesters (PDE) (glycerylphosphorylethanolamine, glycerylphosphorylcholine, glycerylphosphorylserine, and glycerylphosphorylinositol)
4. Phosphomonoesters (PME) (phosphorylethanolamine, phosphorylcholine and glycerylphosphate)
5. Inorganic phosphate (Pi).

The peaks due to PME and PDE are indicators of membrane synthesis. PME is a precursor of membrane phospholipids whilst PDE is mainly from the breakdown products of the membrane. They are both usually elevated when a tumour is metabolically active. It has been suggested that a fall of the PME/PDE ratio indicates a decrease in the rate of phospholipid synthesis, and conversely an increase in this ratio, an increase in synthesis. Thus studies of the ageing process in the normal brain show that with increasing age there is a significant decrease in the levels of PME and a significant increase in levels of PDE (Pettegrew, Keshavan and Minshew, 1993) and that this corresponds to a decreased synthesis and increased breakdown of membrane phospholipids and is perhaps due to loss of dendritic spines and processes that are observed in ageing. These changes are only evident after the age of 50 years and there are no age-related changes in PCr, Pi or ATP.

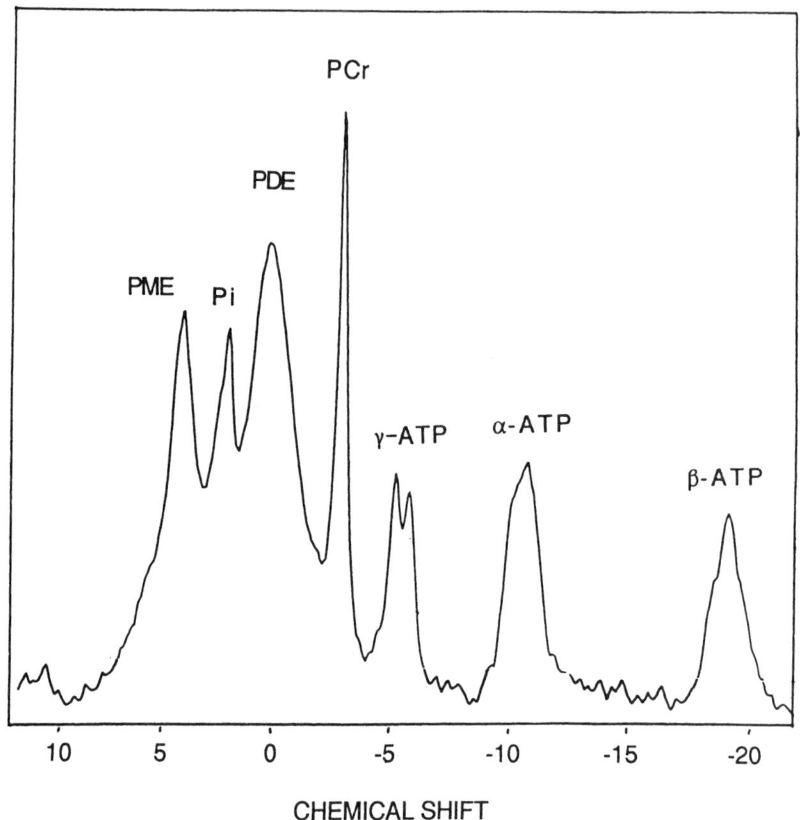

Figure 13.3. *In vivo* phosphorus-31 NMR spectrum of human brain obtained at 1.5 T. Peak assignments are shown for the three resonances of adenosine triphosphate (γ-, α-, β-ATP); phosphocreatine (Pcr); phosphodiesters (PDE); inorganic orthophosphate (Pi); and phosphomonoesters (PME). Chemical shifts in parts per million.

ATP is the energy-containing compound essential for oxidative metabolism, and three separate peaks (γ, α, β) represent signals from the three different phosphorous nuclei within the molecule.

PCr is the most metabolically labile of the brain high-energy phosphates and combines with ADP to form ATP and creatine. ATP in turn is then broken down to ADP and Pi together with the production of energy. The PCr/Pi ratio provides a convenient measure of the energy status of the brain.

Tissue pH has been estimated by measuring the chemical shift between Pi and PCr (Petroff *et al.*, 1985), or between the γ and α peaks of ATP (Pettegrew *et al.*, 1988*a*).

Applications of ^{1}H- and ^{31}P-MRS to the study of neuropsychiatric conditions

Epilepsy

Identifying the epileptic focus in the brain *in vivo* continues to be a challenging procedure that is still associated with a certain amount of uncertainty. In people with temporal lobe seizures approximately 65% have hippocampal sclerosis (Babb and Brown, 1987), and of these about 70% can be detected by MRI techniques. Visual determination of the foci can be difficult, however, when there is bilateral hippocampal involvement. *In vivo* MRS, alone and in combination with MRI, has been used to study the localisation of epileptic foci, especially in relation to surgical excision. Initial MRS studies used ^{31}P but this method provides poor spatial resolution. In spite of this limitation it was found that interictally, seizure foci were alkalotic and thus lateralisation of the seizure foci was possible (Hugg *et al.*, 1992*a,b*; Laxer *et al.*, 1992). Laxer and Garcia (1993) compared MRI, PET and SPECT scanning for preoperative evaluation of patients with epilepsy. Their conclusion was that MRI provided the best anatomical detail and that it contained prognostic information. PET provided useful information in some patients for whom MRI findings were absent or contradictory. Interictal SPECT lacked the specificity to be of use in the preoperative evaluation of refractory patients, whereas ictal SPECT appeared to be useful in temporal and extratemporal lobe epilepsy.

(a) Proton

In 1989 Petroff *et al.* used high field proton NMR spectroscopy to study specimens of histologically normal cerebral tissue from human subjects undergoing neurosurgery for epilepsy with a view to quantifying the cerebral metabolite concentrations. This work was later extended (Peeling and Sutherland, 1993) and it was found that ^{1}H-MRS aided in the diagnosis of the extent of chronic localized encephalitis and the severity of hippocampal gliosis.

Several studies have appeared demonstrating that ^{1}H-MRS can detect reduced levels of NAA in regions of the brain containing the epileptic foci. Vainio *et al.* (1994) have reported a study of seven patients undergoing surgical treatment for intractable temporal lobe epilepsy and compared these to nine normal controls. NAA concentrations were determined both *in vivo* and *in vitro*, on the brain specimen, following surgery. The concentrations of NAA were used to identify the laterality and the extent of the seizure focus. Connelly *et al.* (1994) measured a reduction of 22% in NAA, 15% increase in Cr+PCr and a 25% increase in Cho compounds in the medial temporal lobe ipsilateral to the seizure focus. There were smaller effects in the contralateral temporal lobe. They have suggested that these changes may reflect neuronal loss or damage together with reactive astrocytosis. Using the NAA/(Cr+PCr) ratio they found that this was low in 88% of the patients with 40% showing bilateral effects. On the basis of this ratio they correctly identified lateralization in 15 of the cases with three incorrect. The same group have studied the mesial temporal lobe in 20 children with intractable temporal lobe epilepsy and compared them with 13 normal subjects (Cross *et al.*, 1996). Abnormalities in the NAA/(Cho+Cr) ratio was seen in 75% of the subjects and was correctly lateralising in 55%, with bilateral abnormalities seen in 45%, and incorrectly lateralising in none. Overall they found a unilateral decrease in NAA of about 19% on the side ipsilateral to the seizure focus with a 5% decrease on the contralateral side, suggesting neuronal loss or dysfunction. There was also a bilateral increase of about 18% in creatine and choline consistent with reactive astrocytosis.

Giroud *et al.* (1994) have shown that MRS can detect reduced levels of NAA in epileptic foci even where CT and MRI show no atrophic lesions. In their report three patients with bilateral temporal lobe epilepsy, demonstrated by EEG and sphenoidal electrodes, were studied, and in all three abnormally low levels of NAA were detected bilaterally when compared with matched controls. Some researchers have extended single voxel MRS to chemical shift imaging and demonstrated that metabolite images of diagnostic quality can be produced and that the epileptic focus can be lateralised correctly even in those cases where the MRI appears normal (Layer *et al.*, 1993). Fazekas *et al.* (1995) have explored the role of glutamate in seizure related brain damage. In this case report a patient with continuous motor seizures showed swelling and signal hyperintensity (T2-weighted images) of the contralateral parietotemporal cortex, the thalamus and the ipsilateral cerebellum. MRS of the cortical lesion showed an increase of glutamate and/or glutamine. At a 3 month follow-up the swelling had disappeared but the NAA/Cho ratio was still reduced in the previously affected area.

(b) Phosphorus

Phosphorus magnetic resonance imaging has demonstrated various localised metabolic abnormalities within the epileptogenic region in patients with temporal lobe epilepsy, including alkalosis, increased inorganic phosphate and decreased phosphomonoester levels. In Kuzniecky's study of intractable unilateral temporal lobe epilepsy no differences in pH were detected between the patient group and the controls (Kuzniecky *et al.*, 1992). The phosphocreatine/inorganic phosphate ratio was reduced by 50% in the epileptogenic temporal lobe, and by 35% when compared with the unaffected contralateral temporal lobe. This study reported no differences in the ratio of phosphomonoesters to phosphodiesters between controls and patients. The authors conclude that *in vivo* ^{31}P-MRS yields a distinctive interictal metabolic profile in patients with intractable unilateral temporal lobe epilepsy and may permit noninvasive lateralising evidence of the seizure focus. In a study of eight patients with frontal lobe epilepsy, the epileptogenic region showed interictal alkalosis compared to the contralteral frontal lobe. The inorganic phosphate levels were not increased, but five of the patients had elevated pH and only two showed decreased phosphomonoesters (Garcia *et al.*, 1994).

Schizophrenia, affective disorder and autism

(a) Proton

The majority of studies using proton MRS appear in conference abstracts and fail to show differences in schizophrenics compared with controls (Moore *et al.*, 1992; Nasrallah *et al.*, 1992; Buckley *et al.*, 1993; Yurgelun-Todd *et al.*, 1993). The lack of significant results can be explained by the fact that ratios are routinely used in these studies, with the Cr+PCr signal as the denominator in the ratio calculation. It is assumed that the Cr+PCr signal does not change in the normal or diseased brain, and this assumption has been called into question by a study on a group of 25 schizophrenics and 32 controls looking bilaterally at the hippocampus (Maier *et al.*, 1995). In this study metabolite concentrations were calculated using the brain water signal, as an internal calibrant, from the same volume of interest as the metabolite spectrum. In the schizophrenic group there was a significant reduction of NAA ($P<0.009$), creatine ($P<0.012$) and choline ($P<0.045$) on the left side, whilst smaller losses of choline and creatine were found in the right hippocampus with little or no NAA loss. Figure 13.4 shows the percentage loss in metabolite concentration for left and right hippocampi. The asymmetry of the three metabolites in the normal brain shows a greater concentration on the left side, and this is reversed for NAA in schizophrenia. These abnormalities are found in both males and females

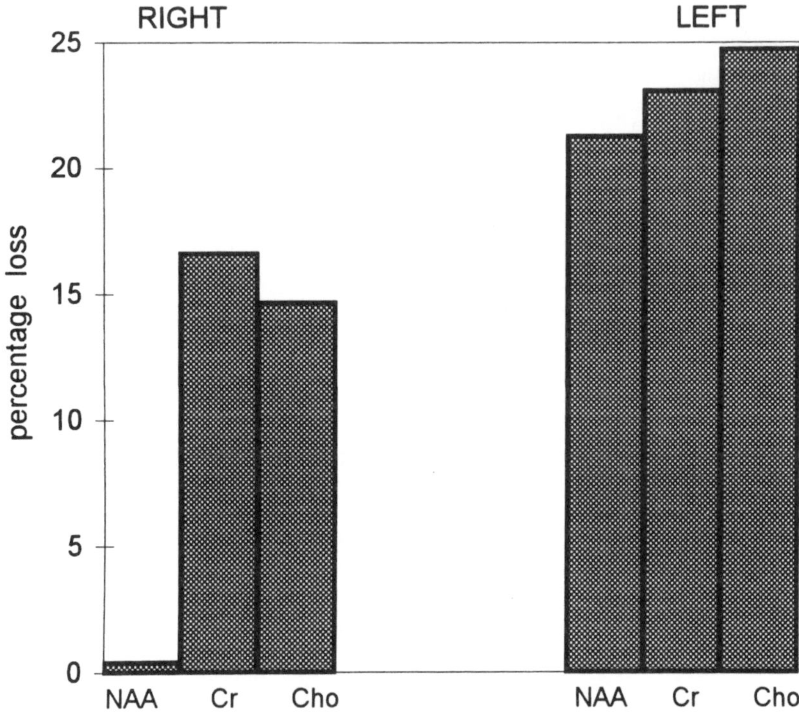

Figure 13.4. Mean group percentage loss of hippocampal metabolites in schizophrenics compared to normal controls. The figure demonstrates the left-sided loss of NAA (*N*-acetyl aspartate) with little or no changes in right-sided NAA, suggesting that changes in creatine and choline are not necessarily related to cell loss.

and are independent of age and neuroleptic medication. A reanalysis of the data using ratios of NAA/(Cr+PCr) and Cho/(Cr+PCr) failed to demonstrate the loss of NAA and choline because of the simultaneous loss of Cr+PCr.

Regressions of NAA, creatine and choline with age showed no difference between the schizophrenic and the control group in rate of change of metabolite concentration, suggesting that there is no progressive pathological process in the schizophrenic group other than normal aging. Figure 13.5 shows this regression for NAA lending weight to the suggestion that schizophrenia is not an illness characterised by progressive neuronal loss. In contrast, Nasrallah *et al.* (1994), report finding a reduction in NAA in the right hippocampal/amygdala region in schizophrenia although absolute quantification was not attempted in this study. Buckley *et al.* (1994) studied the left temporal and frontal lobe regions in 28 schizophrenics and

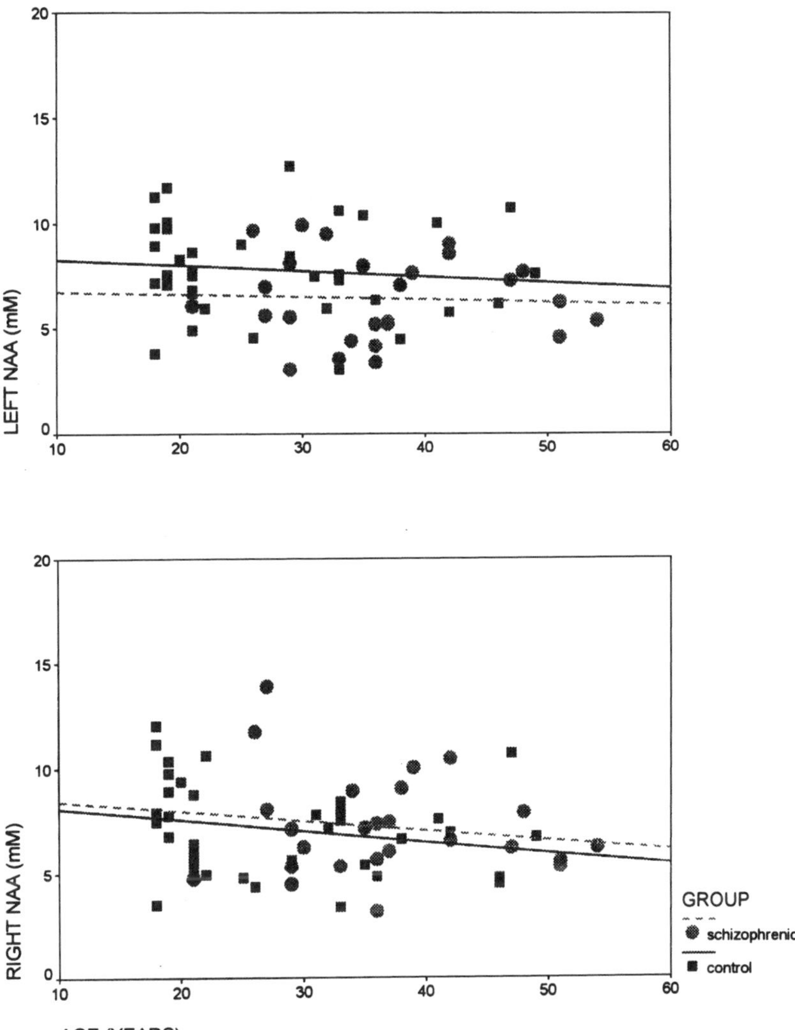

Figure 13.5. Regression plots of left- and right-sided hippocampal NAA (*N*-acetyl aspartate) in both schizophrenics and normal controls. Statistical analysis shows no significant loss in NAA in the two groups over the age range 18–55 years. Reprinted from *Schizophrenia Research*, vol. 22, M. Maier and M.A. Ron, Hippocampal age-related changes in schizophrenia: a proton magnetic resonance spectroscopy study, pp. 5–17, 1996 with kind permission of Elsevier Science – NL, Sara Burgerhartstraat 25, 1055 KV Amsterdam, The Netherlands.

20 normal controls, and found a significant reduction in frontal but not temporal NAA in schizophrenics compared with controls. Frontal choline was also found to be raised in schizophrenics. Renshaw *et al.* (1995) studied the temporal lobe bilaterally in first episode schizophrenics and the NAA/(Cr+PCr) ratio was significantly lower in the psychotic patients. This would suggest that abnormalities in the temporal lobe are present early in schizophrenia. Sharma *et al.* (1992) studied the basal ganglia structure surrounding the anterior horn of the lateral ventricle and the occipital cortex in four bipolar (manic), four schizophrenic and one patient with major depression. Metabolite ratios from the occipital cortex were similar in all patients and controls, Bipolar patients treated with lithium had elevated NAA/(Cr+PCr) in the basal ganglia when compared to normals and these patients also showed elevated Cho/(Cr+PCr) and inositol/(Cr+PCr) ratios. Unfortunately, the small number of subjects in this study and the absence of a statistical analysis of the data make interpretation of the results difficult.

(b) Phosphorus

Pettegrew *et al.* (1991) using phosphorus spectroscopy studied the dorsal prefrontal cortex (DPFC) of 11 drug-naive first episode schizophrenics and found decreased levels of PME and Pi together with increased levels of ATP and PDE, compared to controls. The levels of PCr and ADP did not differ in the two subject groups. It has been suggested that this picture is one of a decreased synthesis and increased breakdown of membrane phospholipids, giving a picture in the schizophrenic brain that is similar to the normal brain in advanced age.

In the developing brain PME tends to increase from the age of 10 to 20 years, then stabilises until the age of 50 and then falls. Corresponding to this, PDE falls between the ages of 10 and 20, stabilises and then increases after the age of 50 (Pettegrew *et al.*, 1993). Hence the picture in schizophrenia is compatible with either premature ageing or an exaggeration of normal programmed regressive events occurring in the neural system sampled. Increased ATP and decreased Pi are consistent with cerebral hypometabolism in the DPFC, and this is in agreement with decreased cerebral blood flow, and glucose utilisation, observed by PET in the same region.

The authors suggest that these findings might also represent a trait marker for schizophrenia as a similar pattern was found in one control who later developed a schizophreniform illness (Keshavan, Pettegrew and

Panchalingam, 1991*b*). Williamson *et al.* (1991) have also suggested that the reduced levels of PME in the DPFC might represent a trait marker as there is no overlap in the range of PME values when compared with controls. However in their work they reported no increase in ATP and a small increase in Pi and PCr in schizophrenics, and this inconsistency in some of the parameters makes it more difficult to decide whether the changes are state or trait markers of the illness. This pattern of metabolite changes was confirmed by Stanley *et al.* (1995), who found decreased levels of PME, together with increased intracellular free magnesium, in drug naive, newly diagnosed medicated and chronic medicated patients. Only the drug naive patients showed an increase in PDE. It would seem that a reduction in precursors of membrane phospholipid are observed during the early and chronic stages of the schizophrenic illness, and breakdown products of membrane phospholipids are increased at the early stage of illness before medication treatment. Shioiri *et al.* (1994) found a direct correlation between the extent of PME reduction in the frontal lobes and negative symptom subscales, supporting the 'hypofrontality hypothesis'. Deicken *et al.* (1994) found higher PDE and lower PCr in both the left and right frontal regions in schizophrenics, with no group differences in left and right parietal regions. They also correlated right frontal PDE and PCr with hostility–suspiciousness and anxiety–depression subscales of the Brief Psychiatric Rating Scale. Keshavan *et al.* (1993) attempted to correlate frontal lobe phospholipid metabolism and cerebral morphology measured by MRI in a group of nine drug naive schizophrenics. Total corpus callosal area was significantly correlated with PDE concentration, and this relation was confined to the genu of the corpus callosum. This relationship was strengthened when females were excluded from the analysis. They suggested that failure of neuronal 'pruning' could interfere with the development of cortical neurones. In addition there is a trend for ventricular size to be associated with lower PME and higher PDE, suggesting that altered membrane metabolites may be associated with nonspecific cerebral atrophy.

The left temporoparietal region of the brain has been studied by O'Callaghan *et al.* (1991) in 18 treated schizophrenics and no significant differences in ^{31}P metabolite levels between patients and controls were evident, although the mean pH was found to be higher in patients ($P<0.07$). There was a significant effect of age on α-ATP and PDE/β-ATP, and an effect of neuroleptic dosage on Pi and Pi/PDE. The difficulty in interpreting data collected with the use of a surface coil is highlighted by this study as it is possible that skin and muscle tissue contaminate the NMR signal. Surface coils are rarely used now and localisation techniques are preferred for spectroscopy (Frahm, Merboldt and Hanicke, 1987).

In 1992 Calabrese *et al.* tested the hypothesis of metabolic asymmetry in temporal lobes of 11 schizophrenic patients. In the controls there was no asymmetry of phosphorous metabolite ratios, pH, or the percentage of total phosphorous signal for individual metabolites. In the schizophrenic group PCr/β-ATP and PCr/Pi appeared to reflect primarily higher ratios on the right side, while the percentage of β-ATP appeared to reflect higher relative concentrations in the left temporal lobe. These results support the hypothesis of an asymmetric distribution of ^{31}P metabolites in the temporal lobe of schizophrenics. An association between the temporal lobe phosphorous metabolism and the severity of psychiatric symptomatology was also found, but because of the very large volumes of interest used in this study, which included brain as well as CSF, these results most likely reflect the left temporal lobe atrophy that is commonly found in schizophrenia. Kato *et al.* (1992) studied 22 patients with bipolar illness (currently depressed), and found that PME and intracellular pH increased significantly in the depressed state compared to the euthymic state. The values in the euthymic state were also significantly lower when compared to age-matched normal controls. In addition PCr was significantly decreased in severely depressed patients when compared to those with mild depression. In a further study the same group (Kato *et al.*, 1994) looked at the relationship between ^{31}P MRS and ventricular enlargement in 40 patients with bipolar disorder and 60 age-matched controls. No correlation was found between imaging and phosphorous spectroscopy, although PME was negatively correlated with age in bipolar disorder. Their conclusion was that the reduction in PME was not related to ventricular enlargement.

Interest has also been shown in autism. Pettegrew's group has studied the dorsal prefrontal cortex of 11 high-functioning autistic young men and compared them to normal controls (Pettegrew, Minshew and Payton, 1989); Minshew *et al.*, 1993). No alteration of brain PME or PDE was seen, but the autistic group had decreased levels of PCr and esterified ends (α-ATP, α-ADP, dinucleotides and diphosphosugars) compared to controls, which is the opposite of what is observed in schizophrenic patients. Decreased levels of PCr in the absence of pH changes suggest increased PCr utilisation and a hypermetabolic state. As neuropsychological, including language, test scores declined in this group so did levels of the most labile high energy phosphate and of membrane building blocks, whereas membrane breakdown products increased. These observations were not the result of age or IQ, and are thought to be consistent with a hypermetabolic energy state and undersynthesis of brain membranes.

Alzheimer's disease and other dementing illnesses

(a) Proton

Kwo-On-Yeun *et al.* (1994) performed *in vitro* NMR on frozen post-mortem brain tissue in Alzheimer's disease (AD) and in normal controls. In AD, reductions were present in the grey matter of the neocortex but not in the white matter. Within the parahippocampal gyrus there were reductions in both tissue types, but only cortical levels correlated with clinical scales of dementia severity. A pattern of closer correlation was observed between dementia severity as measured by the mini mental state examination during life and NAA levels from brain areas of increasing pathological predilection in AD. The authors suggest that reductions in brain NAA correlate with dementia severity during life.

Klunk *et al.* (1992) found lower levels of NAA in perchloric extracts of AD brain, and this correlated with the number of senile plaques and neurofibrillary tangles. GABA levels were also lower in the Alzheimer group, and raised levels of glutamate showed an inverse correlation with NAA. No changes were reported in taurine, aspartate or glutamine. The decreased NAA is believed to reflect neuronal loss and the excess glutamate, together with the reduction in GABA, exposes the neurones to toxic damage. An increase in glutamine and glutamate has been reported in patients with Huntington's disease (Davie *et al.*, 1994*b*), and this finding is consistent with the excitotoxic hypothesis of the disease, which postulates that glutamate or another endogenous excitatory amino acid, acting at one of the glutamate receptor subtypes (kainate, *N*-methyl-D-aspartate and quisqualate), could be involved in the pathogenesis of the disease (DiFiglia, 1990). Miller *et al.* (1993) found that in the parietal and occipital cortices of a group of 11 elderly patients with mild to moderate AD there was a 22% increase in myoinositol (MI) and a 11% decrease in NAA, compared with ten healthy age-matched subjects. The most likely mechanism for the increase in MI is inhibition of the enzyme(s) responsible for conversion of MI to phosphatidyl inositol, and this could affect the polyphosphoinositol second messanger cascade. The results seem to show that the abnormalities in the inositol polyphosphate messanger pathway occur early in the natural history of AD, and this may possibly be used as an early diagnostic test for distinguishing AD from other types of dementia. Shonk *et al.* (1995)

confirmed this finding in a large study of 114 patients with AD or other dementias compared with 98 patients without dementia and 32 healthy control subjects. Reduced levels of NAA and increased levels of MI characterised AD. Patients with other dementias had reduced levels of NAA but normal levels of MI. Following further analyses of ratios of MI/NAA and MI/creatine the authors concluded that proton MRS enables identification of mild to moderate AD with a specificity and sensitivity that suggest clinical utility.

Creutzfeldt–Jakob disease has been studied by Bruhn *et al.* (1991) where a 40% reduction in NAA, a 10% reduction in creatine and a 30% increase in inositol was detected.

Murata *et al.* (1993), looking at white matter around the anterior horn of the lateral ventricle, studied the premature aging in 18 adult Down's syndrome (DS) subjects and analysed the results separately in three age groups (the 20s, 30s and 40s). In the control group there were no age-related changes in the metabolites across the three groups, however in the patients the amount of NAA remained constant throughout the three groups, but the relative amount of choline was significantly increased in the 40s group. No morphological changes were apparent in patients across the age range studied. The authors suggested that in DS patients in the fifth decade, metabolic abnormalities such as degradation and/or rapid synthesis of brain cell membrane may occur prior to neuronal loss and degeneration. This increase in choline is apparently consistent in time with the appearance of senile plaques and neurofibrillary tangles in DS patients after the age of 40.

(b) Phosphorus

Pettegrew *et al.* (1987, 1988*b*,*c*) have shown that Alzheimer's disease (AD) is associated with an increase in brain PME early in the course of the disease followed by an increase in PDE occurring later. Elevation in levels of PME had a negative correlation with the number of senile plaques, whereas the elevation in PDE had a positive correlation with plaque number, and no correlations were found between PME or PDE and neurofibrillary tangles. This suggests that elevation in PME, precursors of membrane phospholipids, occurs early in the disease and that abnormalities in the synthesis of membrane phospholipids are early events in the pathogenesis of AD. In contrast, elevations in PDE, the breakdown products of phospholipids, reflect the degeneration of neural membranes, which correlates with senile plaque formation. The possible mechanism leading to an increase in PME could be secondary to a metabolic block at the rate limiting enzyme (cytidine triphosphate:phosphocholine cytidyltransferase), which is inactivated by phosphorylation and independent evidence exists for the hyperphosphorylation of proteins (tau and MAP-2) in the Alzheimer brain. Nitsch *et al.* (1992), using post-mortem AD brain and chromatography, have shown that there are membrane defects in AD that do not appear in Huntington disease, Parkinson disease or Down's syndrome. It is also interesting that in normal ageing, levels of PME decrease together with increasing PDE, and this is a different picture to the one seen in AD and consequently this process is qualitatively different from normal ageing. Brown *et al.* (1989) studied patients with probable AD and multiple subcortical cerebral infarctions (MSCI). The MSCI group demonstrated elevations of PCr/Pi in both temporoparietal and frontal regions. The AD group showed elevation of PME and the PME/PDE ratio as well as elevation of Pi in the same regions. The study showed that ^{31}P MRS could distinguish MSCI from AD and that the PCr/Pi ratio accurately classified 100% of the MSCI patients and 92% of AD, and that Pi and PME together classified all the MSCI and all but one AD patient. It would seem that ^{31}P MRS is useful in distinguishing AD from MSCI *in vivo*. Recently, Murphy *et al.* (1993) have published results in conflict with those of Pettegrew. In this study both ^{31}P MRS and PET were used to study nine drug free patients with mild to moderate AD and eight matched controls. Significant glucose hypometabolism was found in the AD group but no significant differences in any phosphorous metabolites concentrations or ratios was detected. Nor was there any correlation of phosphorous metabolite level with severity of dementia or glucose metabolism. They concluded that glucose metabolism is reduced early in the disease and that near normal levels of metabolites are maintained in AD. Thus alterations in ATP are not a consequence of reduced glucose metabolism in AD and do not play a significant role in the pathophysiology of the disorder. The only criticism of this study is that spectroscopy was obtained from whole brain coronal slices and consequently regional variations in metabolites may have been missed by looking at such large regions.

Studies of other nuclei

Lithium

In vivo studies of lithium (Li) have provided direct measurement of brain concentration and its relationship to the therapeutic effect. Kato, Takahashi and Inubushi (1991) measured brain Li levels in ten bipolar patients and found that the brain concentrations were half of those measured in serum.

Serial measurements indicated that Li concentrations in the brain increased markedly during manic episodes, while serum concentrations remained unchanged. A similar study by Gyulai *et al.* (1991) confirmed this finding by studying Li concentration in brain, calf muscle and serum. They found that the minimum effective concentration of Li in the brain necessary for maintenance treatment of bipolar disorder is around 0.2–0.3 mEq/L. Brain Li concentrations have also been found to correlate better with serum concentrations than with erythrocyte concentrations (Kato *et al.*, 1993*a*), a result opposite to that found in animals. Alterations in brain phosphorous metabolism as a result of Li therapy has been investigated (Kato *et al.*, 1993*b*) in 17 bipolar patients in manic and euthymic states. Both PME and intracellular pH were higher in the manic state than in the euthymic state, and the values in the euthymic state were lower than in normal controls. It appears that patients with bipolar disorder may have membrane abnormalities present in the euthymic state and that state dependent alterations of catecholaminergic activity may be a secondary phenomenon. However, Stoll *et al.* (1992) have shown that treatment with Li does not alter the overall brain content of choline containing compounds, but it remains possible that a component of these compounds, particularly free choline, is elevated during Li treatment.

Fluorine

A considerable number of drugs used in clinical psychiatry contain fluorine and these can be studied by ^{19}F-MRS (Arndt *et al.*, 1988). Bartels *et al.* (1991) have shown that monitoring of fluorine-containing neuroleptics is possible *in vivo*, and by injecting 37.5 mg of fluphenazine decanoate an NMR signal of that compound was detected in the brain within 30 minutes. Komoroski *et al.* (1990) have measured brain levels of trifluoperazine and found regional differences in concentration, the concentration in the occipital region being 200% larger than the frontal region. However, because a surface coil was used it is possible that muscle and fat contributions are more significant in the occiput than for the frontal lobe. The authors suggested that *in vivo* measurement of neuroleptic levels in the brain might be useful in the study of drug non-response.

Lactate

The basal concentration of lactate in the human brain, measured by ^{1}H-MRS, is found to be 0.6 mM (Hanstock *et al.*, 1988). Various studies of lactate have been performed in patients following stroke, and by infusing ^{13}C-labelled glucose it has been found that the level of lactate is raised for several weeks in the brain following a stroke and that this pool of lactate is constantly being renewed by infiltrating macrophages (Rothman *et al.*, 1991).

Lactate-induced panic has been studied by Dager *et al.* (1994), in eight panic disorder subjects and eight healthy controls. After intravenous infusion of sodium lactate, brain lactate levels were compared to venous levels. Significant rises in brain lactate levels occurred in all subjects but panic patients who responded to lactate had significantly higher brain lactate levels before, during and after the infusion than did the controls or medicated patients who were lactate non-responders. After the infusion the panic patients with lactate-induced panic had prolonged elevation of brain lactate and this appeared to be decoupled from the falling blood levels. Dager *et al.* (1995) have also investigated the effects of hyperventilation on brain lactate in patients with panic disorder, and found that panic disorder subjects exhibited significantly greater rises in brain lactate compared to normal subjects in response to the same levels of hyperventilation.

Carbon-13 (^{13}C)

The natural abundance of ^{13}C is only 1% and consequently studies of this nucleus need the use of exogenous labelled ^{13}C-compounds.

^{13}C is only now being developed for routine human *in vivo* studies although ^{13}C-enriched compounds have already been used to measure various metabolic pathways (Beckmann *et al.*, 1991). ^{13}C-labelled glucose has been used to study cerebral glucose metabolism by infusing the labelled glucose and measuring the turnover rate of the ^{13}C-isotope in the brain glutamate pool (Rothman *et al.*, 1992). Spectroscopic studies of the visual cortex by Rothman show that under visual stimulation the concentration of lactate increases and these results are similar to those obtained by PET.

The future

Studies of the brain by MR techniques provide spatial, chemical and functional information. Brain morphology has been investigated extensively using MRI and has provided important information. Because changes on MRS can be present when no apparent abnormalities are seen on MRI, it is hoped that eventually the use of MRS will complement that of MRI. MRS has already shown itself to be of considerable use in the study of various brain disorders; the dementias, epilepsy, white matter diseases including HIV, inborn errors of metabolism, closed head injury, hepatic encephalopathy, neonatal hypoxia, birth trauma and perinatal encephalopathy have all been studied.

Initially it was hoped that different diseases would be characterised by having a diagnostic MRS ‘fingerprint’. Unfortunately the metabolite profiles have not been sufficiently specific for this to be possible. However the MRS technique has opened the door to the study of brain metabolism, an area not previously accessible easily to neurochemists *in vivo*, and methods of spectral editing are making it easier to detect smaller signals such as those due to GABA (Rothman *et al.*, 1993) and in the future metabolites other than the ones discussed in this chapter will become accessible to MRS measurements.

Already we are able to produce chemical shift images (CSI), which show maps of metabolite distributions in the brain. NAA, creatine and choline maps have been produced and show regional differences in metabolite concentration. As an example, both proton and phosphorous CSI have been done in temporal lobe epilepsy showing abnormalities in neuronal distribution and viability (Hugg *et al.*, 1992, 1993). These can be used to study neuronal markers in the normal and abnormal brain and to develop and modify hypotheses about brain function and choose regions that appear to deserve further study.

References

Arndt, D.C., Ratner, A.V., Faull, K.F. *et al.* (1988). ^{19}F magnetic resonance imaging and spectroscopy of a fluorinated neuroleptic ligand: in vivo and in vitro studies. *Psychiatric Research*, **25**, 73–9.

Arnold, D.L. (1992). Reversible reduction of NAA after acute central nervous system damage. *Society of Magnetic Resonance in Medicine (Book of Abstracts)*, **1**, 643.

Arnold, D.L., Mathews, P.M., Francis, G. and Antel, J. (1990). Proton magnetic resonance spectroscopy of human brain in vivo in the evaluation of multiple sclerosis: assessment of the load of the disease. *Magnetic Resonance in Medicine*, **14**, 154–9.

Austin, S.J., Connelly, A., Gadian, D.G. *et al.* (1991). Localised ^{1}H NMR spectroscopy in Canavan’s disease: a report of two cases. *Magnetic Resonance in Medicine*, **19**, 439–45.

Babb, T.L. and Brown, W.J. (1987). Pathological findings in epilepsy. In *Surgical Treatment of the Epilepsies* (ed. J. Engel Jr), pp. 511–40. New York: Raven Press.

Bartels, M., Gunther, U., Albert, K. *et al.* (1991). ^{19}F nuclear magnetic resonance spectroscopy of neuroleptics: the first in vivo pharmacokinetics of trifluoperazine in the rat brain and the first in vivo spectrum of fluphenazine in the human brain. *Biological Psychiatry*, **30**, 656–62.

Beckmann, N., Turkalj, I., Seeling, J. and Keller, U. (1991). 13-C NMR for the assessment of human brain glucose metabolism in vivo. *Biochemistry*, **30**, 6362–6.

Birken, D.L. and Oldendorf, W.H. (1989). *N*-acetyl-l-aspartic acid: a literature review of a compound prominent in ^{1}H-NMR spectroscopic studies of brain. *Neuroscience and Behavioural Reviews*, **13**, 23–31.

Bloch, R., Hansen, W.W. and Packard, M.E. (1946). Nuclear induction. *Physics Review*, **69**, 127.

Bottomely, P.A., Edelstein, W.A., Foster, T.H. and Adams, W.A. (1985). In vivo solvent-suppressed localized hydrogen nuclear magnetic resonance spectroscopy: a window to metabolism? *Proceedings of the National Academy of Science USA*, **82**, 2148–52.

Breiter, S.N., Arroyo, S., Mathews, V.P. *et al.* (1994). Proton MR spectroscopy in patients with seizure disorders. *American Journal of Neuroradiology*, **15**, 373–84.

Brenner, R.E., Beech, J.S., Williams, S.C.R. *et al.* (1993). Reversibility of the reduction of NAA in diabetic ketoacidosis. *Society of Magnetic Resonance in Medicine (Book of Abstracts)*, **3**, 1559.

Brown, G.G., Levine, S.R., Gorell, J.M. *et al.* (1989). In vivo ^{31}P NMR profiles of Alzheimer's disease and multiple subcortical infarct dementia. *Neurology*, **39**, 1423–7.

Brown, T.R., Kincaid, B.M. and Ugurbil, K. (1982). NMR chemical shift imaging in three dimensions. *Proceedings of the National Academy of Sciences USA*, **79**, 3523–6.

Bruhn, H., Frahm, J., Gyngell, M.L. *et al.* (1989). Cerebral metabolism in man after acute stroke: new observations using localized proton NMR spectroscopy. *Magnetic Resonance in Medicine*, **9**, 126–31.

Bruhn, H., Weber, T., Thorwirth, V. and Frahm, J. (1991). In vivo monitoring of neuronal loss in Creutzfeldt-Jakob disease by proton magnetic resonance spectroscopy. *Lancet*, **337**, 1610–11.

Buckley, P., Moore, C., Larkin, C. *et al.* (1993). ^{1}H magnetic resonance spectroscopy of frontal and temporal lobe metabolism in schizophrenia. *Schizophrenia Research* (Special Issue), 194.

Buckley, P.F., Moore, C., Long, H. *et al.* (1994). ^{1}H-magnetic resonance spectroscopy of the left temporal and frontal lobes in schizophrenia: clinical, neurodevelopmental, and cognitive correlates. *Biological Psychiatry*,.**36**, 792–800.

Calabrese, G., Deicken, R.F., Fein, G. *et al.* (1992). ^{31}Phosphorous magnetic resonance spectroscopy of the temporal lobes in schizophrenia. *Biological Psychiatry*, **32**, 26–32.

Chong, W.K., Sweeney, B., Wilkinson, I.D. *et al.* (1993). Proton spectroscopy of the brain in HIV infection: correlation with clinical immunologic and MR imaging findings. *Radiology*, **188**, 119–24.

Christiansen, P., Toft, P., Larsson, H.B.W. *et al.* (1993). The concentration of *N*-acetyl aspartate, creatine+phosphocreatine, and choline in different parts of the brain in adulthood and senium. *Magnetic Resonance Imaging*, **11**, 799–806.

Connelly, A., Jackson, G.D., Duncan, J.S. *et al.* (1994). Magnetic resonance spectroscopy in temporal lobe epilepsy. *Neurology*, **44**, 1411–17.

Cross, J.H., Connelly, A., Jackson, M.D. *et al.* (1996). Proton magnetic resonance spectroscopy in children with temporal lobe epilepsy. *Annals of Neurology*, **39**, 107–13.

Dager, S.R., Marro, K.I., Richards, T.L. and Metzger, G.D. (1994). Preliminary application of magnetic resonance spectroscopy to investigate lactate-induced panic. *American Journal of Psychiatry*, **151**, 57–63.

Dager, S.R., Strauss, W.L., Marro, K.I. *et al.* (1995). Proton magnetic resonance spectroscopy investigation of hyperventilation in subjects with panic disorder and comparison subjects. *American Journal of Psychiatry*, **152**, 666–72.

Davie, C.A., Barker, G.J., Quinn, N. *et al.* (1994*a*). Proton MRS in Huntington's disease. *Lancet*, **343**, 1580.

Davie, C.A., Hawkins, C.P., Barker, G.J. *et al.* (1994*b*). Serial proton magnetic resonance spectroscopy in acute multiple sclerosis lesions. *Brain*, **117**, 49–58.

de Certaines, J.D., Bovee, W.M.M.J. and Podo, F. (eds.) (1992). *Magnetic Resonance Spectroscopy in Biology and Medicine*. Pergamon Press.

De Stefano, N., Francis, G., Antel, J.P. and Arnold, D.L. (1993). Reversible decreases of NAA in the brain of patients with relapsing remitting multiple sclerosis. *Society of Magnetic Resonance in Medicine (Book of Abstracts)*, **1**, 280.

Deicken, R.F., Calabrese, G., Merrin, E.L. *et al.* (1994). *Biological Psychiatry*, **36**, 503–10.

DiFiglia, (1990). Excitotoxic injury of the neostriatum: a model for Huntington's disease. *Trends in Neurosciences*, **13**, 286–9.

Espanol, M.T., Yang, G.Y., Shimizu, H. *et al.* (1992). Does NAA predict outcome of transient global cerebral ischaemia in rat brain? *Society of Magnetic Resonance in Medicine (Book of Abstracts)*, **2**, 2148.

Fazekas, F., Kapeller, P., Schmidt, R. *et al.* (1995). Magnetic resonance imaging and spectroscopy findings after focal status epilepticus. *Epilepsia*, **36**, 946–9.

Fisher, M., Sotak, C.H., Minematsu, K. and Li, L. (1992). New magnetic resonance techniques for evaluating cerebrovascular disease. *Annals of Neurology*, **32**, 115–22.

Frahm, J., Merboldt, K.D. and Hanicke, W. (1987). Localised proton spectroscopy using stimulated echoes. *Journal of Magnetic Resonance*, **72**, 502–8.

Frahm, J., Bruhn, H., Gyngell, M.L. *et al.* (1989*a*). Localized high-resolution proton NMR spectroscopy using stimulated echoes: initial applications to human brain in vivo. *Magnetic Resonance in Medicine*, **9**, 79–93.

Frahm, J., Bruhn, H., Gyngell, M.L. *et al.* (1989*b*). Localised proton NMR spectroscopy in different regions of the human brain in vivo. Relaxation times and concentrations of cerebral metabolites. *Magnetic Resonance in Medicine*, **11**, 47–63.

Fukuzako, H., Takeuchi, K., Fujimoto, T. *et al.* (1992). ^{31}P magnetic resonance spectroscopy of schizophrenic patients with neuroleptic resistent positive and negative symptoms. *Biological Psychiatry*, **31** (supplement), 204A–295A.

Garcia, P.A., Laxer, K.D., van der Grond, J. *et al.* (1994). Phosphorus magnetic resonance spectroscopic imaging in patients with frontal lobe epilepsy. *Annals of Neurology*, **35**, 217–21.

Gill, S.S., Thomas, D.G.T., Van Bruggen, N. *et al.* (1990). Proton MR spectroscopy of intracranial tumours: in vivo and in vitro studies. *Journal of Computer Assisted Tomography*, **14**, 497–504.

Giroud, M., Walker, P., Bernard, D. *et al.* (1994). Preliminary observations of metabolic characterization of bilateral temporal epileptic focus, using proton magnetic resonance spectroscopy. Three cases. *Neurological Research*, **6**, 481–3.

Graham, S.H., Meyerhoff, D.J., Bayne, L. *et al.* (1994). Magnetic resonance spectroscopy of *N*-acetyl aspartate in hypoxic-ischaemic encephalopathy. *Annals of Neurology*, **35**, 490–4.

Grodd, W., Kraegelch-Mann, I., Peterson, D. *et al.* (1990). In vivo assessment of *N*-acetyl aspartate in brain in spongy degeneration (Canavan's disease) by proton spectroscopy. *Lancet*, **336**, 437–8.

Gyulai, L., Wicklund, S.W., Greenstein, R. *et al.* (1991). Measurement of tissue lithium concentration by lithium magnetic resonance spectroscopy in patients with bipolar disorder. *Biological Psychiatry*, **29**, 1161–70.

Hanstock, C.C., Rothman, D.L., Prichard, J.W. *et al.* (1988). Spatially localized ^{1}H-NMR spectra of metabolites in the human brain. *Proceedings of the National Academy of Sciences USA*, **85**, 1821–5.

Hoult, D.I., Busby, S.J.W., Radda, G.K. *et al.* (1974). Observation of tissue metabolites using phosphorous nuclear magnetic resonance. *Nature*, **252**, 285–7.

Hugg, J.W., Laxer, K.D., Matson, G.B. *et al.* (1992*a*). Lateralization of human focal epilepsy by ^{31}P magnetic resonance spectroscopic imaging. *Neurology*, **42**, 2011–18.

Hugg, J.W., Matson, G.B., Twieg, D.B. *et al.* (1992*b*). Phosphorus-31 MR spectroscopic imaging (MRSI) of normal and pathological human brains. *Magnetic Resonance Imaging*, **10**, 227–43.

Hugg, J.W., Laxer, K.D., Matson, G.B. *et al.* (1993). Neuronal loss localizes focal epilepsy by proton MR spectroscopic imaging. *Annals of Neurology*, **34**, 788–94.

Kato, T., Takashashi, S. and Inubushi, T. (1991). Brain lithium concentration by ^{7}Li- and ^{1}H-magnetic resonance spectroscopy in bipolar disorder. *Psychiatry Research: Neuroimaging*, **45**, 53–63.

Kato, T., Takashi, S., Shioiri, T. and Inubushi, T. (1992). Brain phosphorous metabolism in depressive disorders detected by phosphorous 31 magnetic resonance spectroscopy. *Journal of Affective Disorder*, **26**, 223–30.

Kato, T., Shioiri, T., Inubushi, T. and Takahashi, S. (1993*a*). Brain lithium concentrations measured with lithium 7- magnetic resonance spectroscopy in patients with affective disorders: relationship to erythrocyte and serum concentrations. *Biological Psychiatry*, **33**, 147–52.

Kato, T., Takahashi, S., Shioiri, T. *et al.* (1993*b*). Alterations in brain phosphorous metabolism in bipolar disorders detected by in vivo ^{31}P and ^{7}Li magnetic resonance spectroscopy. *Journal of Affective Disorder*, **27**, 53–9.

Kato, T., Shioiri, T., Murastuta, J. *et al.* (1994). Phosphorus-31 magnetic resonance spectroscopy and ventricular enlargement in bipolar disorders. *Psychiatry Research: Neuroimaging*, **55**, 41–50.

Keshaven, M.S., Kapur, S. and Pettegrew, J.W. (1991*a*). Magnetic resonance spectroscopy in psychiatry: potential, pitfalls and promise. *American Journal of Psychiatry*, **148**, 976–85.

Keshavan, M.S., Pettegrew, J.W. and Panchalingam, K.S. (1991*b*). Phosphorus-31 magnetic resonance spectroscopy detects altered brain metabolism before onset of schizophrenia. *Archives of General Psychiatry*, **48**, 1112.

Keshavan, M.S., Sanders, R.D., Pettegrew, J.W. *et al.* (1993). Frontal lobe metabolism and cerebral morphology in schizophrenia: ^{31}P MRS and MRI studies. *Schizophrenia Research*, **10**, 241–6.

Klunk, W.E., Panchalingam, K., Moossy, J. *et al.* (1992). *N*-acetyl-L-aspartate and other amino acid metabolites in Alzheimer's disease brain: a preliminary proton NMR study. *Neurology*, **42**, 1578–85.

Koller, K.J., Zaczek, R. and Coyle, J.T. (1984). *N*-acetyl-aspartyl-glutamate: regional levels in rat brain and the effects of brain lesions as determined by a new HPLC method. *Journal of Neurochemistry*, **43**, 1136–42.

Komoroski, R.A., Newton, J.E.O., Karson, C. *et al.* (1990). Detection of psychoactive drugs in vivo in humans using ^{19}F NMR spectroscopy. *Biological Psychiatry*, **29**, 711–14.

Kreis, R., Ernst, T. and Ross, B.D. (1993). Development of the human brain: in vivo quantification of metabolite and water content with proton magnetic resonance spectroscopy. *Magnetic Resonance in Medicine*, **30**, 424–37.

Kuzniecky, R., Elgavish, G.A., Hetherington, H.P. *et al.* (1992). In vivo ^{31}P nuclear magnetic resonance spectroscopy of human temporal lobe epilepsy. *Neurology*, **42**, 1586–90.

Kwo-On-Yuen, P.F., Newmark, R.D., Budinger, T.F. *et al.* (1994). Brain *N*-acetyl-L-aspartic acid in Alzheimer's disease; a proton magnetic resonance spectroscopy study. *Brain Research*, **667**, 167–74.

Layer, G., Traber, F., Muller-Lisse, U. *et al.* (1993). 'Spectroscopic imaging'. A new MR technique in the diagnosis of epilepsy? *Radiologie*, **33**, 178–84.

Laxer, K.D. and Garcia, P.A. (1993). Imaging criteria to identify the epileptic focus. Magnetic resonance imaging, magnetic resonance spectroscopy, positron emission tomography scanning, and single photon emission computed tomography. *Neurosurgical Clinics of North America*, **4**, 199–209.

Laxer, K.D., Hubesch, B., Sappey-Marinier, D. and Weiner, M.W. (1992). Increased pH and inorganic phosphate in temporal seizure foci demonstrated by ^{31}P MRS. *Epilepsia*, **33**, 618–23.

Luyten, P.R., Marien, A.J.H., Sijtsma, B. and Den Hollander, J.A. (1986). Solvent-suppressed spatially resolved spectroscopy – an approach to high-resolution NMR on a whole-body MR system. *Journal of Magnetic Resonance*, **67**, 148–55.

Maier, M. (1995), In vivo magnetic resonance spectroscopy: applications in psychiatry. *British Journal of Psychiatry*, **167**, 299–306.

Maier, M., Ron, M.A., Barker, G.J. and Tofts, P. (1995). Proton magnetic resonance spectroscopy: an in vivo method of detecting hippocampal neuronal loss in schizophrenia. *Psychological Medicine*, **25**, 1201–9.

Meyerhoff, D.J., Mackay, S., Poole, N. *et al.* (1994). *N*-acetylaspartate reductions measured by ^{1}H-MRS in cognitively impaired HIV-seropositive individuals. *Magnetic Resonance Imaging*, **12**, 653–9.

Michaelis, T., Merboldt, K.D., Bruhn, H. *et al.* (1993). Absolute concentrations of metabolites in the adult brain in vivo: quantification of localized proton MR spectra. *Radiology*, **187**, 219–27.

Miller, B.L. (1991). A review of chemical issues in ^{1}H-NMR spectroscopy: *N*-acetyl-aspartate, creatine and choline. *NMR in Biomedicine*, **4**, 47–52.

Miller, B.L., Moats, R.A., Shonk, T. *et al.* (1993). Alzheimer disease: depiction of increased cerebral myo-inositol with proton MR spectroscopy. *Radiology*, **187**, 433–7.

Miller, D.H., Austin, S.J., Connelly, A. *et al.* (1991). Proton magnetic resonance spectroscopy of an acute and chronic lesion in multiple sclerosis. *Lancet*, **337**, 58–9.

Minshew, N.J., Goldstein, G., Dombrowski, S.M. *et al.* (1993). A preliminary ^{31}P-MRS study of autism: evidence for undersynthesis and increased degradation of brain membranes. *Biological Psychiatry*, **33**, 762–73.

Moon, R.B. and Richards, J.H. (1973). Determination of intracellular pH by ^{31}P magnetic resonance. *Journal of Biological Chemistry*, **248**, 7246–78.

Moore, C.M., Redmond, O.M., Buckley, P. *et al.* (1992). In vivo proton nmr spectroscopy (STEAM) in patients with schizophrenia. *Society of Magnetic Resonance in Medicine (Book of Abstracts)*, **1**, 1933.

Murata, T., Koshino, Y. and Omori, M. (1993). In vivo proton magnetic resonance spectroscopy study in premature aging in adult Down's syndrome. *Biological Psychiatry*, **34**, 290–7.

Murphy, D.G.M., Bottomley, P.A., Salerno, J.A. *et al.* (1993). An in vivo study of phosphorous and glucose metabolism in Alzheimer's disease using magnetic resonance spectroscopy and PET. *Archives of General Psychiatry*, **50**, 341–9.

Nasrallah, H.A., Skinner, T.E., Schmalbrock, P. and Robitaille, P.M. (1992). In vivo proton magnetic resonance spectroscopy (MRS) of the hippocampus/amygdala region in schizophrenia. *Schizophrenia Research* (Special Issue), 150.

Nasrallah, H.A., Skinner, T.E., Schmalbrock, P. and Robitaille, P.M. (1994). Proton magnetic resonance spectroscopy (^{1}H MRS) of the hippocampal formation in schizophrenia: a pilot study. *British Journal of Psychiatry*, **165**, 481–5.

Nitsch, R.M., Blusztajn, J.K., Anastassios, G. *et al.* (1992). Evidence for a mambrane defect in Alzheimer disease brain. *Proceedings of the National Academy of Science USA*, **89**, 1671–5.

O'Callaghan, E., Redmond, O., Ennis, R. *et al.* (1991). Initial investigation of the left temporoparietal region in schizophrenia by ^{31}P magnetic resonance spectroscopy. *Biological Psychiatry*, **29**, 1149–52.

Okumura, N., Otsuki, S. and Nasu, H. (1959). The influence of insulin hypoglycaemic coma, repeated electroshocks, and chlorpromazine or beta-phenylisopropylmethylamine administration on the free amino acids in the brain. *Journal of Biochemistry*, **46**, 247–52.

Peeling, J. and Sutherland, G. (1993). ^{1}H magnetic resonance spectroscopy of extracts of human epileptic neocortex and hippocampus. *Neurology*, **43**, 589–94.

Petroff, O.A.C., Prichard, J.W., Behar, K.L. *et al.* (1985). Cerebral intracellular pH by ^{31}P nuclear resonance spectroscopy. *Neurology*, **35**, 781–8.

Petroff, O.A.C., Spencer, D.D., Alger, J.R. and Prichard, J.W. (1989). High-field proton magnetic resonance spectroscopy of human cerebrum obtained during surgery for epilepsy. *Neurology*, **39**, 1197–1202.

Pettegrew, J.W., Withers, G., Panchalingam, K. and Post, J.F.M. (1987). ^{31}P nuclear magnetic resonance (NMR) spectroscopy of brain in aging and Alzheimer's disease. *Journal of Neural Transmission*, **24** (Supplement), 261–8.

Pettegrew, J.W., Withers, G., Panchalingam, K. and Post, J.F.M. (1988*a*). Considerations for brain pH assessment by ^{31}P NMR. *Magnetic Resonance Imaging*, **6**, 135–42.

Pettegrew, J.W., Moossy, J., Withers, G. *et al.* (1988*b*). ^{31}P nuclear magnetic resonance study of the brain in Alzheimer's disease. *Journal of Neuropathology and Experimental Neurology*, **47**, 235–48.

Pettegrew, J.W., Panchalingam, K., Moossy, J. *et al.* (1988*c*). Correlation of ^{31}P magnetic resonance spectroscopy and morphological findings in Alzheimer's disease. *Archives of Neurology*, **45**, 1093–6.

Pettegrew, J.W., Minshew, N.J. and Payton, J.B. (1989). ^{31}P NMR in normal IQ adult autistics. *Biological Psychiatry* (Abstract), **25**, 182.

Pettegrew, J.W., Keshavan, M.S., Panchalingam, K. *et al.* (1991). Alterations in brain high energy phosphate and membrane phospholipid metabolism in first episode, drug naive schizophrenics: a pilot study of dorsal prefrontal cortex by in vivo phosphorous-31 nuclear magnetic resonance spectroscopy. *Archives of General Psychiatry*, **48**, 563–8.

Pettegrew, J.W., Keshavan, M.S. and Minshew, N.J. (1993). ^{31}P nuclear magnetic resonance spectroscopy: neurodevelopment and schizophrenia. *Schizophrenia Bulletin*, **19**, 35–53.

Purcell, E.M., Torrey, H.C. and Pound, R.V. (1946). Resonance absorption by nuclear magnetic movements in a solid. *Physics Review*, **69**, 37–8.

Renshaw, P.F., Yurgelun-Todd, D.A., Tohen, M. *et al.* (1995). Temporal lobe proton magnetic resonance spectroscopy of patients with first-episode psychosis. *American Journal of Psychiatry*, **152**, 444–6.

Rothman, D.L., Houseman, A.M., Graham, G.D. *et al.* (1991). Localized proton NMR observation of [3-^{13}C] lactate in stroke after [1-^{13}C] glucose infusion. *Magnetic Resonance in Medicine*, **21**, 302–7.

Rothman, D.L., Novotny, E.J., Shulman, G.I. *et al.* (1992). ^{1}H-[^{13}C] NMR measurements of [4-^{13}C] glutamate turnover in human brain. *Proceedings of the National Academy of Sciences USA*, **89**, 9603–6.

Rothman, D.L., Petroff, O.A.C., Behar, K.L. and Mattson, R.H. (1993). Localized ^{1}H NMR measurements of gamma-aminobutyric acid in human brain in vivo. *Proceedings of the National Academy of Sciences*, **90**, 5662–6.

Sharma, R., Venkatasubramanian, P.N., Baramy, M. and Davis, J.M. (1992). Proton magnetic resonance spectroscopy of the brain in schizophrenic and affective patients. *Schizophrenia Research*, **8**, 43–9.

Shioiri, T., Kato, T., Inubushi, T. *et al.* (1994). Correlations of phosphomonoesters measured by phosphorus-31 magnetic resonance spectroscopy in the frontal lobes and negative symptoms in schizophrenia. *Psychiatry Research*, **55**, 223–35.

Shonk, T.K., Moats, R.A., Gifford, P. *et al.* (1995). Probable Alzheimer disease: diagnosis with proton MR spectroscopy. *Radiology*, **195**, 65–72.

Shulman, R.G., Blamire, A.M., Rothman, D.L. and McCarthy, G. (1993). Nuclear magnetic resonance imaging and spectroscopy of human brain function. *Proceedings of the National Academy of Sciences USA*, **90**, 3127–33.

Stanley, J.A., Williamson, P.C., Drost, D.J. *et al.* (1995). An in vivo study of the prefrontal cortex of schizophrenic patients at different stages of illness via phosphorus magnetic resonance spectroscopy. *Archives of General Psychiatry*, **52**, 399–406.

Stoll, A.L., Renshaw, P.F., Sachs, G.S. *et al.* (1992). The human brain resonance of choline-containing compounds is similar in patients receiving lithium treatment and controls: an in vivo proton magnetic resonance spectroscopy study. *Biological Psychiatry*, **32**, 944–9.

Tedeschi, G., Bertolino, A., Righini, A. *et al.* (1995). Brain regional distribution pattern of metabolite signal intensities in young adults by proton magnetic resonance spectroscopic imaging. *Neurology*, **45**, 1384–91.

Toft, P.B., Christiansen, P., Pryds, O. *et al.* (1994*a*). T1, T2, and concentrations of brain metabolites in neonates and adolescents estimated with H-1 MR spectroscopy. *Journal of Magnetic Resonance Imaging*, **4**, 1–5.

Toft, P.B., Leth, H., Lou, H.C. *et al.* (1994*b*). Metabolite concentrations in the developing brain estimated with proton MR spectroscopy. *Journal of Magnetic Resonance Imaging*, **4**, 674–80.

Vainio, P., Usenius, J.P., Vapalahti, M. *et al.* (1994). Reduced *N*-acetylaspartate concentration in temporal lobe epilepsy by quantitative ^{1}H MRS in vivo. *Neuroreport*, **5**, 1733–6.

Vion-Dury, J., Meyerhoff, D.J., Cozzone, P.J. and Weiner, M.W. (1994). What might be the impact on neurology of the analysis of brain metabolism by in vivo magnetic resonance spectroscopy? *Journal of Neurology*, **241**, 354–71.

Williamson, P., Drost, D., Stanley, J. *et al.* (1991). Localized phosphorus-31 magnetic resonance spectroscopy in chronic schizophrenic patients and normal controls. *Archives of General Psychiatry*, **48**, 578.

Yurgelun-Todd, D.A., Renshaw, P.F., Waternaux, S.A. *et al.* (1993). ^{1}H spectroscopy of the temporal lobes in schizophrenic and bipolar patients. *Society of Magnetic Resonance in Medicine (Book of Abstracts)*, **3**, 1539.

14

The hallucination: a disorder of brain and mind

ANTHONY S. DAVID & GERALDO BUSATTO

Introduction

Hallucinations are a principal feature of psychosis. The usual definition is of a percept in the absence of an external stimulus. To distinguish this further from imagery, a caveat must be added, namely, that the percept is unbidden, outside of conscious control and registered as though in external space. Such a rigid definition would exclude the 'hallucinatory' experiences of most patients seen in psychiatric and neuropsychiatric settings. This is especially so of auditory–verbal hallucinations where patients with established diagnoses of schizophrenia often find it difficult to say whether the 'voice' is inside or outside the head (Junginger and Frame, 1985; Nayani and David, 1996). Sometimes it is only the content of the utterance that persuades the subject of its non-self provenance. Similarly, the normal experience of inner speech seems to shade into the abnormal experience of commenting voices, a classical symptom of schizophrenia.

These aspects together lead to the conclusion that hallucinations, at least those encountered in psychiatric practice, cannot be considered as random 'discharges' from a diseased brain but rather, the distorted output of a complex virtual machine. The hallucination is therefore best considered as a disorder of brain and mind.

Visual versus auditory hallucinations

To what extent does brain damage provide clues to how hallucinations are produced? First of all it is necessary to distinguish between hallucinations in different modalities and with different content. In this chapter we will concentrate on auditory hallucinations but to illustrate some principles, visual hallucinations will also be discussed.

In a review of neurological causes of auditory-verbal hallucinations

(AVHs) (David, 1994*a*), very few instances were found where there was a direct relationship between a focal lesion or a focal electrical event, be it induced or naturally occurring, and the experience of hearing voices. Examples from the classic brain stimulation work of Penfield and colleagues (Penfield and Perot, 1963) were, on closer scrutiny, more often combined audiovisual phenomena and often recognised, apparently, by the subject as memories. Whether the mnemonic colouring is genuine or simply the consequence of extensive temporal lobe depolarisation, is unclear (see Halgren *et al.*, 1978; Gloor, 1990). Similarly, brain lesions causing schizophrenia-like auditory hallucinations in the absence of epilepsy are extremely rare (see Hécaen and Ropert, 1959, for exceptions).

The situation is entirely different for visual hallucinations. Here it would be easier to list the diseases of the brain that are not associated with this phenomenon (see Berrios, 1985). Although visual hallucinations are less prevalent than auditory hallucinations in schizophrenia they are reported in up to 40% of patients (Phillipson and Harris, 1985; Mueser, Bellack and Brady, 1990) and are a prominent feature of late-onset schizophrenia (Howard and Levy, 1994). Complex visual hallucinations are seen in cases of vertebrobasilar insufficiency (Price *et al.*, 1983), so-called peduncular hallucinosis, and Parkinson's disease (Zoldan *et al.*, 1995) suggesting some overlapping or final common neuronal pathway. It appears that any global disruption may give rise to visual hallucinations. One could propose that such disruptions may be *physiological* such as before and after sleep, *diffuse*, such as delirium from metabolic conditions (Lishman, 1987) and *independent of aetiology*, that is vascular, tumours, infections, etc. Thus, it seems that the brain has a *propensity* to produce visual hallucinations in a variety of circumstances – in contradistinction to auditory hallucinations. Furthermore, surveys of the general population, for example the US Epidemiological Catchment area study (N=17 000), find visual hallucinations to be more common than auditory (Tien, 1991). A highly speculative explanation for these trends is that since the visual system is phylogenetically and ontogenetically old and serves as a basis upon which higher and effortful processes have evolved, it is liable to be 'disinhibited' by many factors, unlike the newer auditory-linguistic system. One hypothesis arising from this is that, in signal detection terms, the visual system is more sensitive and perhaps more biased towards false-positive responding than the auditory system. Proving this would require somehow equating stimuli in the two modalities and measuring, for example, cortical evoked responses.

This is not to say that focal lesions that impinge on the visual pathways do not provoke visual phenomena. Again, a disruption at any point on the visual pathways may give rise to hallucinations, including and especially the eye itself.

Broadly, two main hypotheses have been proposed as causative models for visual hallucinations. One is a 'disinhibition' model through which cortical activity experienced as hallucinations is 'released' as a consequence of reduced sensory input (Schultz and Melzack, 1991). This is supported by the observations that 10–30% of blinded individuals experience hallucinations (Lepore, 1990), that hallucinations within a scotoma have long been recognised (Brown, 1985) and that destructive lesions of the optic nerve, chiasm and radiation (Kölmel, 1985) may all result in hallucinations. The alternative 'cerebral irritation' model implies that abnormal cortical excitability in regions associated with visual memory is primary in these experiences. This is supported by the complex visual hallucinations that result from, as noted earlier, experimental stimulation of the temporal lobes (Penfield and Perot, 1963) and which are experienced by patients with temporal (and parietal) lobe epilepsy (Kim *et al.*, 1993; Salanova *et al.*, 1995) and migraine (Arnaud *et al.*, 1986; Panayiotopoulos, 1994) secondary to alterations in occipital perfusion. It is also possible that both disinhibition and irritation processes could operate in a single individual.

The Charles Bonnet syndrome entails the experience of complex visual hallucinations such as colourful, moving animals and figures, in a setting without other signs of psychotic illness. Some visual impairment is frequently demonstrated (or assumed as in elderly cases) (Teunisse *et al.*, 1995). Preliminary neuroimaging research using SPET (see below) has pointed to altered cortical activation (regionally increased cerebral blood flow) in temporal and occipital areas in such patients (Sichart and Fuchs, 1992; Adachi *et al.*, 1994). Of particular interest is a brief report of a man, with vivid visual hallucinations of animals and people secondary to cortical Lewy body disease, by Howard *et al.* (1995) using functional MRI (fMRI) showing that primary and secondary visual areas become relatively unresponsive to exogenous input during complex visual hallucinations.

Of interest in terms of cerebral localisation, are cases where the abnormal perceptual phenomena occur in a hemianopic visual field (Lance, 1976) due to occipital and occipito-parietal lesions in the main (hallucinations do occur in the intact hemifield but this is usually due to allosthaesic palinopsia (Brown, 1985)).

Similarly, of relevance to the release and irritation models is the effect of eye closure. In some cases, closing the eyes abolishes the hallucinations, suggesting that they arise on the basis of the sensory contents of an activated but perhaps noisy 'irritable' visual pathway – which may then be misinterpreted post-hoc 'in the mind's eye'. Where eye closure elicits hallucinations, this clearly supports a release or disinhibition account (Fisher, 1991). The same applies to hallucinations ipsi- or contra-lateral to a field defect.

Visual imagery

Recently, visual imagery in normal subjects has been studied using neuroimaging techniques (Kosslyn *et al.*, 1993, 1995) including fMRI (Le Bihan *et al.*, 1993). Primary and association visual cortex appear to be active during voluntary and induced imagery (Zeki, Watson and Frackowiak, 1993). However, phenomenal awareness may be evoked in the absence of primary cortex activations (Barbur *et al.*, 1993; Roland and Gulyás, 1994). More complex mental manipulation of images involves temporal and parietal regions (Köhler *et al.*, 1995). A neuropsychological study of schizophrenic patients, some of whom had visual hallucinations, showed that they had a normal capacity for image generation within the right hemisphere (David and Cutting, 1992): semantic decisions elicited from the right visual field/left hemisphere resulted in prolonged reaction time. This is compatible with the notion that in hallucinations, mental images may be produced normally but then misinterpreted (perhaps as a result of left hemisphere dysfunction) as coming from outside.

Auditory hallucinations

Hearing impairment

Does the release explanation have relevance to auditory hallucinations? While hearing impairment detected early in life has been found to be a risk factor for schizophrenia *per se* (David *et al.*, 1994; O'Neal and Robins, 1958) a specific pre-morbid link with auditory hallucinations has yet to be established. Several cross-sectional studies have supported an association between deafness and paranoia in the elderly and there have been reports of an association with auditory hallucinations. This is especially clear in the case of unilateral hallucinations (Almeida *et al.*, 1993; Doris *et al.*, 1995; Gordon, 1995). Usually the hallucination occurs on the deaf side although exceptions occur, perhaps where they are drug-induced (Gilbert, 1993). A consistent association has been found between deafness and musical hallucinations (Aizenberg *et al.*, 1991; Khan and Krishnan, 1981). Reviews by Keshavan *et al.* (1992) and Berrios (1990) show that musical hallucinations in non-psychotic individuals almost invariably implicate hearing loss

(Gordon, 1994) sometimes with additional cerebral pathology (Paquier *et al.*, 1992; Fénelon *et al.*, 1993). Recent reports (Fisman, 1991 case 2; Shapiro, Kasem and Tewari, 1991) do not contradict this if one accepts that the onset in old age implies some hearing impairment, whether or not it is obvious. One German case description, of a 52-year-old man, does claim purely central pathology on the basis of white matter lesions on MRI and focally increased metabolism detected using 18-fluorodeoxyglucose PET (Erkwoh *et al.*, 1992) although there was some high-tone loss.

A reduction in central as opposed to peripheral perceptual sensitivity may be implicated in auditory hallucinations. Mathew *et al.* (1993) measured auditory thresholds in schizophrenic patients rated as hallucinators and found that the usual right ear superiority was lost suggesting a left temporal lobe dysfunction.

Laterality

The left hemisphere is of course specialised in linguistic production and analysis. However, the 'non-propositional' nature of some AVHs has suggested the right hemisphere as their source. David (1994a) outlined a series of scientific proofs that would support this. For example an excess of this symptom in left-handed schizophrenics was predicted and has been reported by Tyler, Diamond and Lewis (1995). A corresponding excess of auditory hallucinations in females in general and female schizophrenic patients was also predicted and reported (Bardenstein and McGlashan, 1990; Rector and Seeman, 1992; Tien, 1991). However research utilising the technique of dichotic listening points to *left* hemisphere dysfunction. Dichotic listening entails competition between the right and left hemispheres in the identification of two speech tokens presented simultaneously, one to each ear. The left hemisphere usually 'wins', especially in right handers. This right ear/left hemisphere advantage appears to be attenuated in patients who are hallucination-prone (Green, Hugdahl and Mitchell, 1994; Bruder *et al.*, 1995) and correlates with symptom severity. The possibility remains therefore that relatively intact right hemisphere functioning could support AVHs in schizophrenia.

Language and auditory hallucinations in schizophrenia

As noted earlier, schizophrenic auditory hallucinations have a precise content that is often highly personalised to the voice-hearer (Nayani and David, 1996). It has been suggested that consistency of the semantic content of AVHs leads the voice-hearer to personify the experience (Hoffman *et al.*, 1994). Often a complex relationship develops between the patient and 'the voices' – usually that of the powerless and the powerful respectively (Chadwick and Birchwood, 1994) although some patients come to value their hallucinations (Miller, O'Connor and DiPasquale, 1993). Cultural factors including ethnicity, religion and urbanisation are clearly influential here (see Azhar, Varma and Hakim, 1993) as are the presumbly universal and developmentally timed intra-personal dialogues that we habitually construct (Sinason, 1993; Kohlberg, 1968; see Hermans, 1996).

Various treatment approaches have arisen out of the fact that hallucinations may arise in predictable contexts and provoke a range of coping strategies, some of which reduce their frequency (Falloon and Talbot, 1981; Slade and Bentall, 1988). As well as being of practical value, this work aids the theoretical understanding of the phenomena.

Cognitive and behavioural treatment – recent findings

Margo and co-workers (Margo, Hemsley and Slade, 1981) showed that meaningful and attention demanding verbal material reduced hallucination frequency – presumably by competing for a common neuropsychological resource. Listening to music seems to help some patients either by blocking out the voices or again by diverting attention (Gallagher, Dinan and Baker, 1994). Habituation in response to guided exposure has only a modest effect on AVHs suggesting some difference in the causal mechanisms between these and obsessional ruminations (Persaud and Marks, 1995). A different therapeutic approach has been to target the effect or impact of AVHs such as the distress they cause. Preliminary work (Bentall, Haddock and Slade, 1994; Haddock, Bentall and Slade, 1993) has shown that the effect can be attenuated via modification of cognitive appraisal, by focusing on the characteristics of the voice (perhaps resulting in exposure) but also by encouraging the patient to accept the voices as self-generated (Bentall *et al.*, 1994). Hoffman and Satel (1993) took a psycholinguistic approach based on Hoffman's theory that discourse planning errors lie at the root of hallucinations (Hoffman, 1986). By training four patients to monitor and check their utterances more carefully they showed a reduction in hallucinations in three of them. Finally, we assume the efficacy of acupuncture, both somatic and auricular (Zhengxiu, 1989) in reducing auditory hallucinations depends on attention diversion but would hesitate before ruling out other mechanisms.

Inner speech

The observation that the universal experience of inner speech resembles some AVHs continues to stimulate research of a purely cognitive kind and also, more recently, functional neuroimaging studies. A single case study of a woman with continuous hallucinations in the form of voices addressing and advising her, showed that inner speech – as defined as the process by which phonological representations are maintained in short-term memory – could coexist with AVHs (David and Lucas, 1993). This implies that inner speech may in fact consist of several different processes or that AVHs are not synonymous with inner speech in any simple sense. In contrast a separate case study suggested that thought echo (a pathological experience akin to hearing voices) does appear to be incompatible with effective short-term or working memory (David, 1994b).

A correspondence between subvocal speech and hallucinations was noted by Gould (1949) and periodically since then (see Green and Kinsbourne, 1990, and David, 1994a, for reviews).

Detailed dissection of inner speech into 'inner ear' and 'inner voice' components using the manipulations of articulatory suppression (to block the inner voice) and interference with irrelevant input (to block the inner ear) has been attempted by Smith and colleagues (Smith, Wilson and Reisberg, 1995; but see Macken and Jones, 1995 for an alternative view). In a clever series of experiments Smith *et al.* showed that the verbal transformation effect (that is the sensation that when a word like 'life' is repeated over and over it turns into 'fly'); parsing meaningful letter strings (e.g. N-M-E=enemy) and imaging familiar tunes, all rely on a partnership between inner ear and inner voice. Moreover, Smith *et al.* (1995) claim that deciding whether words ending with the letter 's' are pronounced with the unvoiced /s/ as in cats or the voiced /z/ as in dogs relies entirely on the inner voice, while deciding whether pseudo-homophones such as 'phyte' sound like real words, relies on neither! The evidence points to the distinctiveness of these components although this is not yet unequivocal (Gupta and Mac Whinney, 1995).

It would be revealing to apply these paradigms to hallucinating subjects in the manner of David and Lucas (1993). The verbal transformation effect has been used in this context and most recent findings suggest that hallucinators are no more prone to the effect than controls. However, Haddock *et al.* (1993) demonstrated that if it is suggested to subjects that on listening to say, 'tress' repeated over and over, they should hear new words, all report more transformations (e.g. stress, dress) but especially the hallucinators who report, in addition, hearing other words (e.g. caressed, Christ, etc).

A novel approach to understanding how internally generated words might arise 'spontaneously' comes from neural network computer simulations (Hoffman *et al.*, 1995), 'trained' to recognise a limited set of words in grammatical sentences. When connections within the network are reduced, fewer words are detected and more are misidentified. Of most interest is the apparent recognition of words during input-pauses (i.e. 'computer hallucinations') and this occurs especially in conditions of increased phonetic noise. Once this has happened, the artificial hallucinations recur, much like real ones (Chaturvedi and Sinha, 1990). Such patterns of activation are described as parasitic foci (Hoffman and McGlashan, 1993).

None of these cognitive models explain the typically abusive content of AVHs of schizophrenia. As schizophrenia researchers Jan Stevens and Jim Gold once noted, if AVHs stem from inner speech, '. . . why would anyone talk to themselves that way?' (Stevens and Gold, 1991). It would be premature to conclude that people do not talk to themselves that way and researchers have been devising ways to study this using prompted sampling of thoughts (Kosslyn *et al.*, 1990; Hurlburt, Happé and Frith, 1994; Hoffman *et al.*, 1996). Whyte (1995) in an unpublished study asked nine normal volunteers to keep a diary of all instances of inner speech over 24 hours. A total of 176 instances of auditory imagery were recorded, of which 159 (90%) were verbal. Most (67%) entries were self-directed. Almost all were in the person's own voice (88.5%) with the remainder either their own plus another (4.5%) or another person's voice (7%). Terms of abuse were occasionally noted although these were other-directed or simple exclamations. A second-person form of address was common but no one reported a third-person voice.

Neuroimaging and inner speech

The techniques of functional neuroimaging have been applied to inner speech with the expressed intent of contrasting this with AVHs (see below). McGuire and colleagues at the Institute of Psychiatry and MRC Cyclotron Unit in London carried out a series of experiments on normal and schizophrenic subjects. In the first of these the neural correlates of inner speech in the form of generating internally the experience of 'hearing' a simple sentence in one's own inner voice and in a different alien voice, were examined using positron emission tomography (PET) in normal volunteers (McGuire *et al.*, 1996*b*). The scanning procedure utilised a slow bolus technique with $H_2{}^{15}O$, which has a short half-life, to measure radioactivity per pixel in 90 s epochs during each experimental condition. Each was contrasted with the other and with a simpler baseline task of reading single words, with a total of 12 experimental blocks. The sentences had to be generated around personal adjectives, some of which were derogatory (e.g. stupid; idiot), into a sentence such as, *you are (an)* . . ., in order to mimic the content of common AVHs in schizophrenia. Subjects were well practised before undergoing scanning and did not exhibit overt speech. It was found that the inner speech (own voice) condition minus the baseline task activated a highly localised region of the left inferior frontal gyrus approximately corresponding to Broca's area, an area normally active during overt speech. During the inner speech (alien voice) condition, a much wider area of positive (increased blood flow) and negative (decreased blood flow) activation was detected. The positive activation extended to most of the peri-Sylvian areas, the left pre-frontal region and the supplementary motor area (SMA). Hence it appears that, in this experiment, 'normal' inner speech involves the recruitment of a relatively specific and, presumably, purely output system corresponding to the inner voice while imagining speech in an alien voice involves areas traditionally associated with language input (i.e. sensory) systems as well as more in the way of motor programming (SMA). However, this distinction may in part be an over simplification since both passive reading and inner speech probably evoke some imagistic sensory processing which, in the subtraction, cancelled out.

PET studies in patients with schizophrenia will be reviewed below but at this point it is informative to discuss the companion paper by McGuire *et al.* (1995), which contrasted schizophrenic patients who frequently suffer from AVHs when ill (n=6), with patients who seldom or never suffered in this way (n=6). The main finding was that the hallucination-prone group failed to activate left temporal regions, in particular, the middle temporal gyrus, during the alien voice generation task when compared with the non-hallucination group of patients. On the basis of human and animal physiological research the authors interpret activation of the left middle temporal regions as signalling self-generated speech (see McGuire *et al.*, 1996*b*). The failure of this mechanism could thus result in the auditory image being attributed to an outside agent.

This external ascription is especially likely to occur, if the voice is unlike one's own inner voice. The problem of deciding who spoke rather than what has been said falls under the rubric of source monitoring (Johnson, Foley and Leach, 1988). Hallucinations can therefore be conceived of as failures of source monitoring. The advantage of this approach is that it proposes a monitor that operates with a simple range of algorithms based on such things as the sensory qualities of memories. Let us say that a remembered speech segment fails to attract a 'tag' denoting its source, then an operation is triggered which runs: if the memory is vivid, then I probably said it. A fading memory trace may therefore be mislabelled as 'other'. Some empirical evidence for such a process underlying AVHs has been found (Bentall, Baker and Havers, 1991).

Indirect psychological evidence for a failure in self-monitoring comes from examining speech repairs, especially when these occur rapidly, often within a word, before external acoustic feedback can have come into play. Leudar, Thomas and Johnston (1994) found that internal error detection occurred much less commonly in schizophrenic patients compared with normal controls. However, there was no difference between patients with and without AVHs as classified according to PSE ratings (Wing, Cooper and Sartorius, 1974).

Structural neuroimaging

Relating hallucinations to anatomical parameters has been attempted in a number of recent studies. The aim is, presumably, *not* to show that various brain structures expand and contract with the waxing and waning of this particular symptom but to show a structural correlate of the propensity to develop hallucinations given the presence of a psychotic disorder. The first successful attempt to relate auditory hallucinations to a localised cerebral region was by Barta and colleagues at the Johns Hopkins Hospital (Barta *et al.*, 1990), who reported a negative correlation between superior temporal gyrus (STG) volume and the severity of AVHs during the course of the illness – as gleaned from case records. Both sides were implicated but the correlation with the left STG was the stronger. Attempts to replicate this have so far been unsuccessful. Shenton and colleagues (1992) showed that the volume of this same region (especially the posterior part) correlated inversely with the severity of thought disorder. Other workers have concentrated on the related area, the planum temporale, but again, relationships with thought disorder only and a lack of the normal planum asymmetry have been found. Unfortunately the significant correlations with thought disorder found by Vita *et al.* (1995) and Petty *et al.* (1995) were in opposite directions to each other.

The only other finding of note comes from a CT scan study of 33 schizophrenic patients with persistent auditory hallucinations (Cullberg and Nybäck, 1992). A positive association between severity and size of the third ventricle was demonstrated. This points to diencephalic structures, which Davison and Bagley implicated in their review of organic conditions, giving rise to auditory hallucinations in the context of schizophrenia-like syndromes (Davison and Bagley, 1969).

The functional anatomy of schizophrenic hallucinations: PET and SPET studies

Using positron emission tomography (PET) and single photon emission tomography (SPET) it is possible to measure, in living human subjects, either regional glucose metabolism or regional cerebral blood flow (rCBF), both of which provide indices of regional neuronal activity (Frackowiak *et al.*, 1980; Sokoloff, 1981). PET can provide images of spatial resolution of 5 mm or less. PET tracers are labelled with short-lived isotopes, such as $C^{15}O_2$ and $H_2{}^{15}O$ for the rapid assessment of rCBF, and ^{18}F-fluorodeoxyglucose (^{18}F-FDG) for measuring glucose metabolism. Although SPET is less sensitive, equipment is easily operable and tracers have longer half-lives than those for PET, avoiding the need for a nearby cyclotron (Verhoeff *et al.*, 1992).

Most PET and SPET resting studies in schizophrenia reported in the 1980s consisted of case-control comparisons addressing the presence of frontal cortical hypoactivity ('hypofrontality') in chronic patients with prominent negative symptoms (Wolkin *et al.*, 1985; De Lisi *et al.*, 1989). However, a few studies with acute unmedicated patients, in which hallucinations were presumably a prominent feature (Sheppard *et al.*, 1983; Early *et al.*, 1987; Wiesel *et al.*, 1987) not only failed to find 'hypofrontality' but also detected group differences involving other brain areas. Thus measuring rCBF with PET, Early *et al.* (1987) found increased activity in a left pallidal region in acute psychotic patients compared to controls. Investigating a similar group, Wiesel *et al.* (1987) reported increased glucose metabolism in the left caudate. These studies were the first to hint at the possibility that hallucinations and other positive symptoms of schizophrenia might be associated with distinct patterns of brain activity.

This notion has been supported by several subsequent studies. De Lisi *et al.* (1989) detected increased metabolism in the temporal cortex of chronic schizophrenic patients in comparison to healthy controls, which was significantly correlated with scores for hallucinations from the Brief Psychiatric Rating Scale (BPRS) but temporal activity also correlated with other symptoms. Investigating an heterogeneous sample of schizophrenic patients with ^{15}O-rCBF PET Liddle *et al.* (1992) demonstrated that three different symptom clusters (Liddle, 1987) were each significantly related to a distinct functional brain system. Whereas negative symptoms correlated negatively with rCBF in the left pre-frontal and parietal cortices and 'disorganisation' correlated positively with anterior cingulate rCBF, the subsyndrome of 'reality distortion' (hallucinations/delusions) was specifically associated with increased rCBF in the left medial temporal and ventral striatal regions. Using a similar strategy, Kaplan *et al.* (1993) also found a direct association between hallucinations/delusions and left temporal activity as measured with PET and the ^{18}F-FDG method. Finally, a ^{99m}Tc-HMPAO SPET study by Ebmeier *et al.* (1993) reported trends toward a positive association between 'reality distortion' and caudate rCBF, a finding that has been recently extended by Vita *et al.* (1995).

Other recent PET and SPET studies have concentrated on the investigation of patients with hallucinations as the most prominent and persistent feature. Using ^{99m}Tc-HMPAO SPET, Musalek *et al.* (1989) studied healthy controls and patients with chronic, treatment-resistant hallucinations. Auditory hallucinations were associated with increased rCBF in the anterior basal ganglia and the medial temporal region bilaterally, as well as rCBF reductions in frontal cortical areas. Using ^{123}I-IMP SPET, Matsuda *et al.* (1988) reported increased tracer uptake in the left superior temporal gyrus in hallucinating schizophrenics compared to non-hallucinating patients. Finally, Cleghorn *et al.* (1992) studied 22 unmedicated schizophrenic patients with chronic auditory hallucinations using PET and the ^{18}F-FDG method, and found significant correlations between the intensity of these symptoms and glucose metabolism in the striatum and anterior cingulate regions.

The studies reviewed so far implicate abnormal functioning of a network involving temporal, striatal and possibly anterior cingulate regions in the genesis of hallucinations in schizophrenia. These findings fit well with the neuropsychological model of schizophrenic symptoms proposed by Frith and Done (1988). This postulates that hallucinations and other positive symptoms result from an internal monitoring deficit that renders patients unable to recognise intended self-generated acts as such. Based on anatomical and behavioural studies in animals, Frith and Done proposed as likely sites for this monitoring deficit the parahippocampal gyrus and the anterior cingulate cortex, via which information about intentions generated in the prefrontal cortex reaches a 'monitoring centre' in the hippocampus. The anatomical organisation of the striatum is also compatible with a role for this region in internal monitoring circuits. There are massive interconnections between the basal ganglia and cortical areas (Parent and Hazrati, 1995), and a direct excitatory projection from the hippocampus to the ventral striatum has also been identified (Kelley and Domesick, 1982).

The latter, a site implicated in schizophrenia pathophysiology (Gray *et al.*, 1991), may be important in relaying information from the hippocampal monitoring centre to other cortical regions.

A new dimension to the imaging studies described here has been added by the incorporation of cognitive activation tasks during the period of rCBF/glucose metabolism measurement with SPET or PET. The activation of neural systems involved in the performance of relevant tasks may bring out specific correlations between regional activity and symptoms that would not be detectable at rest. Busatto *et al.* (1995) measured rCBF with ^{99m}Tc-HMPAO SPET in 18 schizophrenic patients and 16 healthy controls during a paired-associates verbal memory task. It was found that patients with a recent history of hallucinations had rCBF increases to the left basal ganglia during the memory challenge, whereas non-hallucinating patients and healthy controls tended to show reduced rCBF to that area. Using the same technique, Rubin and colleagues (1991, 1994) measured rCBF in a large group of unmedicated schizophrenic patients compared to healthy controls during performance of the Wisconsin Card Sorting Test (WCST). Left basal ganglia rCBF increases, not seen in controls, were present in the patient group, and were positively correlated with BPRS scores for positive symptoms (Rubin *et al.*, 1994). Both paired-associate memory tasks and the WCST involve selection of appropriate/inhibition of inappropriate responses according to external contingencies, and are likely to engage the internal monitoring system described above (Frith and Done, 1988). Thus rCBF activation studies provide further evidence that increased basal ganglia activity may be a brain dysfunctional correlate of monitoring deficits underlying hallucinatory phenomena in schizophrenia (see also Ellis, Young and Critchley, 1989).

Many of the functional imaging studies reviewed above (Cleghorn *et al.*, 1990; Cleghorn *et al.*, 1992; Liddle *et al.*, 1992; Rubin *et al.*, 1994; Busatto *et al.*, 1995) assessed the presence of hallucinations with retrospective rating scales, covering periods of up to a month before scanning. Their findings therefore relate to the *tendency* to produce hallucinations, but say little about the functional brain systems involved in the actual *occurrence* of this psychotic phenomenon. The latter question has been specifically investigated in a ^{99m}Tc-HMPAO SPET study by McGuire, Shah and Murray (1993). Using a powerful test–retest design, these authors measured rCBF in 12 male schizophrenic patients during the experience of hallucinations and after psychotic remission. The hallucinatory state was associated with greater blood flow in language-related areas, significantly so in a region approximately corresponding to Broca's area and as a trend, in the anterior cingulate and left temporal cortices. Using a similar design, Suzucki *et al.* (1993) serially scanned two schizophrenics and three schizophreniform patients during and after remission of auditory hallucinations with ^{123}I-IMP SPET, and found increased rCBF in the left auditory association cortex in the hallucinatory state.

Neurotransmitter studies

PET and SPET techniques can also be applied to map the distribution of receptors for several transmitters in the living human brain, after the administration of radio-labelled ligands that selectively bind to specific receptor populations (Sedvall *et al.*, 1986). The investigation of dopamine D_2 receptors is of obvious interest to the study of hallucinations, given the proposed relationship between excessive dopamine transmission and positive symptoms (Crow, 1982). However, most PET and SPET studies using D_2-selective ligands could not detect binding abnormalities in acute, drug-naïve psychotic patients (Farde *et al.*, 1990; Pilowsky *et al.*, 1994), and also failed to identify relationships between D_2 binding and the severity of hallucinations (Martinot *et al.*, 1991, 1994).

The availability of benzodiazepine receptor ligands for PET and SPET permits the assessment of $GABA_A$ receptors, the main subtype of GABA receptors in the brain, in living schizophrenic patients. This is also of relevance to the study of hallucinations, given the interactions between the inhibitory transmitter GABA and dopamine in the brain (Dewey *et al.*, 1992) and the clinical evidence that benzodiazepines may be effective against positive symptoms of schizophrenia (Delini-Stula and Berdah-Tordjman, 1995). Busatto *et al.* (1997) recently conducted a ^{123}I-Iomazenil SPET study with 15 schizophrenic patients and 12 healthy controls, and found weak evidence of reduced $GABA_A$ binding in several cortical regions in the schizophrenic group. Interestingly, the intensity of hallucinations and delusions was more strongly related to diminished $GABA_A$ binding specifically in the left medial temporal region. These results reiterate the role of medial temporal abnormalities in the genesis of hallucinations, and suggest that diminished GABAergic inhibition is a posssible neurochemical correlate of the excessive medial temporal activity seen in association with hallucinations in schizophrenia (Liddle *et al.*, 1992; Kaplan *et al.*, 1993).

Receptors of the 5-HT_2 subtype may be particularly relevant to the pathophysiology of visual hallucinations. *In vitro* ligand binding studies and behavioural studies in animals strongly suggest that the hallucinogenic properties of LSD and mescaline are mediated by 5-HT_2 receptor stimulation (Pierce and Peroutka, 1989; Dewey *et al.*, 1992). Atypical antipsychotics with strong 5-HT_2 antagonistic properties seem to be particularly effective in the treatment of organic psychoses with prominent visual hallucinations (Meco *et al.*, 1994). Neuroreceptor imaging studies of 5-HT systems have been limited by the lack of selective ligands (Stocklin, 1992). Recently, however, SPET and PET radioligands with high selectivity for 5-HT_2 receptors have been piloted in baboons and healthy human subjects with promising results (Abi-Dargham *et al.*, 1995; Sadzot *et al.*, 1995). Future *in vivo* imaging studies using these compounds in psychotic subjects may clarify the relationship between 5-HT_2 receptor abnormalities and hallucinations.

'Capturing' auditory hallucinations

Few neuroimaging studies can claim to have captured the transient neurological changes coincident with the experience of an auditory hallucination. McGuire *et al.*'s SPET study mentioned above comes closest in its comparison of patients on two occasions: while hallucinating and some weeks later after treatment. The HMPAO technique provides a kind of 'freeze frame' image of rCBF during patient signalled hallucinations. However PET and fMRI have a temporal resolution in the range of tens of seconds and have been applied successfully in patients with prominent hallucinations. Silbersweig *et al.* (1995) published in the journal *Nature* a case study of a man with multi-modal hallucinations with additional data from a further five medicated patients with more conventional schizophrenic auditory hallucinations. Averaging PET blood flow data on the group during periods of scanning in which they indicated, by means of a button press, when they were 'hearing voices', showed common areas of increased activation concentrated in the sub-cortex such as the thalamus, striatum and amygdala. More widespread cortical activity was seen in the single case in visual and auditory areas. It is possible that the subcortical activation reflected common affective responses (or precursors) to hallucinations while the implementation of the phenomenal experience relied on a number of cortical systems that varied from subject to subject, perhaps as a reflection of content.

An fMRI study

Functional MRI is the latest technique to be applied to the understanding of AVHs. Research at the Institute of Psychiatry has made use of new

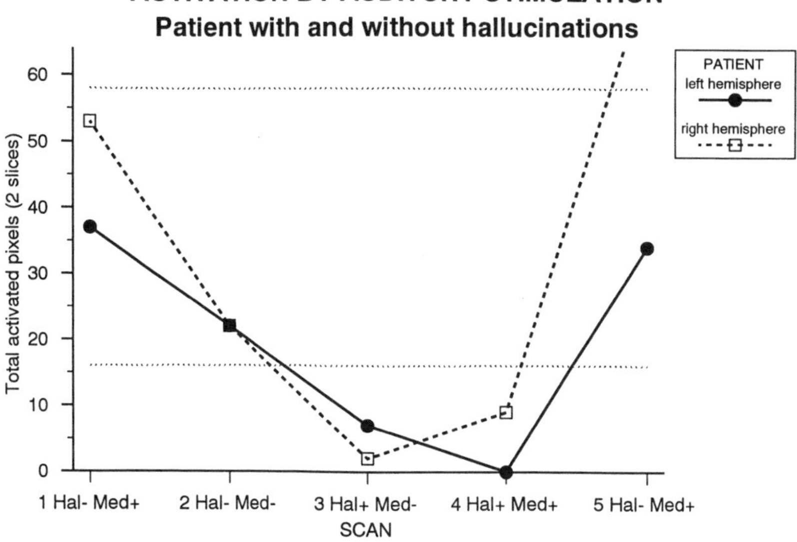

Figure 14.1. The graph plots the total number of auditorially activated pixels in each cerebral hemisphere for axial slices going through the auditory association cortices. The normal range (between dotted lines) is derived from six healthy volunteers. The patient's left (solid line) and right (dashed line) hemispheres show normal levels of activation in sessions 1, 2 and 5 when he was not hallucinating but significantly subnormal levels in sessions 3 and 4 when he was hearing voices continuously. Hal, hallucination; Med, medication.

statistical image analysis methods such as time series regression and spatial connectivity testing (Bullmore *et al.*, 1996; see Chapter 13). David and colleagues (1996) reported a single case study incorporating a 2 × 2 factorial design of hallucinations and drug treatment. The patient was a middle-aged man with a long history of paranoid schizophrenia and, at times, continuous AVHs – attributed to good and evil spirits.

When admitted to the Maudsley Hospital, London, his treatment was changed to the atypical neuroleptic, risperidone. This abolished his hallucinations although he remained deluded. Shortly after this he had the first of five fMRI, studies when taking risperidone 3 mg twice daily. One month later, he was refusing all medication but remained virtually hallucination free and agreed to have a second fMRI scan. After a further month he was experiencing florid and continuous AVHs. He declined medication but acquiesced to further study. After about two months the patient was readmitted as an emergency having stated his intention to commit suicide by jumping from Westminster Bridge, at the behest of 'the voices'. Risperidone was reinstated and after one week he was scanned for the fourth time, prior to any significant alleviation in his symptoms. The fifth and final scan was performed nine months later when the patient was stable, hallucination-free and established on medication (see Figure 14.1).

Echoplanar MR brain images were acquired using a 1.5 tesla GE Signa system retrofitted with Advanced NMR hardware using a standard head coil. Axial slices 5 mm thick were obtained, positioned to include the visual and auditory cortex. Ten images depicting BOLD contrast (Kwong *et al.*, 1992) were acquired with an in-plane resolution of 3 mm in 3 s.

Sensory stimulation took the form of overlapping periodic presentation of auditory and visual material. Auditory stimulation was prerecorded text read aloud via headphones at a constant volume sufficient to overcome ambient machine noise, and occurred for 39 s alternating with 39 s of silence. The patient was simply asked to listen to the speech. Visual stimulation was a regular patterned array of red flashing diodes at 8 Hz delivered using lightproof goggles, which was switched off and on every 30 s. The different periodicity of the visual and auditory stimuli allowed us to distinguish modality-specific activation in BOLD signal using the time series regression method.

Visual activation was normal in all five studies. Auditory-verbal activation was less prominent than visual in scans 1 and 2 (little or no hallucinations) and virtually disappeared in scans 3 and 4 during hallucinations, returning strongly in scan 5. In the non-hallucinating state, activation can be located in the superior temporal lobe (a region normally activated by speech). Activation in response to speech in the non-hallucinating state was mapped in three dimensions onto the space corresponding to the Talairach reference system. This was found to be centred on the middle portion of the superior temporal gyrus (STG) extending posteriorly, and middle temporal gyrus (MTG) [Brodmann's Area (BA) 21/22 and BA 42]. These regions are considered to be auditory association areas.

The marked attenuation of bilateral auditory activation in the hallucinating state, regardless of medication status, is striking. This was interpreted as indicating physiological competition for a common neural substrate or, alternatively, psychological competition for a common attentional resource, by the hallucinations. This was a modality-specific effect since visual activation was unchanged in the face of auditory hallucinations. Taken with the earlier study of visual hallucinations (see above, Howard *et al.*, 1995), it is possible to conclude that hallucinations exert a localised, modality-specific effect on sensory and association cortex, at least in terms of inducing a local increase in oxygenated blood flow. Note that hallucinations in other sensory modalities may not demonstrate this phenomenon: for example, olfactory hallucinations did not impair olfactory identification in one study (Kopala, Good and Honer, 1994). Such evidence from fMRI studies of visual and auditory hallucinations could be construed as being the physiological equivalent of the Perky effect, that is, the ability of imagery to block (or compete with) exogenous sensory input (Craver-Lemley and Reeves, 1992). That such a mechanism may be implicated in hallucinations was first suggested 100 years ago in the journal *Science* (Scripture, 1896).

The data suggest that auditory association cortex is active during schizophrenic auditory hallucinations. Other cortical and subcortical regions may also be implicated in such hallucinations, as in Silbersweig *et al.*'s study (1995). However, since these were not prominently activated in our paradigm we cannot infer their attenuation. Complementary work using the highly sensitive technique of magneto-encephalography (Tiihonen *et al.*, 1992) showed that early auditory evoked potentials were inhibited during hallucinations, again pointing to subcortical involvement. The above case study gives an indirect 'negative image' of the cortical implementation of AVHs. FMRI has also been used to detect the presence and absence of hallucinations within a five minute scanning sequence, in the same patient (Woodruff *et al.*, 1995) on the basis of changes in BOLD signal. The authors further showed that areas active during the experience of auditory hallucinations overlapped with those responsive to external speech in the absence of hallucinations, particularly on the right side. This implies that the final common pathway to experiencing auditory hallucinations involves areas that subserve normal speech perception. Further, it supports the idea that auditory hallucinations involve right auditory cortical regions (see p. 340), which are involved in the processing of the prosodic aspects of speech (see McGuire *et al.*, 1996*a*).

Conclusions

What then can we say about hallucinations with the backing of at least some evidence? Visual hallucinations and auditory hallucinations have different aetiologies but probably share some common mechanisms (they occur both in schizophrenia and, for example, some individuals with Charles Bonnet syndrome: Patel, Keshavan and Martin, 1987). The role of sensory defects in inducing hallucinations seems stronger for visual but may still apply to auditory hallucinations, especially those of music. These clues do not constitute an explanation. AVHs, the main focus of this chapter, are constructed within narrow parameters of form and content. So far, a model within language production and reception, and monitoring provides the best explanatory framework. Inner speech may be involved in the generation of AVHs (from McGuire *et al.*, 1993) but may not be abnormal in itself. Auditory imagery, that is a sensory component, is intuitively central to the experience of hallucinations and recent fMRI studies support this. Either a distortion of the image itself (its prosody, pitch or timbre), its apparent coherence (Hoffman *et al.*, 1994) or ego-alien content (Nayani and David, 1996) or defect in self-monitoring (or combination of all of these) leads to a misattribution of the source. This mislabelling requires more precise cognitive dissection. Is it transient? If so, how does the deficit interact with content? From an anatomical point of view, auditory hallucinations appear to involve primary and association auditory areas (Woodruff *et al.*, 1995; David *et al.*, 1996), with middle temporal (McGuire *et al.*, 1995) and subcortical areas (Silbersweig *et al.*, 1995; Busatto *et al.*, 1996) acting perhaps as a gating mechanism to facilitate or disinhibit auditory activation – in the same way as sensory deficits. The multistage process sketched above, based on many strands of evidence, is perhaps the most developed for any of the psychotic symptoms (see Frith, 1995). Nevertheless, hallucinations will continue to tax researchers and will require the continued and combined understanding of brain and mind.

Acknowledgements

The authors wish to thank Phil McGuire and Peter Woodruff for comments on the manuscript and Martin Whyte for his data on inner speech in normal subjects. We are also grateful to Patsy Mott for her work on the chapter.

References

Abi-Dargham, A., Terriere, D., Zea-Ponce, Y. *et al.* (1995). [^{123}I]5-R91150: a new SPECT tracer for the serotonin $5HT_{2A}$ receptors. *Journal of Nuclear Medicine*, **36**, 164P.

Adachi, N., Nagayama, M., Anami, K. *et al.* (1994). Asymmetrical blood flow in the temporal lobe in the Charles Bonnet syndrome: serial neuroimaging study. *Behavioural Neurology*, **7**, 97–9.

Aizenberg, D., Dorfman-Etrog, P., Zemishlany, Z. and Hermesh, H. (1991). Musical hallucinations and hearing deficit in a young non-psychotic female. *Psychopathology*, **24**, 45–8.

Almeida, O., Forstl, H., Howard, R. and David, A. (1993). Unilateral auditory hallucinations. *British Journal of Psychiatry*, **162**, 262–4.

Arnaud, J.L., Rose, F.C., Diamond, S. and Arnaud, P. (1986). Visual hallucinations and migraine. *Functional Neurology*, **1**, 473–9.

Azhar, M.Z., Vrma, S.L. and Hakim, H.R. (1993). Phenomenological differences of hallucinations between schizophrenic patients in Penang and Kelatan. *Medical Journal of Malaysia*, **48**, 146–52.

Barbur, J.L., Watson, J.D.G., Frackowiak, R.S.J. and Zeki, S. (1993). Conscious visual perception without V1. *Brain*, **116**, 1293–302.

Bardenstein, K.K. and McGlashan, T.H. (1990). Gender differences in affective, schizoaffective, and schizophrenic disorders: a review. *Schizophrenia Research*, **3**, 159–72.

Barta, P.E., Pearlson, G.D., Powers, R.E. *et al.* (1990). Auditory hallucinations and smaller superior temporal gyral volume in schizophrenia. *American Journal of Psychiatry*, **147**, 457–62.

Bentall, R., Baker, G. and Havers, S. (1991). Reality monitoring and psychotic hallucinations. *British Journal of Clinical Psychology*, **30**, 213–22.

Bentall, R.P., Haddock, G. and Slade, P.D. (1994). Cognitive behavior therapy for persistent auditory hallucinations. From theory to therapy. *Behavior Therapy*, **25**, 51–66.

Berrios, G.E. (1985). Hallucinosis. In *Neurobehavioural Disorders* (ed. J.A.M. Frederiks), pp. 561–72. North Holland: Elsevier Science Publishers.

Berrios, G. (1990). Musical hallucinations: a historical and clinical study. *British Journal of Psychiatry*, **156**, 188–94.

Brown, J.W. (1985). Hallucinations. Imagery and the microstructure of perception. In *Handbook of Clinical Neurology* (ed. P.J. Vinken, G.W. Bruyn, H.L. Klawans and J.A.M. Fredericks), pp. 351–72. Amsterdam & New York: Elsevier Science Publishers.

Bruder, G., Rabinowics, E., Towey, I. *et al.* (1995). Smaller right ear (left hemisphere) advantage for dichotic fused words in patients with schizophrenia. *American Journal of Psychiatry*, **152**, 932–5.

Bullmore, E., Brammer, M., Williams, S.C.R. *et al.* (1996). Statistical methods of estimation and inference for functional MR image analysis. *Magnetic Resonance in Medicine*, **35**, 261–77.

Busatto, G.F., David, A.S., Costa, D.C. *et al.* (1995). Schizophrenic auditory hallucinations are associated with increased regional cerebral blood flow during verbal memory activation in a study using single photon emission computed tomography. *Psychiatry Research*, **61**, 255–64.

Busatto, G.F., Pilowsky, L.S., Costa, D.C. *et al.* (1997). Reduced in vivo benzodiazepine receptor binding correlates with severity of psychotic symptoms in schizophrenia. *American Journal of Psychiatry*, **154**, 56–63.

Chadwick, P. and Birchwood, M. (1994). The omnipotence of voices: a cognitive approach to auditory hallucinations. *British Journal of Psychiatry*, **164**, 190–201.

Chaturvedi, S. and Sinha, V. (1990). Recurrence of hallucinations in consecutive episodes of schizophrenia and affective disorder. *Schizophrenia Research*, **3**, 103–6.

Cleghorn, J.M., Garnett, E.S., Nahmias, C. *et al.* (1990). Regional brain metabolism during auditory hallucinations in chronic schizophrenia. *British Journal of Psychiatry*, **157**, 562–70.

Cleghorn, J.M., Franco, S., Szechtman, B. (1992). Toward a brain map of auditory hallucinations. *American Journal of Psychiatry*, **149**, 1062–9.

Craver-Lemley, C. and Reeves, A. (1992). How visual imagery interferes with vision. *Psychological Review*, **99**, 633–49.

Crow, T.J. (1982). Two syndromes of schizophrenia? *Trends in Neurosciences*, **5**, 351–4.

Cullberg, J. and Nybäck, H. (1992). Persistent auditory hallucinations correlate with the size of the third ventricle in schizophrenic patients. *Acta Psychiatrica Scandinavia*, **86**, 469–72.

David, A.S. (1994*a*). The neuropsychology of auditory-verbal hallucinations. In *The Neuropsychology of Schizophrenia* (ed. A. David and J. Cutting), pp. 269–312. Hove, East Sussex: Lawrence Erlbaum Associates.

David, A.S. (1994*b*). Thought echo reflects the activity of the phonological loop. *British Journal of Clinical Psychology*, **33**, 81–3.

David, A.S. and Cutting, J.D. (1992). Visual imagery and visual semantics in the cerebral hemispheres in schizophrenia. *Schizophrenia Research*, **8**, 263–71.

David, A.S. and Lucas, P. (1993). Auditory–verbal hallucinations and the phonological loop: a cognitive neuropsychological study. *British Journal of Clinical Psychology*, **32**, 431–41.

David, A., Malmberg, A., Lewis, G. *et al.* (1994). Are there neurological and sensory risk factors for schizophrenia? *Schizophrenia Research*, **14**, 247–51.

David, A., Woodruff, P.W.R., Howard, R. *et al.* (1996). Auditory hallucinations inhibit exogenous activation of auditory association cortex. *Neuroreport*, **7**, 932–6.

Davison, K. and Bagley, C.R. (1969). Schizophrenia-like psychoses associated with organic disorders of the central nervous system. In *Current Problems in Neuropsychiatry*, (ed. R.N. Herrington), pp. 113–84. Ashford, Kent: Hedley Brothers.

De Lisi, L.E., Buchsbaum, M.S., Holcomb, H.H. *et al.* (1989). Increased temporal lobe glucose use in chronic schizophrenic patients. *Biological Psychiatry*, **25**, 835–51.

Delini-Stula, A. and Berdah-Tordjman, D. (1995). Benzodiazepines and GABA hypothesis of schizophrenia. *Journal of Psychopharmacology*, **9**, 57–63.

Dewey, S.L., Smith, G.S., Logan, J. *et al.* (1992). GABAergic inhibition of endogenous dopamine release measured in vivo with ^{11}C-raclopride and positron emission tomography. *Journal of Neuroscience*, **12**, 3773–80.

Doris, A., O'Carroll, R.E., Steele, J.D. and Ebmeier, K.P. (1995). Single photon emission computed tomography in a patient with unilateral auditory hallucinations. *Behavioural Neurology*, **8**, 145–8.

Early, T.S., Reiman, E.M., Raichle, M.E. and Spitznagel, E.L. (1987). Left globus pallidus abnormality in never-medicated patients with schizophrenia. *Proceedings of the National Academy of Sciences, USA*, **84**, 561–3.

Ebmeier, K.P., Blackwood, D.H., Murray, C. *et al.* (1993). Single photon emission computed tomography with ^{99m}Tc-exametazime in unmedicated schizophrenic patients. *Biological Psychiatry*, **33**, 487–95.

Ellis, A.W., Young, A.W. and Critchley, E.M.R. (1989). Intrusive automatic or nonpropositional inner speech following bilateral cerebral injury. *Aphasiology*, **3**, 581–5.

Erkwoh, R., Ebel, H., Kachel, F. *et al.* (1992). Musical and verbal hallucinations correlated to electroencephalographic and PET-findings. Case report. *Nervenarzt*, **63**, 169–74.

Falloon, I.R. and Talbot, R.E. (1981). Persistent auditory hallucinations: coping mechanisms and implications for management. *Psychological Medicine*, **11**, 329–39.

Farde, L., Wiesel, F.A., Stone-Elander, S. *et al.* (1990). D_2 dopamine receptors in neuroleptic-naive schizophrenic patients. A positron emission tomography study with [^{11}C] raclopride. *Archives of General Psychiatry*, **47**, 213–19.

Fénelon, G., Marie, S., Ferroir, J.-P. and Guillard, A. (1993). Musical hallucinations: 7 cases. *Revue Neurologique (Paris)*, **149**, 8–9.
Fisher, C.M. (1991). Visual hallucinations on eye closure associated with atropine toxicity. A neurological analysis and comparison with other visual hallucinations. *Canadian Journal of Neurological Science*, **18**, 18–27.
Fisman, M. (1991). Musical hallucinations: report of two unusual cases. *Canadian Journal of Psychiatry*, **36**, 609–11.
Frackowiak, R.S.J., Lenzi, G.L., Jones, T. and Heather, J.D. (1980). Quantitative measurement of regional cerebral blood flow and oxygen metabolism in man using ^{15}O and positron emission tomography: theory, procedure and normal values. *Journal of Computer Assisted Tomography*, **4**, 727–36.
Frith, C. (1995). Functional imaging and cognitive abnormalities. *Lancet*, **346**, 615–20.
Frith, C.D. and Done, C.J. (1988). Towards a neuropsychology of schizophrenia. *British Journal of Psychiatry*, **153**, 437–43.
Gallagher, A.G., Dinan, T.G. and Baker, L.J.V. (1994). The effects of varying auditory input on schizophrenia hallucinations: a replication. *British Journal of Medical Psychology*, **67**, 67–75.
Gilbert, G.J. (1993). Pentoxifyline-induced musical hallucinations. *Neurology*, **43**, 1621–2.
Gloor, P. (1990). Experimental phenomena of temporal lobe epilepsy. *Brain*, **133**, 1673–94.
Gordon, A.G. (1994). Musical hallucinations. *Neurology*, **44**, 986–7.
Gordon, A.G. (1995). Schizophrenia and the ear. *Schizophrenia Research*, **17**, 289–90.
Gould, L.N. (1949). Auditory hallucinations and subvocal speech. *Journal of Nervous and Mental Disease*, **109**, 418–27.
Gray, J.A., Feldon, J., Rawlins, J.N.P. *et al.* (1991). The neuropsychology of schizophrenia. *Behavioral and Brain Sciences*, **14**, 1–84.
Green, M.F. and Kinsbourne, M. (1990). Subvocal activity and auditory hallucinations: clues for behavioural treatment. *Schizophrenia Bulletin*, **16**, 617–25.
Green, M.F., Hugdahl, K. and Mitchell, S. (1994). Dichotic listening during auditory hallucinations in patients with schizophrenia. *American Journal of Psychiatry*, **151**, 357–62.
Gupta, P. and MacWhinney, B. (1995). Is the articulatory loop articulatory or auditory? Re-examining the effects of concurrent articulation on immediate serial recall. *Journal of Memory and Language*, **34**, 63–88.
Haddock, G., Bentall, R.P. and Slade, P.D. (1993). Psychological treatment of chronic auditory hallucinations: two case studies. *Behavioural and Cognitive Psychotherapy*, **21**, 335–46.
Haddock, G., Slade, P.D. and Bentall, R.P. (1995). Auditory hallucinations and the verbal transformation effect: the role of suggestions. *Personality and Individual Differences*, **19**, 301–6.
Halgren, E., Walter, R.D., Cherlow, D.G. and Crandall, P.H. (1978). Mental phenomena evoked by human electrical stimulation of the human hippocampal formation and amygdala. *Brain*, **101**, 83–117.
Hécaen, H. and Ropert, R. (1959). Hallucinations auditives au cours de syndromes neurologiques. *Annales Médico-Psychologiques*, **1**, 257–306.
Hermans, H.J.M. (1996). Voicing the self: from information processing to dialogical interchange. *Psychological Bulletin*, **119**, 31–50.

Hoffman, R. (1986). Verbal hallucinations and language production processes in schizophrenia. *Behavioural and Brain Sciences*, **9**, 503–48.

Hoffman, R.E. and McGlashan, T.H. (1993). Parallel distributed processing and the emergence of schizophrenic symptoms. *Schizophrenia Bulletin*, **19**, 119–40.

Hoffman, R.E. and Satel, S.L. (1993). Language therapy for schizophrenic patients with persistent 'voices'. *British Journal of Psychiatry*, **162**, 755–8.

Hoffman, R.E., Oates, E., Hafner, J. *et al.* (1994). Semantic organization of hallucinated 'voices' in schizophrenia. *American Journal of Psychiatry*, **151**, 1229–30.

Hoffman, R.E., Rapaport, J., Ameli, R. *et al.* (1995). A neural network simulation of hallucinated 'voices' and associated speech perception impairments in schizophrenic patients. *Journal of Cognitive Neuroscience*, **7**, 479–96.

Hoffman, R.E., Docherty, N.M., Oates, E. *et al.* (1996). Semantic organization of hallucinated 'voices' in schizophrenia: II. Comparison with normal 'thought samples'. (Submitted).

Howard, R. and Levy, R. (1994). Charles Bonnet syndrome plus: complex visual hallucinations of Charles Bonnet syndrome type in late paraphrenia. *International Journal of Geriatric Psychiatry*, **9**, 399–404.

Howard, R., Williams, S., Bullmore, E. *et al.* (1995). Cortical response to exogenous visual stimulation during visual hallucinations. *Lancet*, **345**, 70.

Hurlburt, R.T., Happé, F. and Frith, U. (1994). Sampling the form of inner experience in three adults with Asperger syndrome. *Psychological Medicine*, **24**, 385–95.

Johnson, M.K., Foley, M.A. and Leach, K. (1988). The consequence for memory of imagining in another person's voice. *Memory and Cognition*, **16**, 337–42.

Junginger, J. and Frame, C.L. (1985). Self-report of the frequency and phenomenology of verbal hallucinations. *Journal of Nervous and Mental Disease*, **173**, 149–55.

Kaplan, R.D., Szetchman, H., Franco, S. *et al.* (1993). Three clinical syndromes of schizophrenia in untreated subjects: relation to brain glucose activity measured by positron emission tomography (PET). *Schizophrenia Research*, **11**, 47–54.

Kelley, A.E. and Domesick, V.B. (1982). The distribution of the projection from the hippocampal formation to the nucleus accumbens in the rat. An anterograde- and retrograde-horseradish peroxidase study. *Neuroscience*, **7**, 2321–5.

Keshavan, M.S., David, A.S., Steingard, S. and Lishman, W.A. (1992). Musical hallucinations: a review and synthesis. *Neuropsychiatry, Neuropsychology and Behavioural Neurology*, **3**, 211–23.

Khan, A.M. and Krishnan, V.H.R. (1981). Unilateral auditory hallucinations – a case report. *Irish Journal of Psychological Medicine*, **8**, 136–7.

Kim, S.M., Park, C.H., Intenzo, C.M. and Zhang, J. (1993). Brain SPECT in a patient with post-stroke hallucinations. *Clinical Nuclear Medicine*, **18**, 413–16.

Kohlberg, L., Yaeger, J. and Hjertholm, E. (1968). Private speech: four studies and a review of theories. *Child Development*, **39**, 691–736.

Köhler, S., Kapur, S., Moscovitch, M., Winocur, G. and Houle, S. (1995). Dissociation of pathways for object and spatial vision: a PET study in humans. *Neuroreport*, **6**, 1865–8.

Kölmel, H.W. (1985). Complex visual hallucinations in the hemianopic field. *Journal of Neurology, Neurosurgery, and Psychiatry*, **48**, 29–38.

Kopala, L.C., Good, K.P. and Honer, W.G. (1994). Olfactory hallucinations and olfactory identification ability in patients with schizophrenia and other psychiatric disorders. *Schizophrenia Research*, **12**, 205–11.

Kosslyn, S.M., Seger, C., Pani, J.R. and Hillger, L.A. (1990). When is imagery used in everyday life? A diary study. *Journal of Mental Imagery*, **14**, 131–52.

Kosslyn, S.M., Alpert, N.M., Thompson, W.L. *et al.* (1993). Visual mental imagery activates topographically organized visual cortex: PET investigations. *Journal of Cognitive Neuroscience*, **5**, 263–87.

Kosslyn, S.M., Thompson, W.L., Kim, I.J. and Alpert, N.M. (1995). Topographical representations of mental images in primary visual cortex. *Nature*, **378**, 496–8.

Kwong, K.K., Belliveau, J.W., Chesler, D.A. *et al.* (1992). Dynamic magnetic resonance imaging of human brain activity during primary sensory stimulation. *Proceedings of the National Academy of Sciences, USA*, **89**, 5675–9.

Lance, J.W. (1976). Simple formed hallucinations confined to the area of a specific visual field defect. *Brain*, **99**, 719–34.

Le Bihan, D., Turner, R., Zeffiro, T.A. *et al.* (1993). Activation of human primary visual cortex during visual recall: a magnetic resonance imaging study. *Proceedings of the National Academy of Sciences, USA*, **90**, 11 802–5.

Lepore, F.E. (1990). Spontaneous visual phenomena with visual loss: 104 patients with lesions of retinal and neural afferent pathways. *Neurology*,**40**, 444–7.

Leudar, I., Thomas, P. and Johnston, M. (1994). Self-monitoring in speech production: effects of verbal hallucinations and negative symptoms. *Psychological Medicine*, **24**, 749–61.

Liddle, P.F. (1987). Schizophrenic syndromes, cognitive performance and neurological dysfunction. *Psychological Medicine*, **17**, 49–58.

Liddle, P.F., Friston, K.J., Frith, C.D. *et al.* (1992). Patterns of cerebral blood flow in schizophrenia. *British Journal of Psychiatry*, **160**, 179–86.

Lishman, W.A. (1987). *Organic Psychiatry. The Psychological Consequences of Cerebral Disorder*, 2nd edition. Oxford & London: Blackwell Scientific Publications.

Macken, W.J. and Jones, D.M. (1995). Functional characteristics of the inner voice and the inner ear: single or double agency? *Journal of Experimental Psychology: Learning, Memory, and Cognition*, **21**, 436–48.

Margo, A., Hemsley, D.R. and Slade, P.D. (1981). The effects of varying auditory input on schizophrenic hallucinations. *British Journal of Psychiatry*, **139**, 122–7.

Martinot, J.L., Paillere-Martinot, M.L., Loc'h, C. *et al.* (1991). The estimated density of D_2 striatal receptors in schizophrenia. A study with positron emission tomography and ^{76}Br-bromolisuride. *British Journal of Psychiatry*, **158**, 346–50.

Martinot, J.L., Paillere-Martinot, M.L., Loc'h, C. *et al.* (1994). Central D_2 receptors and negative symptoms of schizophrenia. *British Journal of Psychiatry*, **164**, 27–34.

Mathew, V.M., Gruzelier, J.H. and Liddle, P.F. (1993). Lateral asymmetries in auditory acuity distinguish hallucinating from nonhallucinating schizophrenic patients. *Psychiatry Research*, **46**, 127–38.

Matsuda, H., Gyobo, T., Masayasu, I. and Hisada, K. (1988). Increased accumulation of *N*-isopropyl-(I-123) *p*-iodoamphetamine in the left auditory area in a schizophrenic patient with auditory hallucinations. *Clinical Nuclear Medicine*, **13**, 53–5.

McGuire, P.K., Shah, G.M.S. and Murray, R.M. (1993). Increased blood flow in Broca's area during auditory hallucinations in schizophrenia. *Lancet*, **342**, 703–6.

McGuire, P.K., Silbersweig, D.A., Wright, I. *et al.* (1995). Abnormal monitoring of inner speech: a physiological basis for auditory hallucinations. *Lancet*, **346**, 596–600.

McGuire, P.K., Silbersweig, D.A. and Frith, C.D. (1996*a*). Functional neuroanatomy of verbal self-monitoring. *Brain*, **119**, 907–17.

McGuire, P.K., Silbersweig, D.A., Murray, R.M. *et al.* (1996*b*). The functional anatomy of inner speech and auditory imagery. *Psychological Medicine*, **26**, 29–38.

Meco, G., Alessandria, A., Bonifati, V. and Giustini, P. (1994). Risperidone for hallucinations in levodopa-treated Parkinson's disease patients. *Lancet*, **343**, 1370–1.

Miller, L.J., O'Connor, E. and DiPasquale, T. (1993). Patients' attitudes toward hallucinations. *American Journal of Psychiatry*, **150**, 584–8.

Mueser, K.T., Bellack, A.S. and Brady, E.U. (1990). Hallucinations in schizophrenia. *Acta Psychiatrica Scandinavica*, **82**, 26–9.

Musalek, M., Podreka, I., Walter, H. *et al.* (1989). Regional brain function in hallucinations: a study of regional cerebral blood flow with ^{99m}Tc-HMPAO-SPECT in patients with auditory hallucinations, tactile hallucinations and normal controls. *Comprehensive Psychiatry*, **30**, 99–108.

Nayani, T.H. and David, A.S. (1996). The auditory hallucination: a phenomenological survey. *Psychological Medicine*, **26**, 177–89.

O'Neal, P. and Robins, L.N. (1958). Childhood patterns predictive of adult schizophrenia: a 30-year follow-up study. *American Journal of Psychiatry*, **115**, 385–91.

Panayiotopoulos, C.P. (1994). Elementary visual hallucinations in migraine and epilepsy. *Journal of Neurology, Neurosurgery, and Psychiatry*, **57**, 1371–4.

Paquier, P., van Vugt, P., Bal, P. *et al.* (1992). Transient musical hallucinosis of central origin: a review and clinical study. *Journal of Neurology, Neurosurgery, and Psychiatry*, **55**, 1069–73.

Parent, A. and Hazrati, L.N. (1995). Functional anatomy of the basal ganglia. I. The cortico-basal ganglia-thalamo-cortical loop. *Brain Research Reviews*, **20**, 91–127.

Patel, H.C., Keshavan, M.S. and Martin, S. (1987). A case of Charles Bonnet syndrome with musical hallucinations. *Canadian Journal of Psychiatry*, **32**, 303–4.

Penfield, W. and Perot, P. (1963). The brain's record of auditory and visual experience: a final summary and conclusion. *Brain*, **86**, 568–693.

Persaud, R. and Marks, I. (1995). A pilot study of exposure control of chronic auditory hallucinations in schizophrenia. *British Journal of Psychiatry*, **167**, 45–50.

Petty, R.G., Barta, P.E., Pearlson, G.D. *et al.* (1995). Reversal of asymmetry of the planum temporale in schizophrenia. *American Journal of Psychiatry*, **152**, 715–21.

Phillipson, O.T. and Harris, J.P. (1985). Perceptual changes in schizophrenia: a questionnaire survey. *Psychological Medicine*, **15**, 859–66.

Pierce, P.A. and Peroutka, S.J. (1989). Hallucinogenic drug interactions with neurotransmitter receptor binding sites in human cortex. *Psychopharmacology*, **97**, 118–22.

Pilowsky, L.S., Costa, D.C., Ell, P.J. *et al.* (1994). D_2 dopamine receptor binding in the basal ganglia of antipsychotic-free schizophrenic patinets. An ^{123}I-IBZM single photon emission computerised tomography study. *British Journal of Psychiatry*, **164**, 16–26.

Price, J., Whitlock, F.A. and Hall, R.T. (1983). The psychiatry of vertebrobasilar insufficiency with report of a case. *Psychiatria Clinica*, **16**, 414–17.

Rector, N.A. and Seeman, M.V. (1992). Auditory hallucinations in women and men. *Schizophrenia Research*, **7**, 233–6.

Roland, P.E. and Gulyás, B. (1994). Visual representations of scenes and objects: retinotopical or non-retinotopical? *Trends in Neurosciences*, **17**, 294–7.

Rubin, P., Holm, S., Friberg, L. *et al.* (1991). Altered modulation of prefrontal and subcortical brain activity in newly diagnosed schizophrenia and schizophreniform disorder. A regional cerebral blood flow study. *Archives of General Psychiatry*, **48**, 987–95.

Rubin, P., Holm, S., Madsen, P.L. *et al.* (1994). Regional cerebral blood flow distribution in newly diagnosed schizophrenia and schizophreniform disorder. *Psychiatry Research*, **53**, 57–75.

Sadzot, B., Lemaire, C., Maquet, P. *et al.* (1995). Serotonin 5HT2 receptor imaging in the human brain using positron emission tomography and a new radioligand, [^{18}F]altanserin: results in young normal controls. *Journal of Cerebral Blood Flow and Metabolism*, **15**, 787–97.

Salanova, V., Andermann, F., Rasmussen, T. *et al.* (1995). Parietal lobe epilepsy. Clinical manifestations and outcome in 82 patients treated surgically between 1929 and 1988. *Brain*, **118**, 607–27.

Schultz, G. and Melzack, R. (1991). The Charles Bonnet syndrome: 'phantom visual images'. *Perception*, **20**, 809–25.

Scripture, E.W. (1896). Measuring hallucinations. *Science*, **3**, 762–3.

Sedvall, G., Farde, L., Persson, A. and Wiesel, F.-A. (1986). Imaging of neurotransmitter receptors in the living human brain. *Archives of General Psychiatry*, **43**, 995–1005.

Shapiro, C.M., Kasem, H. and Tewari, S. (1991). My Music – a case of musical reminiscence diagnosed courtesy of the BBC. *Journal of Neurology, Neurosurgery, and Psychiatry*, **54**, 88–9.

Shenton, M.E., Kikinis, R., Jolesz, F.A. *et al.* (1992). Abnormalities of the left temporal lobe and thought disorder in schizophrenia: a quantitative magnetic resonance imaging study. *New England Journal of Medicine*, **327**, 604–12.

Sheppard, G., Gruzelier, J., Manchanda, R. *et al.* (1983). ^{15}O positron emission tomographic scanning in predominantly never-treated acute schizophrenic patients. *Lancet*, **322**, 1448–52.

Sichart, U. and Fuchs, T. (1992). Visuelle Halluzinationen bei älteren Menschen mit reduziertem Visus: das Charles Bonnet-syndrom. *Klin. Mbl. Augenheilk*, **200**, 224–7.

Silbersweig, D.A., Stern, E., Frith, C. *et al.* (1995). A functional neuroanatomy of hallucinations in schizophrenia. *Nature*, **378**, 176–9.

Sinason, M. (1993). Who is the mad voice inside? *Psychoanalytic Psychotherapy*, **7**, 207–21.

Slade, P. and Bentall, R. (1988). *Sensory Deception: A Scientific Analysis of Hallucination*. London: Croom Helm.

Smith, J.D., Wilson, M. and Reisberg, D. (1995). The role of subvocalization in auditory imagery. *Neuropsychologia*, **33**, 1433–54.

Sokoloff, L. (1981). Localization of functional activity in the central nervous system by measurement of glucose utilization with radioactive deoxyglucose. *Journal of Cerebral Blood Flow and Metabolism*, **1**, 7–36.

Stevens, J.R. and Gold, J.M. (1991). What is schizophrenia? *Behavioral and Brain Sciences*, **14**, 50–1.

Stocklin, G. (1992). Tracers for metabolic imaging of brain and heart. Radiochemistry and radiopharmacology. *European Journal of Nuclear Medicine*, **19**, 527–51.

Suzucki, M., Yuasa, S., Minabe, Y. *et al.* (1993). Left superior temporal blood flow increases in schizophrenic and schizophreniform patients with auditory hallucinations: a longitudinal case study using ^{123}I-IMP SPET. *European Archives of Psychiatry and Clinical Neuroscience*, **242**, 257–61.

Teunisse, R.J., Cruysberg, J.R., Verbeek, A. and Zitman, F.G. (1995). The Charles Bonnet syndrome: a large prospective study in The Netherlands. A study of the prevalence of the Charles Bonnet syndrome and associated factors in 500 patients attending the University Department of Ophthalmology at Nijmegan. *British Journal of Psychiatry*, **166**, 254–7.

Tien, A.Y. (1991). Distributions of hallucinations in the population. *Social Psychiatry and Psychiatric Epidemiology*, **26**, 287–92.

Tiihonen, J., Hari, R., Naukkarinen, H. *et al.* (1992). Modified activity of the human auditory cortex during auditory hallucinations. *American Journal of Psychiatry*, **149**, 255–7.

Tyler, M., Diamond, J. and Lewis, S. (1995). Correlates of left-handedness in a large sample of schizophrenic patients. *Schizophrenia Research*, **18**, 37–41.

Verhoeff, N.P.L.G., Buell, U., Costa, D.C. *et al.* (1992). Basics and recommendations for brain SPECT. *Nuclear Medicine*, **31**, 114–31.

Vita, A., Dieci, M., Giobbio, G.M. *et al.* (1995). Language and thought disorder in schizophrenia: brain morphological correlates. *Schizophrenia Research*, **15**, 243–51.

Whyte, M.B. (1995). Auditory, imagery in normal subjects and psychiatric patients with auditory hallucinations. Unpublished BSc Dissertation, King's College School of Medicine and Dentistry, London.

Wiesel, F.A., Wik, G., Sjogren, I. *et al.* (1987). Regional brain glucose metabolism in drug free schizophrenic patients and clinical correlates. *Acta Psychiatrica Scandinavica*, **76**, 628–41.

Wing, J.K., Cooper, J.E. and Sartorius, N. (1974). *Measurement and Classification of Psychiatric Symptoms*. Cambridge: Cambridge University Press.

Wolkin, A., Jaeger, J., Brodie, J.D. *et al.* (1985). Persistence of cerebral metabolic abnormalities in chronic schizophrenia as determined by positron emission tomography. *American Journal of Psychiatry*, **142**, 564–71.

Woodruff, P., Brammer, M., Mellers, J. *et al.* (1995). Auditory hallucinations and perception of external speech. *Lancet*, **346**, 1035.

Zeki, S., Watson, J.D.G. and Frackowiak, R.S.J. (1993). Going beyond the information given: the relation of illusory motion to brain activity. *Proceedings of the Royal Society of London (Biology)*, **2252**, 215–22.

Zhengxiu, S. (1989). Observation on the curative effect of 120 cases of auditory hallucination treated with auricular acupuncture. *Journal of Traditional Chinese Medicine*, **9**, 176–8.

Zoldan, J., Friedberg, G., Livneh, M. and Melamed, E. (1995). Psychosis in advanced Parkinson's disease: treatment with ondansetron, a 5-HT$_3$ receptor antagonist. *Neurology*, **45**, 1305–8.

Index